T0146254

Natural Disasters and Public Health

Natural Disasters and Public Health

HURRICANES KATRINA, RITA, AND WILMA

Edited by Virginia M. Brennan

The Johns Hopkins University Press

Baltimore

The introduction and chapters 2–25 appeared in a special issue of *Journal of Health Care for the Poor and Underserved* (18.2), May 2007.

The Johns Hopkins University Press
2715 North Charles Street
Baltimore, Maryland 21218-4363
www.press.jhu.edu

ISBN 10:   0-8018-9199-X
ISBN 13:   978-0-8018-9199-1

Library of Congress Control Number: 2008936107

A catalog record for this book is available from the British Library.

Special discounts are available for bulk purchases of this book. For more information, please contact Special Sales at 410-516-6936 or specialsales@press.jhu.edu.

The Johns Hopkins University Press uses environmentally friendly book materials, including recycled text paper that is composed of at least 30 percent post-consumer waste, whenever possible. All of our book papers are acid-free, and our jackets and covers are printed on paper with recycled content.

To my parents,
John Joseph Brennan
and
Eileen Frances Fitzgerald Brennan

Contents

Acknowledgments

This work would not have been possible without the guidance and support of my public health mentors, Rueben C. Warren and Bailus Walker, nor without the support of Wayne J. Riley and Meharry Medical College. Bill Breichner, Journals Manager at the Johns Hopkins University Press (JHUP), was instrumental in the creation of this book, as he has been for every issue of the *Journal of Health Care for the Poor and Underserved* since we joined JHUP in 2004. I would also like to thank Suzanne Flinchbaugh, Assistant Acquisitions Editor, and Linda Forlifer, Assistant Managing Editor, at JHUP for their help with this book.

The friendship, hard work, and contributions of my Meharry colleagues and coworkers Hershell Warren, Robert S. Levine, Kimyona Roberts, Irwin Goldzweig, Erin Boyd, Saqi Maleque, Kondra Williams, Robin Griffin, Subhankar Mukhopadhyay, Agodi Umeukeje, and Nathaniel Briggs make every day one when I want to go to work. Finally, I am ever grateful to my companion in joys and sorrows, Jim Waechter.

Natural Disasters and Public Health

Introduction
Hurricanes Katrina and Rita:
Professionally Fulfilling, Personally Painful

Wayne J. Riley, MD, MPH, MBA, FACP

My experiences with Hurricanes Katrina and Rita were both professional and personal. As a New Orleans–born physician, I was honored to be among the health care professionals and the legions of volunteers in Houston and Harris County, Texas, who contributed to the coordination and provision of medical care during a time of national crisis. The mobilization of health care and disaster medicine resources in Houston and Harris County was, perhaps, surpassed only by the city of New York's response, post-9/11. It was, indeed, Houston's finest hour.

When the first planeloads of evacuees arrived in Houston on August 31, 2005, few of us could imagine how my adopted hometown would be changed, likely forever, and how we would be tested as a community. I could not guess then how gratifying it would be to care for some of my fellow New Orleanians who, overnight, became both my patients and my neighbors.

On a personal level, the arrival of my parents, two adult siblings, one niece and one nephew at my family home in Houston created new and unexpected "up close and personal" interactions that challenged us all. Indeed, the Riley family "Feng Shui" soon became unbalanced. In the blink of an eye, the census in our four-bedroom household went from four to twelve. My sister and her husband and their two kids lost their home and all of their possessions to Hurricane Katrina. My parents' home in New Orleans was heavily damaged and rendered uninhabitable, until just recently, due to extensive wind damage and a proliferation of mold. They, too, lost most of their personal possessions.

To add insult to injury, my semi-retired father, Emile Edward Riley, Jr., M.D. (Meharry '60), arrived at our doorstep in poor health after an 18-hour journey by car that normally took five and one-half hours. Within a month and a half—just after Hurricane Rita bore down on the southeast Texas coast—he would enter a Houston hospital and suffer a massive stroke that would leave him profoundly dysarthric and hemiplegic for the rest of his days. This turn of events was particularly painful to me, as my dad was and is my first hero (his Katrina-damaged Meharry diploma adorns a wall in my office). These dialectical experiences, seared into my consciousness forever,

DR. WAYNE RILEY is President and CEO of Meharry Medical College. Previously, he was vice-president for health affairs and governmental relations at Baylor College of Medicine in Houston and chairman of the Harris County Hospital District Medical Board.

are not unlike those encountered by many others in the aftermath of two mighty Gulf Coast storms.

Houston's and Harris County's Finest Hour

As the vice-president for health affairs and governmental relations at Baylor College of Medicine in Houston and chairman of the Harris County Hospital District Medical Board, I was among a small group of medical staff leaders that sprang into action when evacuees began to arrive in the city. We quickly decided that the best venues available to create a local "Katrina Clinic" were the aging and somewhat mothballed "eighth wonder of the world"—the Houston Astrodome—and the downtown George R. Brown Convention Center.

On August 31, 2005, the first trickle of evacuees began to arrive at both sites. A mere two days later, a torrent in excess of 20,000 people flooded both facilities (over 200,000 came to Houston, overall). Many had not changed clothes or had much food in days. More important to the health care team, many had no access to their medications or to routine dialysis, nor did they have medical records or even pill bottles to authenticate their prescription needs. Their medical and dental providers back home could not be reached because, like the Houston evacuees, the caregivers, too, had fled the floodwaters to find refuge in communities across the region and around the nation.

To coordinate care and to make quick decisions about how best to organize what seemed like an impossible task, representatives of Houston Mayor Bill White's office; the county executive, Robert Eckels; Harris County Hospital District's CEO, David Lopez, and the health care infrastructure of Texas Medical Center; and, the city of Houston came together at a makeshift command center.

The needs were many: sphygmomanometers to take blood pressure readings; glucometers to test blood glucose levels; metered dose inhalers for asthmatics and emphysemics; insulin; syringes; ambulatory oxygen tanks; and tetanus vaccine, to name just a few. The most important of the city's considerable health care assets to step forward was the Harris County Hospital District—the hospital and community clinic safety net for residents of Harris County. The full medical, nursing, and ancillary staff of the District was deployed. Everything imaginable—from portable X-ray machines, ultrasound equipment, IV fluids, and most everything else we normally expect in a hospital—was placed at our disposal.

Resident physicians and faculty from both Baylor College of Medicine and University of Texas–Houston Health Science Center descended on the Astrodome and the downtown Convention Center to provide care. Shift assignments were made and coordinated by a designated "Katrina Medical Director" from the Baylor faculty.

I personally worked more than five 12-hour shifts in those early days, directly treating patients alongside community physicians and supervising the work of house staff and other volunteer physicians, nurses, and dentists. I tended patients suffering with just about every imaginable problem—from toothaches to respiratory ailments to sore throats to advancing coronary artery disease.[1]

I gained a new appreciation during those long but fulfilling days for the men and women of our uniformed and armed forces who provide such services on a routine basis all over the world. The work was both exhilarating and exhausting. And while videotape loops showing looting and civil disorder flashed regularly on TV sets around the globe, the decency, civility, gratitude, and genuine appreciation of the many thousands of New Orleans residents evacuated to Houston found no such audience.

I will always remember the many words of thanks and the hugs I received from countless evacuees after tending to their medical needs. It made me proud to be a healer and to assist in ameliorating their misery. It also made me proud to be a native of New Orleans.

My Beloved New Orleans and Family: The Challenges Ahead

As a proud native of the Crescent City, I have often reflected on the lessons learned from my post-hurricane experiences and on the challenges ahead. New Orleans will likely never be the same. In some ways that is desirable and in others it is regrettable. Nonetheless, the rebirth and renewal of a great American city is underway, albeit stuttering and frustratingly feckless at times. As part of that renewal, the medical, dental, and health care renaissance of New Orleans should and must be a national priority. The challenges are many and seemingly intractable. However, the collective resolve of this nation's health care leaders is needed to vitiate the movement to address the health care of those who will return, over time, to contribute to that renewal. In my view, such resolve is a national and international imperative.

Personally, my post-Katrina visits to New Orleans to address family recovery are still very poignant. As a young man just out of Yale University, before I began my itinerant journey on the path to becoming a physician-educator and health care administrator, I returned home and devoted five years of my life to serving the city of my birth on the staff of New Orleans' first African American mayor. I love and still miss New Orleans. Since my departure in the late 1980s, New Orleans has been the setting, in an existential way, for nurturing family connections and connectedness. The city is part of me and part of who I am. That is why I will always cherish the opportunity I had to serve it, in yet another manner, as a physician in those sweltering days of late summer 2005.

Four months after Katrina and Rita, on the beautiful morning of January 31, 2006, my father succumbed to complications from his stroke and passed away. It would be just a short three months later when I would be approached about the opportunity to lead his *alma mater*, Meharry.

I now view my leadership of Meharry Medical College as a very special calling to continue serving New Orleans and the entire Gulf Coast community by preparing young men and women to contribute to the biomedical science, public health, medical, and dental workforce of that recovering region. For I know that future generations of Meharry graduates, like my father and many others before him, will continue to migrate to the Gulf region to address the stark disparities in medical and dental care that existed before and that exist even more so now after two great storms.

In this volume, readers will find a superb set of papers that cogently analyze the extant health care infrastructure and workforce in New Orleans; highlight the challenges and tasks ahead; take stock of the progress to date; and amplify the clarion call

Chapter 1
Hurricanes Katrina, Rita, and Wilma and the Medically Underserved

Virginia M. Brennan, PhD, MA

The least intense of the three big storms of the fall of 2005 in the United States was the most catastrophic in terms of lives lost and damage wreaked: Hurricane Katrina made landfall on the U.S. Gulf Coast on August 29, 2005. It took over 1,800 lives, ranking third highest in U.S. history after the Galveston Hurricane of 1900 and the Lake Okeechobee Hurricane of 1928, and caused about $81 billion in damages.[1] Remarkable for the destruction wrought, Katrina and its aftermath have earned a prominent place in U.S. history because of the spotlight they shone on the low-income, minority populations of the Gulf Coast and the inadequate government preparation and response to the disaster. This book is about public health as it concerns these medically underserved populations in and around the hurricane season of 2005.

Hurricane Rita, the fourth strongest hurricane ever recorded in the Atlantic Basin, directly struck Louisiana and Texas (also affecting Arkansas, Mississippi, and the Florida Keys) shortly after Hurricane Katrina, first making landfall in the United States on September 23, 2005.[2] Responsible for as many as 111 deaths in Texas alone (in part due to 98° heat in areas under emergency evacuation, as well as to a catastrophic fire on a bus carrying elderly evacuees in Texas),[3] Rita gave birth to at least 90 tornadoes in Alabama, Mississippi, Louisiana, and Arkansas. The health of the elderly was particularly affected.[3] A pre-landfall storm surge caused by Rita compounded the problems with New Orleans's already overwhelmed infrastructure when it breached the levee on the Industrial Canal that partially protected the predominantly low-income, African American Ninth Ward of the city.[2,4]

Hurricane Wilma, the strongest storm ever recorded in the Atlantic Basin, hit the southwestern coast of Florida as a Category 3 hurricane on October 24, 2005, and quickly moved across the southern portion of the state. At least 62 deaths due to Wilma were recorded overall (35 in the United States); financially, Wilma was the third costliest hurricane in U.S. history, behind Katrina (September 2005) and Andrew (August 1992). The population and infrastructure of numerous counties were seriously damaged by the 10 tornadoes that formed out of Wilma.[5] Over three million people in Florida lost power. Like Katrina and Rita, Wilma fell hard on medically underserved people, in this case the rural residents of Hendry County (near Lake Okeechobee).[6] Overall, 15

VIRGINIA M. BRENNAN *is the editor of the* Journal of Health Care for the Poor and Underserved *and a faculty member at Meharry Medical College.*

tropical storms in the Atlantic Basin became hurricanes in 2005, a record surpassing the previous high set in 1969, with 12 hurricanes.[7]

Public health scholarship outlines what to expect when hurricanes strike.[8-13] Hurricanes pose serious threats to health because they can kill, and cause catastrophic injuries; they also destroy or impair the health care infrastructure, with long-lasting consequences for access to primary and acute care.[8] Drowning is far and away the greatest cause of death due to hurricanes (approximately 90% of all deaths caused directly by hurricanes are by drowning), although this proportion declines as early warning systems and effective evacuation get people out of harm's way.[10,14,15] (Only 40% of deaths in Louisiana due to Hurricane Katrina, for example, were by drowning.)[16] Morbidity associated with hurricanes typically includes mental trauma (known to last as long as five years post-hurricane), injuries, gastrointestinal conditions, other infectious diseases, and skin conditions;[10,11,13] unsurprisingly, these were found among evacuees and rescue workers in 2005.[16-23] (See chapters 11, 14, and 15 in this volume.) Lack of sanitation, lack of clean water, and lack of food plague efforts to assist large numbers of survivors.[13,20,24] The evacuation of long-term and critical care patients is especially difficult, making it of central importance for preparedness plans, particularly for densely populated urban areas;[10] this was one of the ways that New Orleans, especially, appears to have been ill-prepared for Katrina (see chapters 8 and 9 in this volume).[25-29] Racial and ethnic minority communities in the United States (including African Americans,* Hispanics, American Indians, and some Asian/Pacific Islander groups) are known to be more vulnerable to disasters than other communities are, for a wide range of reasons, including linguistic and cultural barriers, community isolation, housing patterns, and the quality of buildings in minority communities.[12]

Hurricane Alley, 2005

Hurricanes Katrina, Rita, and Wilma are not simple examples for studying public health in the context of natural disasters. Katrina, especially, was strongly characterized by the complexities introduced by a large impoverished population being directly affected. While this complexity is all too familiar globally,[30] seeing it on their own shores shocked and frightened many in the United States. The wreckage wrought by storms always inspires awe and sorrow and an impulse to help survivors; the widespread crisis wrought by poverty and a failed governmental response to the hurricanes of 2005 also inspired shame and anger.

New Orleans is a low-lying city, known for its vulnerability to catastrophes caused by water, whether from the Atlantic or from the Mississippi.[1,31] In 2005, it was extremely

---

* The terms *African American* and *Black* are used interchangeably in this chapter, with the caveat that *Black* may encompass people of African descent not born in the United States. The terms *White* and *Anglo* are also used interchangeably. (All of these four terms presuppose that their referents are *non-Hispanic*.) In the book, the terms *Hispanic* and *Latino* are also used interchangeably. The reason for this abundance of names is that individual authors in this volume, or whose work is referred to herein, use different labels. While principled distinctions (concerning race, ethnicity, and the social construction of demographic categories) can be drawn among them, I do not draw any here.

vulnerable in other ways, too: As the Center for American Progress points out, Louisiana and Mississippi are the two states in the union with the greatest proportion of residents living in poverty. While the national proportion of people living in poverty is 13.1%, prior to Katrina it was 23% in New Orleans and 21.6% in Mississippi. More than 90,000 people in the Katrina- and Rita-affected areas of Louisiana, Mississippi, and Alabama had incomes below $10,000 per year. The affected regions also had far greater proportions of African Americans than did the nation as a whole (67.9% New Orleans, 37.2% Mississippi, 26% Alabama, vs. 12–13% nationally), and the median incomes of these African Americans were 40% lower than those of Whites in the same areas. Compared with national averages, far greater proportions of the populations in Louisiana, Mississippi, and Alabama were enrolled in Medicaid and greater proportions in New Orleans and Mississippi lacked health insurance entirely. Finally, much larger proportions of the elderly in these areas were disabled (56.4% New Orleans, 52% Mississippi, 46% Alabama, vs. 39.6% nationally).[32,33] The rurality of the areas hardest hit by Hurricane Wilma coincided with comparable vulnerabilities in their population.[6]

The rest of this introduction provides an overview of the central public health concerns associated with the hurricanes of 2005, especially Katrina. The concerns addressed are chronic illness; the roles of race, ethnicity, and class; health care infrastructure; mental health; and the government response. In each section, the chapters of the present volume that address the concern at hand are noted.

Chronic Illness

After Katrina, in light of the demographic profile sketched above and known health disparities between low-income minority group members and the overall national population,[28,34] health officials expected many storm-related deaths due lack of medicine and treatment for chronic illness.[35] At the evacuation centers, mobile clinics, and Federal Emergency Management Agency (FEMA) trailer parks, chronic illness was the overwhelming source of immediate demands among evacuees. (See chapters 5, 11, 14–16, 18, and 21 in this volume.)

In some cases, the technology necessary to treat chronic illness was wiped out by the storm. The Centers for Medicare and Medicaid Services set out, for example, to find the 5,800 or so dialysis patients in storm-ravaged areas; Andrew Cohen of the Ochsner Clinic Foundation in New Orleans reported concerns that 50% or more of patients who had been receiving dialysis treatment in New Orleans had not been located 10 days after the storm.[36] Katrina closed or seriously damaged 94 kidney dialysis clinics in storm-affected areas; 27 remained closed as of January 2006.[37] Surviving dialysis patients were found to suffer psychosocial effects from the disaster.[38]

More often, however, it was the common chronic illnesses disproportionately suffered by low-income and minority populations nationwide[28,34] that challenged the post-disaster system: people with diagnosed hypertension, heart disease, diabetes, and asthma presented with worsened conditions due to lack of care after the storm, seeking acute care, ongoing care, and refills of lost prescription medications.[16,18,20,23,26,39–45] In evacuation centers in Louisiana in September and October 2005, 31% of medical encounters were for the care of chronic conditions;[20] 55.7% of households surveyed in the New Orleans area during the period of October 17–22, 2005, included at least one member with a chronic medical condition;[41] 42% of evacuees in San Antonio in September 2005 reported a household member with a chronic condition, and 28% reported a household member with a mental or physical disability.[46] More than two years after Katrina, residents of FEMA trailer parks in Mississippi showed worsened chronic health needs and mental health needs, along with their deepening poverty.[45] Notably, high hurricane exposure among pregnant women was associated with worse birth outcomes.[47]

Race, Ethnicity, and Class

In this section we will be looking further at differences in vulnerability to disasters along racial, ethnic, and class lines, where *class* variously refers to differences between groups in terms of income, education, resources, and employment or some combination of these. In the cases of Hurricanes Katrina and Rita, the racial/ethnic groups most widely affected are Blacks and Whites, as well as American Indians and Louisiana Cajuns, while many Hispanic people were at risk from Hurricane Wilma and from the terrible hurricane of 1992, Andrew (which led to some important research that will be touched on here).*

It will be helpful to lay out some statistics to set the scene that played out in the fall of 2005 along the Gulf Coast. Millions evacuated due to Hurricane Katrina alone, over 780,000 were officially displaced, and over 200,000 homes were destroyed. More than 80% of New Orleans was flooded.[28] An estimated 240,000 people, mostly from Louisiana, evacuated to Houston during the week after Katrina struck. An estimated 24,000 of them were sheltered in a temporary evacuation center at the Astrodome.[19] (See the introduction to this volume.) Overall, more than 200,000 people congregated in evacuation centers in at least 18 states after Katrina struck, a number that rose higher when Rita quickly followed.[4]

Members of racial and ethnic minority groups, people in rural areas, and people of low socioeconomic status (SES) stand at heightened risk of harm from disasters.[6,12,30,35,48,49] In Hurricane Katrina, we have the starkest kind of evidence of this: 51% of the dead were Black, while 41% were White. In Orleans Parish, the mortality rate among Blacks was 1.7 to 4 times higher than the rate among Whites. [16†]

---

* See chapters 21 and 22 for work on emergency preparedness among Hispanic populations. See chapter 24 for an intervention by the National Institute of Environmental Health Sciences at the University of Texas to deliver medical supplies and environmental outreach survey teams to people living on the bayous in south Terrebonne and LaFourche Parishes in Louisiana after Hurricane Rita. These parishes on the southern wetlands and bayous of Louisiana are home to the Native United Houma Nation, others of Louisiana Cajun culture, and small-boat shrimp fishermen from a variety of racial and ethnic groups, including Vietnamese. Also see Sullivan's documentary, listed at the end of this volume, which presents results of the group's environmental outreach.

† It is important, too, to note that the elderly were disproportionately represented among the dead: 49% of those who died as a result of Hurricane Katrina were 75 years of age or older.[16] Also note that Orleans Parish is the most impoverished, by many measures, in the New Orleans metropolitan area. See chapter 10 for graphs of poverty, infant mortality, birth outcomes, houses without access to vehicles, and women as heads of households with children in Orleans Parish.

Why this greater mortality among Black people? A number of reasons, though almost certainly not all, are known. One is that overlapping low-income and minority groups tend to live in less sturdy buildings than wealthier people, buildings that are themselves highly vulnerable to damage from hurricane force winds and storm surges.[50] Among people who don't evacuate, the ones in weaker structures are more at risk; among those who do evacuate, the ones whose home is a weaker structure are more likely to become homeless. (For much more on the *geography of stress*, see chapter 10.)

Second, for reasons that are not entirely understood, there are racial and class differences in who evacuates, with minority and lower-income groups less likely to evacuate than Anglo and higher-income groups.[51] Additionally, households with elderly members are less likely than average to evacuate, while those with children are more likely to do so.[51] Among sampled residents of evacuation centers in 2005, most of whom were Black (93%) and low income, 32% said that their source of information about the evacuation order (most often, television programs) did not give clear information about how to evacuate.[18,29,44] (On communication during disasters, see also chapters 17, 19, 21, and 22.)

Among those surveyed who did not evacuate, 34% explained their decision not to do so as the result of not having a car or other way to leave, while 12% said they were physically unable to leave or that they had to care for someone who was unable to leave. Of the same group of people who did not evacuate, 42% said they *could not* have done so. (Another major reason people chose not to evacuate, from Hurricane Katrina as from other storms, was the belief that the storm would not turn out to be as bad as it was.)[18,44,51] Spence et al. (chapter 17 in this volume) discuss failure to evacuate among the disabled.

Evacuation centers in general are the refuge of those with nowhere else to go once their own home is gone or out of reach.[46] This means they do not have the means to rent a motel room, apartment, or house and do not have family, friends, or acquaintances outside their hometown with whom they might stay. This was the profile of the residents of evacuation centers in 2005, who were overwhelmingly low-income, Black evacuees who had lived their whole lives in the City of New Orleans.[18,44] While evacuation centers are vital, they pose hazards of their own, especially when they are very large,[30] poorly staffed, or poorly equipped. New Orleans residents who first fled to the mass temporary shelters set up at the Superdome and the New Orleans Convention Center reported threatening conditions there: 34% of those surveyed who had spent time there reported having been threatened with violence (while 14% of other evacuees surveyed reported this). Shelters are where the health disorders for which disasters are known show up: skin rashes, diarrhea, vomiting, upper respiratory infections, and pneumonias were widespread among evacuees and rescue personnel, especially diarrhea.[17,19,21,22]

The simple act of evacuating can cause its own serious problems, as displacement and homelessness have profound psychosocial effects on adults and children.[13,30,42] (For two personal accounts, see chapter 25 in this volume.) It is well established that breaking up family groups is a major contributor to mental and emotional problems for evacuees,[49] yet breakup is precisely what happened to many of the evacuees who landed in large Katrina shelters: 53% of those surveyed in Houston shelters were separated from immediate family members at the time of the survey (September 10–12, 2005).[18,44]

After leaving mass evacuation centers, some people went to FEMA-supplied trailers; these, too, became nests of trouble, in a perfect example of what Robert Bullard has christened *environmental (in)justice*. Among other things, direct health threats to residents of FEMA trailers arose from toxic levels of formaldehyde, which were discovered in 2007.[52-54] Among surveyed residents in FEMA-subsidized community settings in Louisiana in February 2006[42] and in FEMA trailer parks in Mississippi more than two years after Katrina and Rita,[45] mental health was or had become a major problem for both adults and children; both adults and children suffered from high rates of chronic health conditions and poor access to care.[42,45] We note all of this while bearing in mind that the people involved—people of low SES and members of racial and ethnic minority groups—were already at a major health disadvantage compared with average Americans. (See chapters 2, 10, 21, and 24 in this volume for more on environmental justice issues.)

Still-standing residences in the storm-ravaged areas also became sources of health problems. Seven weeks after Katrina, three after Rita, the Centers for Disease Control and Protection (CDC) conducted a survey of homes in Orleans and Jefferson Parishes: 20% were without running water (over 50% in impoverished Orleans Parish), over 60% lacked electricity and garbage removal, and over 43% lacked telephones (70% in Orleans Parish).[41] The CDC report on homes in Hancock County, Mississippi, shows 33% lacking trash removal, 37% without functioning toilets, 41% without electricity, and 49% having problems with mosquitoes.[24] Mold, strongly linked to respiratory infections, became a widespread problem in the New Orleans area after Katrina. Of the homes surveyed by the CDC, 46% had visible mold damage, a problem that "is likely to be ongoing."[55] Weisler et al. write of the ravaged city, "The often contaminated flood waters covering much of New Orleans for almost two months contained a mix of raw sewage, bacteria, millions of gallons of heavy metals, pesticides and toxic chemicals, raising concerns for residents and cleanup workers" (p. 585).[56]

Thus far, we have seen that the health of low-income and minority group members is more vulnerable to disaster due to building design and construction, settlement patterns, a tendency not to evacuate, over-representation in emergency housing (evacuation centers and FEMA-sponsored trailers), and disaster-related toxicity in their homes, as well as pre-existing health conditions. We cannot stop, though, without also enumerating additional structural factors—woven into the country's socioeconomic system—that put these groups at increased risk of harm from disasters. These factors are homeowner's insurance, government recovery loan programs, and employment. (For more in this area, see chapter 26 in this volume.)

Minority group members and people with low incomes are more likely to rent than own their own homes and thus are much less likely than other groups to be insured against catastrophic damage to their homes. Among those surveyed in evacuation centers in 2005, 33% owned their own homes and 64% rented (albeit many for many years in the same place); the homes of 55% of the group surveyed had been destroyed and those of 29% had been seriously damaged.[18] (See chapter 10 in this volume.)

Even among homeowners, there is a slight tendency for Blacks to be less likely to have such insurance than Whites,[50] but the stinger comes in looking at Black and White insured homeowners: there is a very strong tendency for Blacks in this group to be insured by a small company, while Whites are very likely to be insured by one of three major national insurance companies. Furthermore, homeowners who are insured by the so-called *big three* tend to report receiving fair settlements after disasters, while those insured by smaller companies tend not to, in part because the smaller companies often offer less extensive coverage and are more likely to fail once a major disaster strikes their policyholders.[50] Peacock and Girard suggest that this pattern of insurance coverage, which they documented after Hurricane Andrew in South Florida in 1992, may be due to redlining by the big three insurance companies (i.e., to a practice of marking predominantly Black neighborhoods as areas of no commercial interest). Bullard argues that the same is true in New Orleans in the wake of Hurricane Katrina.[57] Additionally, families who have low incomes are more likely to lack personal resources (such as insurance, savings, working cell phones, and usable credit cards) with which to recover from disasters.[18,44,58]

Government assistance programs also seem to serve majority-group people who are better off more effectively than they serve low-income minority group members. Long-term analyses of the aftermath of Hurricane Andrew demonstrate that low-SES minority group members tend to apply for (and, thus, to receive) Small Business Administration (SBA) loans less often than wealthier Whites, despite patently greater need of assistance.[59] After the hurricanes of 2005, it appears, even applying didn't pay off, as Robert Bullard reports:

> The Small Business Administration has processed only a third of the 276,000 home loan applications it has received. However, the SBA has rejected 82 percent of the applications it received, a higher percentage than in most previous disasters. Well-off neighborhoods like Lakeview [in New Orleans] have received 47 percent of the loan approvals, while poverty-stricken neighborhoods have gotten 7 percent. Middle-class black neighborhoods in the eastern part of the city have lower loan rates (p. 1).[57]

Finally, on the negative side of the race and class ledger of structural factors, we find large, documented differences between Blacks and Whites after Katrina with respect to employment. Recalling that evacuation centers are the refuge of last resort, it is unsurprising to learn that, among evacuees in September 2005 in San Antonio shelters, 51% of the heads of households surveyed reported having jobs in unskilled occupations (such as food service, manual labor, housekeeping, and retail sales), 21% reported skilled occupations, 10% reported being unemployed, 11% on disability, and 8% retired.[46] Additionally, in an analysis of a Gallup/Red Cross poll conducted among 1,200 Katrina survivors one month after the storm, Elliott and Pais found that Black workers were nearly four times as likely as White workers to have lost their jobs; they also found that Black people with household incomes of $10,000 to $20,000 were twice as likely as Black people with household incomes of $40,000 to $50,000 to have lost their jobs.[60] (Also see chapter 14 in this volume.)

Over and above the pre-existing disparities in health and the structural factors that contribute to the vulnerability to disaster among minority and low-income groups, in the case of Hurricane Katrina massive failure on the part of government, especially the federal government, to provide timely and effective assistance to those who ended up in evacuation centers has bred widespread distrust of government efforts in those communities, a fact that may well lessen the effectiveness of future evacuation messages. Seventy-six percent of those surveyed in an evacuation center shortly after Katrina thought that the government response was inexcusably slow, 70% disapproved of President Bush's handling of the crisis, 58% disapproved of Gov. Kathleen Babineaux Blanco's handling of it, and 53% disapproved of Mayor Ray Nagin's handling of it. Additionally, 68% of respondents affirmed the statement that the federal government would have responded more quickly to rescue people trapped by floodwaters if more of them had been wealthier and White rather than poorer and Black. Sixty-one percent affirmed that their experiences in Hurricane Katrina had led them to believe that the government does not care about people like them. Note, too, that 25% of those surveyed did not hear an order to evacuate and that, of these, 62% did not believe the government had issued an evacuation order and 11% reported not knowing it had done so.[18,44,61] (Also see chapter 7 in this volume on distrust among survivors.)

In contrast, community-based organizations and independent organizations of health care providers get positive marks for their efforts to assist those with scant resources of their own, although the scale is so much smaller than what is needed from the government that one cannot substitute for the other. Nevertheless, it is important to recognize such examples of effective agents and interventions as these:

- the Baylor School of Medicine faculty who staffed the medical clinics at the Astrodome to treat evacuees (see the introduction to this volume);
- the heroic efforts of New Orleans clinicians who stayed in the city through the storm to care for those too ill to leave;[25,26]
- Catholic Charities' Operation Starfish, designed with the recognition that African American and Latino populations tend to rely on family members for shelter and support, which helped family members who were separated maintain and re-establish contact with one another (see chapter 26 in this volume);
- other Catholic Charities services, ranging from mental health care and crisis counseling to financial and material assistance as well as housing help and assistance negotiating the FEMA bureaucracy (see chapter 26);
- the Common Ground Clinic, started by volunteers in a mosque in the Algiers section of New Orleans, and the temporary HIV Outpatient Clinic (HOP) staffed by clinicians from Charity Hospital;[62]
- the *action medics*, who provided no-strings care to survivors in New Orleans in the aftermath of Katrina;[63]
- *incite! women of color against violence*, who established a locally run clinic, with special attention to women suffering the effects of violence;[64]
- the pharmacy program at Xavier University (see chapter 4);
- the nursing program at Dillard University (see chapter 3);
- Operation Assist mobile medical clinics (a program jointly operated by the Children's Health Fund and the Columbia University Mailman School of Public Health—see chapter 11);[42,43,65]
- United Way's 2-1-1 hotline for social service referrals, which handled thousands of calls from evacuees around the country (see chapter 26);

- the revival of the Bridge House substance abuse treatment agency in New Orleans (see chapter 23 in this volume); and
- the Hurricane Choir, organized among evacuees and survivors in Baton Rouge, Louisiana, by an Australian choral leader (see chapter 13 in this volume).

Some successes involved the collaboration of distant health departments, including the dental care provided to evacuees in Washington, D.C., through the combined efforts of the District of Columbia and the Mississippi departments of health (see chapter 5 in this volume). Others were organized specifically to address the needs of people of color and people living in poverty. For example, the *Katrina Health Coalition—All Healers Mental Health Alliance*, begun by Dr. Lucille Norville Perez, former president of the National Medical Association and then director of health for the NAACP, united clinicians seeking "to organize a long-term, culturally competent response to the mental health needs of people in the United States, especially people of color and people living in poverty affected by all hazards and disasters."

We cannot close this section on race, ethnicity, and class without noting the great strength many vulnerable evacuees, especially African Americans, derived from their spiritual lives. Religion was deemed "very important" by 80% of respondents to a *Washington Post*/Kaiser/Harvard survey and was found to be the primary source of strength for 85% of the Black participants in the Gallup/Red Cross poll analyzed by Elliott and Pais.[18,44,60] Chapter 12, "Wading in the Waters: Spirituality and Older Black Katrina Survivors," in the present volume, speaks to this.*

The Health Care Infrastructure in New Orleans

Before September 2005, New Orleans's large impoverished population relied heavily on Charity Hospital, one of the nation's oldest public hospitals for both primary care and acute care.[69] † Charity opened in 1736 with a bequest from a French sailor and shipbuilder, Jean Louis, to found a hospital for the indigent of New Orleans. Originally, it was known as L'Hôpital des Pauvres de la Charité and occupied premises in the French Quarter. Now it is located on Tulane Avenue, across Interstate 10 from the Louisiana State University (LSU) Health Sciences Center.

Charity and its sister, University Hospital, sustained severe damage from Hurricane Katrina and the flooding that followed. Although Charity was the region's only Level I trauma center and the only major safety-net hospital in the city,[69,70] its future and that of University Hospital remain in question, with many advocating replacing the cavernous old buildings with a series of community-based clinics.[33,71] Three years after Katrina, LSU's Health Sciences Center hopes to build a new large medical facility to replace both of the old hospitals. All of these are still solutions on paper, though, and there are a lot of questions, including uncertainties about staffing medical facilities with a decimated health

---

*For additional work on the roles race and class played in the hurricane season of 2005 and its aftermath, see Dyson, Hartman and Squires, and Potter.[66-68]

†The other contender for the title is Bellevue Hospital in New York.

professional workforce. What happened at Charity and other institutional care facilities in New Orleans during the Katrina disaster, and what was lost, concern us here.

Many in the evacuation centers had been regular visitors to Charity and safety-net clinics in New Orleans: of those surveyed in the *Washington Post*/Kaiser/Harvard study introduced above, 66% had gotten their medical care at a hospital or clinic, and 54% of these had gotten it at Charity Hospital.[18] Before Katrina, New Orleans was home to 7,000 HIV-infected people, 3,000 of whom received care in a clinic at Charity.[62] Ninety safety-net clinics were in operation in Orleans Parish before the storm, and only 19 six months later.[72] (See the Jackie Judd/Kaiser Family Foundation documentaries, "Voices of the Storm," listed at the end of this volume.) Karras and Hemenway (chapter 16 in this volume) demonstrate the harm to adult sickle cell patients brought on by Charity's closure. In short, the safety net system of this high-poverty city was brought to its knees by the hurricanes.[25,28,33]

Conditions at Charity Hospital from August 28 through September 2, 2005, when patients and staff were finally evacuated by boatmen from the Louisiana Department of Wildlife and Fisheries, were surely worse than any nightmare. The flood crippled the hospital's emergency generators, so the lights and air conditioning were out; soon after, the toilets filled up, and there was no water for hand-washing. Elevators were out of commission, leaving staff to carry critically ill patients down stairs. Health care professionals and patients rose to the occasion with dedication and élan, but the situation was past desperate. A few times, they heard nearby gunfire while evacuating the emergency-room dock. Unable to get a response to their crying need for assistance, they finally got word out to the public through a reporter from CNN.[25,26,72,73]

Long-term care patients in nursing homes and hospitals were another source of sore concern, as clinicians struggled with the necessity to triage their patients in the absence of training in that critical type of emergency decision making. Two hundred fifty patients were stranded at Memorial Hospital after Katrina, and 34 of them died. Of the 34 dead, 24 had been in a long-term care unit operated by LifeCare Hospitals, which rented the space from Memorial's owner, Tenet Healthcare. Caregivers were accused of having euthanized at least 4 of these 24 patients with heavy doses of morphine and midazolam, charges on which a grand jury refused to indict.[72-74] Overall, 215 patients and residents in hospitals and nursing homes died due to Katrina.[56]

Why weren't the hospitals evacuated ahead of time? Many patients did get out, but others—recovering from surgery, debilitated, reliant on mechanical assistance, newborn, mentally incapacitated, or otherwise non-ambulatory—did not. In part, as Gray and Hebert (chapter 8 in this volume) explain, this was due to the lack of a state or city plan, an insufficient number of vehicles, and an insufficient number of destinations where such complex cases could be safely sent. Home health agencies serving the poorest low-income African American and elderly patients in Orleans Parish had a mixed record when it came to the evacuation of their clients. Of the agencies studied by Kirkpatrick and Bryan, only those who evacuated their patients well *before* the City of New Orleans called for mandatory evacuation succeeded in safely caring for these most vulnerable patients, avoiding long waits on the highways and finding ample space in hotels or shelters. (See chapter 9 in this volume.)

In the immediate aftermath of the hurricanes, functioning medical care facilities in the hurricane-stricken region were busy. The CDC, fulfilling one of its central functions during disasters, conducted surveillance at 8 hospitals and 19 acute care clinics (staffed by Disaster Medical Assistance Teams, or DMATs, then under FEMA's direction but since returned to the Department of Health and Human Services) in Jefferson, Orleans, Plaquemines, St. Bernard, St. Charles, and St. Tammany Parishes during the three weeks after Hurricane Rita. Nearly 17,500 case reports were completed, 51.6% for illness, 26% for injury, and 22% for non-acute care (such as prescription refills). The CDC reports that the proportions of illness and injury were similar immediately after Katrina.[22,27]

Even after the hospital crisis entered its "chronic phase" in the spring of 2006, Berggren and Curiel report that the city's hospital capacity was very low, that hospitals had been required to provide huge amounts of uncompensated care (since so many people lost jobs and, with them, health insurance; because of the heavy burden of chronic disease among the poor; and because of the number of transient workers in town), and that health care had become "unacceptably primitive" (p. 1549).[26] Common among the problems clinicians faced were complications from untreated chronic conditions (especially hypertension, diabetes, and AIDS) and mental health problems.[26,75] Medical and prescription records had been destroyed during the storm; laboratory tests were still being sent out of town to be analyzed; microbiologic testing was unavailable; psychiatric patients brought in by police were sometimes sent to facilities as far as 150 miles away.[56,62,76]

Both the storm and these disheartening conditions led to one of the most predictable of the critical infrastructure problems: the health professional workforce shrank with breathtaking speed after the storms and grew increasingly small thereafter. The majority of primary care physicians left New Orleans and, by March 2006, only one quarter of them had returned.[28] A year after Katrina, possibly as few as 35% of the primary care physicians of New Orleans (primary care physicians being most likely to accept Medicaid) had returned.[71] Touro Infirmary, New Orleans's only community-based not-for-profit faith-based hospital (in operation since 1852), was paying a 50–100% premium to nurses willing to re-locate to the city.[26] Among other disincentives, health care professionals and staff wishing to work in New Orleans faced and continue to face a severe hurricane-induced housing shortage.[37]

The other big blow to the health infrastructure of storm-affected regions was to the capacity of hospitals, clinics, and long-term care institutions. While there are 3.26 hospital beds per 1,000 people in the United States as a whole, in New Orleans after the storm the ratio was 1.99/1,000;[26] 2,000 of the usual 4,400 hospital beds were functional.[26,72] Only 3 of 10 acute care hospitals in Orleans Parish were operational in June 2006, most with limited capacity.[28]

Psychiatric capacity also fell precipitously: By August 2006, 77 psychiatric beds (outside of the VA and Louisiana State facilities) were operational in New Orleans, compared with 460 before the storm. In the metropolitan area (Orleans, Chalmette, Jefferson, and St. Bernard Parishes), the number had fallen 57%, from 668 to 289.[77] These shortages are almost inconceivable when considered along with the massive mental and emotional health problems that spring from any disaster[9,11,30,49,78,81] and that have been demonstrated to plague survivors of the hurricanes of 2005.[21,38,42,56,65,71,77,79–84] Wang et al., for example, report that approximately a third of the Hurricane Katrina survivors who needed it received mental health care and that even the care that was delivered was inadequate.[81] The World Health Organization, comparing pre-Katrina and post-Katrina populations in the affected areas, found that both severe and mild-moderate mental illness had almost doubled since the storm.[83] (Also see chapters 6, 10, 12, 13, 18, 19, and 23 in this volume.)

In an update, Lamberg reports that shortages of facilities and clinicians in New Orleans persist, three years after the storm, as do high rates of mental illness: among survivors, more than 62.5% of preschoolers and over 50% of some groups of adults, for example, suffer from post-traumatic stress disorder.[84]

Government Response and Policy Recommendations

The agency that has been most widely criticized for its slow and inadequate response to the hurricanes of 2005 is FEMA; both the delay in delivering relief in the form of food, water, and shelter and the frequent inadequacy of that relief once it came have made a lasting impression on the national psyche.[85]* Seidenberg (chapter 26 in this volume) addresses FEMA in some detail. Other parts of the federal health response functioned better than FEMA: the CDC conducted surveillance, and the U.S. Public Health Service and military provided vital services during the emergency phase.† Not long after Katrina, a policymaking group, facilitated by the Public Health Service, developed "A Framework for Rebuilding."[26]

The papers in this volume, as well as the other literature reviewed here, yield some clear implications for public health policy for disasters. These policy recommendations follow.

Some problematic facets of federal disaster planning should be corrected in the short term. First, it is vital that chronic illness and dental health should be part of disaster planning. (See the discussion of chronic illness above and, for dental care, chapters 5 and 15 in this volume.) In the absence of thorough-going national health care reform, we must ensure adequate funds and personnel to meet the extensive chronic and dental health care needs of people most likely to spend time in government-run evacuation centers and temporary housing, as well as those who return to damaged homes, possibly without jobs. The issues here pile up, but a good model for funding care in the first six months after a disaster is New York's Disaster Relief Medicaid, which was

---

* An expression has entered English, "a Katrina moment," to denote the point at which someone demonstrates that he or she is badly out of touch with the general consensus, and his or her popularity is beginning a precipitous decline. The television commentator Chris Matthews used the expression this way in September 2008, speaking of Sen. John McCain, who had just offered the opinion that the fundamentals of the economy were sound, at a time when major banks were failing: *This might have been his Katrina moment,* Matthews said of McCain's remark.

† By September 7, 2005, the CDC's Agency for Toxic Substances and Disease Registry (ATSDR) had sent nearly 200 members of the U.S. Public Health Service Commissioned Corps, CDC Epidemic Intelligence officers, and federal civilian employees to the region to carry out vital public health functions.[86]

established after the attacks of September 11, 2001. Disaster Relief Medicaid waived requirements for an extensive application or documentation (the application form was a single page). That program served nearly 350,000 people in the 4 months after the attacks.[70] Underlying issues here need attention as well: state-to-state variability in Medicaid requirements, the exclusion of most impoverished adults, and difficult documentation requirements are among the structural features that make it hard to adapt Medicaid to disaster situations.[28,70,85]

Second, funding care doesn't ensure that there will be health care providers ready to do the job. Among the problems are concerns about the licensing of professionals who come from out of state to serve during the disaster phase; 35% of states currently do not allow for this.[87] There are similar concerns about mobile clinics and hospitals.[88] One approach to addressing this builds on existing programs: the federal government might consider recruiting additional personnel for the National Health Service Corps to serve for a period of years in areas that lose health care personnel due to disasters.

Third, mental health care needs must be seriously addressed as part of disaster relief planning. One reason that access to psychiatric care for survivors of the hurricanes has been so severely limited are provisions regarding its funding contained in the 1974 federal law, the Robert T. Stafford Emergency Relief and Emergency Assistance Act, which was intended to fund supplements to U.S. state and local emergency response. The Stafford Act restricts disaster funding for mental health to crisis care, effectively to short-term crisis counseling. Many agree that this must be amended to allow the Substance Abuse and Mental Health Services Agency (SAMHSA) to support longer-term mental health care by area professionals and prescription medication as fundamental parts of disaster relief.[37,45,56,84]

Fourth, electronic medical and prescription records might have prevented a great deal of the disorder and failure to meet health care needs that were observed after the 2005 hurricanes. (See chapters 16 and 20 in this volume for more on this.) If records were accessible at a distance, providers in emergency situations would be able to treat survivors far more effectively, and survivors would be able to take more control over their own health care. See chapter 2 (in this volume) for more on needed policy changes, especially concerning environmental justice.

The immediate congressional response to Hurricane Katrina was the proposed Grassley-Baucus bill, the Emergency Health Care Relief Act, which would have provided survivors of the hurricane with health services for at least five months. However, fiscal conservatives in Congress, with the support of the Bush administration, greatly reduced the bill's scope, ultimately providing inadequate assistance for medical care and not addressing the health system problems. Furthermore, the allocation of block grant funding by the executive branch was severely delayed, leading to some of the serious problems we have reviewed here (including significant mental health problems in adults and children).[70,85] In December 2006, President Bush signed into law the Pandemic and All-Hazards Preparedness Act (PAHPA), a law designed to improve national preparation for disasters. This law places the Department of Health and Human Services (DHHS) (rather than the Department of Homeland Security) in charge of federal public health and emergency medical responses to emergencies, authorizing it to oversee all health personnel during emergencies, including volunteers. However, as

Hodge et al. point out, the law leaves several critical matters unaddressed, including the connection between DHHS and state, local, and tribal entities; the question of licensing and protecting from liability for volunteer health care professionals (noted above); and how limited resources are to be allocated during a health emergency.[89] Until more explicit and comprehensive legislation than these is in place, the federal government will remain ill-prepared for major disasters.

Nieburg et al., offering lessons learned about disaster preparedness from work abroad, argue that, "because the United States is less subject to political instability and resource limitations than most developing countries, we should be able to manage population displacements reasonably well. The insufficient response to Hurricane Katrina seems to have been due largely to a lack of appropriate planning (p. 1548)."[30] While this may be true of the raw elements of successful public health management of some of the immediate needs during disasters—ensuring safety, sanitation, food and water, shelter, tracking of individuals, and communication for displaced people—it doesn't begin to address the many weighty problems of the underserved in the context of the hurricanes of 2005 that we have reviewed here. Pre-existing health disparities, environmental injustice before and after the storms, widespread chronic health problems, disparities in literacy and housing, a tattered health care safety net, a piecemeal health insurance system that fails to meet the needs of many in middle-income as well as low-income groups, and mental health consequences of the disaster all cry out for long-lasting and systemic solutions. Short of those, however, disaster preparedness in the United States must encompass plans that take these conditions into account and at a minimum keep from making them worse. Rosenbaum describes the public health system consequences of Hurricane Katrina this way:

> Emergency medical personnel—both volunteers and those deployed under the 2002 Public Health and Bioterrorism Preparedness and Response Act—could offer short-term assistance, but volunteer clinicians on emergency deployment were clearly in no position to address evacuees' long-term health care needs. The emerging picture by mid-September [2005] was one of devastated state economies and community health infrastructures, long-term joblessness and deepening poverty and dislocation, and a lasting disconnect from health insurance (p. 438).[70]

Reform that ensures universal health coverage would assure health care professionals and hospitals of being paid for their services and survivors of receiving needed care, and that would be a start.

Notes

1. Knabb RD, Rhome JR, Brown DP. Tropical cyclone report: Hurricane Katrina, 23–30 August 2005. Miami: National Hurricane Center, 20 December 2005.
2. Knabb RD, Brown DP, Rhome JR. Tropical cyclone report: Hurricane Rita, 18–26 September 2005. Miami: National Hurricane Center, 17 March 2006.
3. Zachria A, Patel B. Deaths related to Hurricane Rita and mass evacuation. Chest. 2006 Oct 24;130(4):124S.
4. CDC. Public health response to Hurricanes Katrina and Rita—Louisiana, 2005 (Introduction). MMWR. 2006 Jan 20;55(2):29–30.

5. Pasch RJ, Blake ES, Cobb HD, et al. Tropical cyclone report: Hurricane Wilma, 15–25 October 2005. Miami: National Hurricane Center, 12 January 2006.

6. CDC. Rapid needs assessment of two rural communities after Hurricane Wilma—Hendry County, Florida, Nov. 1–2, 2005. MMWR. 2006 Apr 21;55(15):429–31.

7. CDC. Public health response to Hurricanes Katrina and Rita—United States, 2005. MMWR. 2006 Mar 10;55(9):229–31.

8. Lechat MF. The public health dimensions of disasters. Int J Mental Health. 1990 19:70–9.

9. Myers D. Disaster response and recovery: a handbook for mental health professionals. DHHS publication (SMA) 94–3010. Rockville, MD: National Institute of Mental Health, 1994

10. Malilay J. Tropical cyclones. In: Noji EK, ed. The public health consequences of disasters. New York: Oxford University Press, 1997;207–27.

11. Gerrity ET, Flynn BW. Mental health consequences of disasters. In: Noji EK, ed. The public health consequences of disasters. New York: Oxford University Press, 1997;101–21.

12. *Fothergill A, Maestas EG, Darlington JD. Race, ethnicity and disasters in the United States: a review of the literature. Disasters.* 1999 Jun;23(2):156–73.

13. Schultz JM, Russell J, Espinel Z. Epidemiology of tropical cyclones: the dynamics of disaster, disease, and development. Epidemiol Rev. 2005;27:21–35.

14. CDC. Public health response to Hurricanes Katrina and Rita—Louisiana, 2005 (Introduction). MMWR. 2006 Jan 20;55(2):29–30.

15. CDC. Mortality associated with Hurricane Katrina—Florida and Alabama, August–October 2005. MMWR. 2006 Mar 10;55(9):239–42.

16. Brunkard J, Namulanda G, Ratard R. Hurricane Katrina deaths, Louisiana, 2005. Disaster Med Public Health Prep. 2008 Aug 27 [e-pub ahead of print].

17. CDC. Infectious disease and dermatologic conditions in evacuees and rescue workers after Hurricane Katrina—multiple states, Aug.–Sept., 2005. MMWR. 2005 Sept 26;MMWR 54(Dispatch): 1–4.

18. Morin R, Deane C, Altman DE, et al. The Washington Post/Kaiser Family Foundation/Harvard University survey of Hurricane Katrina evacuees. Kaiser Family Foundation Publ. #7401. Menlo Park, CA: Henry J. Kaiser Family Foundation, Sept. 2005.

19. CDC. Norovirus outbreak among evacuees from Hurricane Katrina—Houston, Texas, September 2005. MMWR. 2005 Oct 14;54:1016–8.

20. CDC. Two cases of toxigenic vibrio cholera O1 infection after Hurricanes Katrina and Rita—Louisiana, October 2005. MMWR. 2006 Jan 20;55(2):31–2.

21. CDC. Surveillance in hurricane evacuation centers—Louisiana, Sept.–Oct. 2005. MMWR. 2006 Jan 20;55(2):32–5.

22. CDC. Surveillance for illness and injury after Hurricane Katrina—three counties, Mississippi, Sept. 5–Oct. 11, 2005. MMWR. 2006 Mar 10;55(9):231–4.

23. CDC. Morbidity surveillance after Hurricane Katrina—Arkansas, Louisiana, Mississippi, and Texas, September 2005. MMWR. 2006 July 7;55(26):727–31.

24. CDC. Rapid community needs assessment after Hurricane Katrina—Hancock County, Mississippi, Sept. 14–15, 2005. MMWR. 2006 Mar 10;55(9):234–6.

25. Berggren R. Unexpected necessities—inside Charity Hospital. NEJM. 2005 Oct 13;353(15):1550–3.

26. Berggren RE, Curiel TJ. After the storm—health care infrastructure in post-Katrina New Orleans. NEJM. 2006 Apr 13;354(15):1549–52.

27. CDC. Injury and illness surveillance in hospitals and acute-care facilities after Hurricanes Katrina and Rita—New Orleans area, Louisiana, Sept. 25–Oct. 15, 2005. MMWR. 2006 Jan 20;55(2):35–8.

28. Rudowitz R, Rowland D, Shartzer A. Health care in New Orleans before and after Hurricane Katrina. Health Affairs. 2006 Aug 29;25(5):w393–w406.

29. Arrieta MI, Foreman RD, Crook ED, et al. Insuring continuity of care for chronic disease patients after disaster: key preparedness elements. Am J Med Sci. 2008 Aug;336(2):128–33.

30. Nieburg P, Waldman RJ, Krumm DJ. Evacuated populations—lessons from foreign refugee crises. NEJM. 2005 Oct 13;353(15):1547–9.

31. Barry J. Rising tide: the great Mississippi flood and how it changed America. New York: Simon and Schuster, 1997.

32. Center for American Progress. Who are Katrina's victims? Washington, DC: Center for American Progress, 2005 Sept 6. Available at www.americanprogress.org/kf/katrinavictims.pdf.

33. Zuckerman S, Coughlin T. After Katrina: rebuilding opportunity and equity in the *new* New Orleans. Washington, DC: Urban Institute, 2006 Feb.

34. Smedley BD, Stith AY, Nelson AR, eds. Unequal treatment: confronting racial and ethnic disparities in health care. Institute of Medicine Report. Washington, DC: National Academies Press, 2003.

35. Payne JW. At risk before the storm struck: prior health disparities due to race, poverty multiply death, disease. Washington Post, 2005 Sept 13.

36. Cohen A. Hurricane Katrina: lethal levels. NEJM. 2005 Oct. 13;353(15):1549.

37. Kutner NG. Health needs, health care, and Katrina. In: Brunsma DL, Overfelt D, Picou S, eds. The sociology of disaster: perspectives on a modern catastrophe. Plymouth, UK: Rowman & Littlefield Publ., Inc., 2007;203–16.

38. Hyre AD, Cohen AJ, Kutner N, et al. Psychosocial status of hemodialysis patients one year after Hurricane Katrina. Am J Med Sci. 2008 Aug;336(2):94–8.

39. Greenough PG, Kirsch TD. Public health response—assessing needs. NEJM. 2005 Oct 13;353(15):1544–6.

40. Waknine Y. Highlights from MMWR: CDC Katrina evacuation center surveillance and more. Medscape Med News. 2006 Jan 20.

41. CDC. Assessment of health-related needs after Hurricanes Katrina and Rita—Orleans and Jefferson Parishes, New Orleans area, Louisiana, October 17–22, 2005. MMWR. 2006 Jan 20;55(2):38–41.

42. Abramson D, Garfield R. On the edge: children and families displaced by Hurricanes Katrina and Rita face a looming medical and mental health crisis. A report of the Louisiana Child & Family Health Study, based on a February 2006 household survey of families living in FEMA-subsidized community settings in Louisiana. New York: National Center for Disaster Preparedness and Operation Assist, 2006 Apr 17.

43. Dewan S. Evacuee study finds declining health. New York Times. 2006 Apr 18.

44. Brodie M, Weltzien E, Altman D, et al. Experiences of Hurricane Katrina evacuees in Houston shelters: implications for future planning. AJPH. 2006 May;96(5):1402–8.

45. Shebab N, Anastario MP, Lawry L. Access to care among displaced Mississippi residents in FEMA travel trailer parks two years after Katrina: serious deficits in services—especially for mental health—remain for Mississippi Gulf Coast residents displaced by the hurricanes of 2005. Health Affairs. 2008 Aug 29;27(5):w416–w429.

46. CDC. Rapid assessment of health needs and resettlement plans among Hurricane Katrina evacuees—San Antonio, Texas, Sept. 2005. MMWR. 2006 Mar 10;55(9):242–4.

47.   Xiong X, Harville EW, Mattison DR, et al. Exposure to Hurricane Katrina, post-traumatic stress disorder and birth outcomes. Am J Med Sci. 2008 Aug;336(2):111–5.

48.   Peacock WG, Morrow BH, Gladwyn H, eds. Hurricane Andrew: ethnicity, gender, and the sociology of disasters. New York: Routledge, 1997.

49.   Norris FH. 50,000 disaster victims speak: an empirical review of the empirical literature, 1981–2001. Washington, DC: National Center for PTSD and Center for Mental Health Services (SAMHSA), 2001 Sept.

50.   Peacock WG, Girard C. Ethnic and racial inequalities in hurricane damage and insurance settlements. In: Peacock WG, Morrow BH, Gladwyn H, eds. Hurricane Andrew: ethnicity, gender, and the sociology of disasters. New York: Routledge, 1997;171–90.

51.   Gladwyn H, Peacock WG. Warning and evacuation: a night for hard houses. In: Peacock WG, Morrow BH, Gladwyn H, eds. Hurricane Andrew: ethnicity, gender, and the sociology of disasters. New York: Routledge, 1997;52–74.

52.   Associated Press. FEMA suspends use of disaster trailers. 2007 Aug 2.

53.   Associated Press. FEMA to start testing air quality in trailers by Dec. 19. 2007 Dec 12.

54.   Mitka M. Capitol health call: FEMA and formaldehyde. JAMA. 2008 Mar 12;299(10):1124.

55.   CDC. Health concerns associated with mold in water-damaged homes after Hurricanes Katrina and Rita—New Orleans area, October 2005. MMWR. 2006 Jan 20;55(2):41–4.

56.   Weisler RH, Barbee JG, Townsend MH. Mental health and recovery in the Gulf Coast after Hurricanes Katrina and Rita. JAMA. 2006 Aug 2;296(5):585–8.

57.   Bullard RL. Katrina and the second disaster: a twenty-point plan to destroy Black New Orleans. Atlanta: Environmental Justice Resource Center (Clark Atlanta University), 2005 Dec 23. Available at www.ejrc.cau.edu/Bullard20PointPlan.html (last seen Sept. 18, 2008).

58.   Grenier GJ, Morrow BH. Before the storm: the socio-political ecology of Miami. In: Peacock WG, Morrow BH, Gladwyn H, eds. Hurricane Andrew: ethnicity, gender, and the sociology of disasters. New York: Routledge, 1997;36–51.

59.   Dash N, Peacock WG, Morrow BH. And the poor get poorer: a neglected Black community. In: Peacock WG, Morrow BH, Gladwyn H, eds. Hurricane Andrew: ethnicity, gender, and the sociology of disasters. New York: Routledge, 1997;206–25.

60.   Elliott JR, Pais J. Race, class, and Hurricane Katrina: social differences in human responses to disaster. Soc Sci Res. 2006;35:295–321.

61.   Quinn SC. Hurricane Katrina: a social and public health disaster (letter). AJPH. 2006 Feb;96(2):204.

62.   Berggren R. Adaptations. NEJM. 2006 Apr 13;354(15):1550–1.

63.   Benham R. The birth of the clinic: action medics in New Orleans. In: South End Press Collective, eds. What lies beneath: Katrina, race, and the state of the nation. Cambridge, MA: South End Press, 2007;69–79.

64.   Bierria A, Liebenthal M, Incite! Women of Color against Violence. To render ourselves visible: women of color organizing and Hurricane Katrina. In: South End Press Collective, eds. What lies beneath: Katrina, race, and the state of the nation. Cambridge, MA: South End Press, 2007;31–47.

65.   Children's Health Fund and National Center for Disaster Preparedness, Columbia University. Responding to an emerging humanitarian crisis in Louisiana and Mis-

sissippi: urgent need for a health care "Marshall Plan." New York: Children's Health Fund and National Center for Disaster Preparedness, Columbia University, 2006 Apr 17.

66. Dyson ME. Come Hell or high water: Hurricane Katrina and the color of disaster. New York: Perseus (Basic Civitas Books), 2006.

67. Hartman G, Squires GD, eds. There is no such thing as a natural disaster: race, class, and Hurricane Katrina. New York: Routledge, 2006.

68. Potter H, ed. Racing the storm: racial implications and lessons learned from Hurricane Katrina. Lanham, MD: Lexington Books, 2007.

69. Connolly C. New Orleans health care: another Katrina casualty. Washington Post, 2005 Nov 25.

70. Rosenbaum S. U.S. health policy in the aftermath of Hurricane Katrina. JAMA. 2006 Jan 26;295(4):437–40.

71. Perry M, Dulio A, Artiga S, et al. Voices of the storm: health experiences of low-income Katrina survivors. Kaiser Family Foundation publication #7538. Menlo Park, CA: Henry J. Kaiser Family Foundation, 2006 Aug 8.

72. Curiel T. Murder or mercy? Hurricane Katrina and the need for disaster training. NEJM. 2006 Nov 16;355(20):2067–9.

73. Okie S. Dr. Pou and the hurricane—implications for patient care during disasters. NEJM. 2008 Jan 3;358(1):1–5.

74. Pou AM. Hurricane Katrina and disaster preparedness (letter). NEJM. 2008 Apr 3;358(14):1524.

75. Krousel-Wood MA, Islam T, Muntner P, Stanley E, Phillips A, et al. Medication adherence in older patients with hypertension after Hurricane Katrina: implications for clinical practice and disaster management. Am J Med Sci. 2008 Aug;336(2):99–104.

76. Lamberg L. Katrina survivors strive to reclaim their lives. JAMA. 2006 Aug 2;296(5):499–502.

77. Voelker R. In post-Katrina New Orleans, efforts under way to build better health care. JAMA. 2006 Sept 20;296(11):1333–4.

78. Norris FH, Perilla JL, Riad JK, et al. Stability and change in stress, resources, and psychological distress following natural disaster: findings from Hurricane Andrew. Anxiety Stress Coping. 1999;12(4):363–96.

79. The Carter Center Mental Health Program. Disaster mental health after Hurricane Katrina: November 8 and 9, 2006. Atlanta: Carter Center, 2006.

80. Voelker R. Post-Katrina mental health needs prompt group to compile disaster medicine guide. JAMA. 2006 Jan 18;295(3):259–60.

81. Wang PS, Gruber MJ, Powers RE, et al. Mental health service use among Hurricane Katrina survivors in the eight months after the disaster. Psychiatr Serv. 2007 Nov;58(11):1403–11.

82. Saulny S. A legacy of the storm: depression and suicide. New York Times. 2006 June 21.

83. Kessler RC, Galea S, Jones RT, et al. Mental illness and suicidality after Hurricane Katrina. Geneva: World Health Organization, 2008.

84. Lamberg L. Katrina's mental health impact lingers: patients face shortages of facilities, clinicians. JAMA. 2008 Sept 3;300(9):1011–3.

85. Lambrew JM, Shalala DE. Federal health policy response to Hurricane Katrina: what it was and what it could have been. JAMA. 2006 Sept 20;296(11):1394–7.

86. CDC. Hurricane Katrina response and guidance for health-care providers, relief workers, and shelter operators. MMWR Weekly. 2005 Sept 9; MMWR 54(35): 877.

87. Boyajian-O'Neill LA, Gronewald LM, Glaros AG, et al. Physician licensure during disasters: a national survey of state medical boards (research letter). JAMA. 2008 Jan 9/16;299(2):169–71.

88. Voelker R. Mobile hospital raises questions about hospital surge capacity. JAMA. 2006 Apr 5;295(13):1499–503.

89. Hodge JG, Gostin LO, Vernick JS. The Pandemic and All-Hazards Preparedness Act: improving public health emergency response. JAMA. 2007 Apr 18;297(15):1708-11.

Chapter 2
Katrina Perspectives on the Environment and Public Health

Bailus Walker Jr., PhD, MPH
Rueben Warren, DDS, MPH, DrPH

An appreciation for the devastation that can be caused by natural disasters, including hurricanes and floods, has been developing for many decades. For the United States, hurricanes and floods are the leading sources of disaster-related fatalities. Hurricanes and floods usually raise a broad range of environmental health issues (e.g., housing, water quality, waste water disposal, hygiene, and sanitation) as well as issues of risk assessments and risk communication, and Katrina was no exception. It was a plain and painful reminder that environmental exposures arise because of natural variations, such as naturally occurring extremes in weather, and climate change. The environmental exposures of greatest interest here are due to human interventions, which in recent years have attracted the most attention in the public health community.

Risk Factors

Hurricane Katrina, which made landfall near New Orleans on August 29, 2005, elevated into sharp relief a number of factors conducive to the development of a broad range of environmental risks for disease and premature death. These elements include biological, physical, and ecological factors, as well as social, political, and economic factors. When these factors converge, as they did in the case of Katrina, the risk for disease, disability, and premature death is far greater than any single factor would predict. Thanks to major investments in research, we have a better (though not complete) understanding not only of the physical dimensions of the environment that are toxic but also of a broad range of related conditions in the social, economic, and political environments that are factors in increasing the risk of adverse health conditions. Understanding these factors, as they may relate to the ramifications of Katrina, requires an understanding of the broad setting in which the hurricane slammed New Orleans.

Katrina did not arrive alone. It came during a period defined by the interplay of at least four forces, sketched in fairly broad strokes in the following sections of this paper. They formed the broad context for daily events relevant to the health and welfare of the

*BAILUS WALKER is Professor of Environmental and Occupational Medicine and of Health Policy, Howard University College of Medicine. **RUEBEN WARREN** is the Associate Director for the Institute for Faith Health Leadership at the Interdenominational Theological Center and Adjunct Professor, Department of Community Medicine/Preventive Medicine, Morehouse School of Medicine.*

people disproportionately affected by the hurricane. At the same time, these forces suggest that the consequences of Katrina were, like those of many other natural disasters, exacerbated by inadequacies in the human response.

The observations that follow grow from our experience in New Orleans years before Katrina roared onto the Gulf Coast and our visits to the area in the weeks afterward. We had informal discussions with our academic colleagues and civic leaders in New Orleans and we reviewed volumes of governmental and relief agency reports, and Congressional testimony. We also talked with some of the displaced residents who were transported to Washington, D.C., from hurricane-ravaged areas. In addition, one of us (BW) co-chaired a group discussion of public health impacts of Katrina, a meeting of scientists and engineers convened by the National Academy of Sciences in Washington, D.C.

Environmental Justice

First, when the hurricane struck, the fallout was still in the air from earlier debates about the fact that minority and low-income communities bear a disproportionate share of the hazards caused by the nation's air, water, and waste pollution problems. Intellectual support for this argument came from studies and scholarly analyses that found that municipal and hazardous landfills, incinerators, abandoned toxic waste dumps, and heavy vehicular traffic routes are located primarily in minority and low-income neighborhoods.[1-2] Other studies presented conflicting evidence as to whether a disproportionate burden exists, especially with respect to choosing sites for polluting waste facilities.[3-4] There were also debates about environmental epidemiology, including issues such as statistical biases, uncertainties, and other methodological weaknesses of epidemiological studies.[5] And there were, and still are, controversies surrounding the health outcomes of exposure to low doses of environmental toxins.[6-7]

These issues surfaced again in the context of efforts to communicate risk of environmental exposure of affected groups in New Orleans. The longstanding debate in recent years has been fueled by renewed attention to the concept of *hormesis*, that is, that exposure to small amount of a dangerous substance can stimulate the body's defenses and may be beneficial.[8]

Setting aside the controversies, *environmental justice* has to do with more than documenting uneven exposure of different population groups to environmental hazards. It is also about raising awareness of and sensitivity to the issues and about achieving fairness in federal, state, and local environmental health policy decision-making. Environmental justice also has to do with whether communities have a voice in decisions that affect their health, environment, and quality of life, such as economic growth and development of neighborhoods. Communities where residents cannot devote all of their time to reading and analyzing environmental laws and regulations may not have the background information to make informed decisions. In addition, minority and low-income residents may lack guidance to navigate complex issues such as environmental risk calculations; they also may lack contacts and other resources to take political action necessary to effect change for their benefit. Minority and low-income groups often face further barriers because of subtle, as well as overt, housing discrimination and underrepresentation in governmental (executive and legislative) offices where policy is formulated and implemented.

Encouragingly, environmental justice gained enough momentum and had broad enough support to prompt an Executive Order issued by President Clinton placing environmental justice on the national political agenda.[9] While progress has been made, much more remains to be done to bring to full fruition the objectives of the executive order, or as President Clinton stated as he issued the order, "to ensure that all communities and persons across this nation live in a safe and healthful environment." That objective had not been achieved when Katrina disrupted efforts to achieve parity in New Orleans.[9]

Poverty

Second, Katrina's arrival was also a period in which social distress appeared to be worsening, as severe poverty had increased by 20% between 2000 and 2004.[10] As the discussions about this increase evolved, they reinforced again and again our understanding of how and why socioeconomic status has a strong, pervasive, and even increasing, impact on human health. Socioeconomic status shapes people's experience of, and exposure to, virtually all psychosocial and environmental risk factors for health—past, present, and future—and these in turn operate through a very broad range of physiological mechanisms to influence the course of virtually all major causes of disease and health. Thus, in the end, the socioeconomic position itself is a fundamental cause of individual and population health, and a fundamental lever for improving health in American society. Here, it bears repeating: the weight of evidence makes clear that the economically disadvantaged—the group disproportionately affected by Katrina—are the most vulnerable to the health effects of environmental problems. The economically disadvantaged are typically more heavily exposed to environmental stressors because of residential and occupational location and have fewer resources for taking protective or adaptive actions. There is also ample evidence that the various social and political influences on population vulnerability to environmental stressors include poverty, political inefficiency, and environmentally destructive growth and community development.[11]

Public Health System

Third, at the same time the bleak trends in poverty were being debated, both before Katrina and now, in the post-Katrina period, there was high anxiety about the nation's ability to detect, prevent, and control emerging and resurging diseases, a number of which are preventable through appropriate levels of immunizations.[12] (We should note here that Louisiana had relatively low immunization rates prior to Katrina.[13])

Enmeshed in these concerns was the recognition that progress has been mixed in strengthening public health agencies' capacities to address environmental problems, in building ties to the mental health field, and in meeting the health care needs of the medically indigent. In fact, a number of assessments have concluded that public health systems are severely overtaxed and have long been in decline. For instance, the Institute of Medicine reports that the U.S. public health infrastructure has suffered years of neglect and that the overall shortage of qualified public health workers makes it difficult to meet the demand imposed by an outbreak of infectious diseases alone. Addressing essentially the same issue, another Institute of Medicine committee studying the future of public health in the 21st century, concluded that public health systems suffer from grave under-funding, political neglect, and continuous exclusion from the very forum in which their expertise and leadership are most needed to ensure an effective public health system.[12,14] This problem was recognized by the Bush administration following the anthrax scare in 2001, which underscored the poor abilities of federal and local health agencies to respond to bioterrorism or epidemic threats. Since then, Congress has approved some $3.7 billion to strengthen the nation's public health system.

However, a subsequent study by *Trust for America's Health* (the Trust) a non-profit, non-partisan organization working to make disease prevention a national priority, found that many essential improvements have not yet been achieved.[7] The report revealed that state public health agencies are facing fundamental structural problems that threaten the nation's ability to respond to a large public health emergency. The Trust concluded that the full-scale effort to fix the nations public health system comprehensively is falling short. In the Trust's scoring system of state preparedness to respond to public health emergencies (0 was the lowest possible score, and 10 was the highest), Louisiana scored 5. Moreover, the state did not provide at least 50% of federal capacity-building funds directly to local health departments, usually among the first responders during a public health emergency such as Katrina. In fairness, it should be noted that Louisiana was not the worst in the scoring system: the District of Columbia scored 3 and Wisconsin scored 2. Concerned about these developments, the U.S. Conference of Mayors report that major cities feel shut out of state planning process for public health preparedness and the conference claims that state priorities do not reflect local concerns.[15-16]

These assessments are jarring because Katrina, and recent outbreaks of diseases such as avian flu, severe acute respiratory syndrome (SARS), mumps and the Ebola virus—diseases that pay no heed to geographical boundaries—demonstrate the continuing need for an effective public health system. Moreover, the early detection of, and response to, increasingly diverse public health threats will depend on the capacity of and expertise in the public health system at every level. In this connection, the limited resources available to many local health departments make the involvement of the state necessary to implement state health laws adequately. Often overlooked is the fact that states and their local subdivisions retain the primary responsibility for health under the U.S Constitution. Local health departments, however, have for a long time represented two competing ideas at work: the belief that the most proximate form of government is the most effective and possibly most efficient, and the pragmatic judgments that the state needs a decentralized delivery system to produce the appropriate services. The two reasons are often confused when considering how or why the states should support the operations of local health departments. The distinction is sometimes blurred in debates that the local level is where health services actually come into contact with the people; this is the real firing line. Moreover, after all the federal and state aid has been provided, the technical advice heard, and regulation and policy guidelines duly observed, it is the local health department that delivers the health services. (Disclosure: the authors have had leadership responsibilities in state and local health departments.)

Advances in Science

Fourth, when Katrina struck, American life in general was being rapidly and continuously transformed by scientific and technological progress. Indeed, the ongoing revolution in science was of unprecedented magnitude, accelerating dramatically, and promised almost unlimited opportunity for the betterment of humankind. Despite tremendous progress, translating this knowledge into effective prevention and treatment for major afflictions has been slower than anticipated. For example, sorting out the uncertainties surrounding elements of the deceptively simple equation—*gene + environment = outcome*—requires years. Doing so is important, given the pervasiveness of disorders that have both genetic and environmental components (e.g., atherosclerosis, lung disease, obesity). How to turn biomedical science knowledge into practical outcomes must be an increasing focus of attention of the public health and medical communities.

Equally important are the advances in the physical sciences that have enabled weather forecasting (e.g., predicting hurricanes) to become more and more precise. Improved forecasting has been aided by computer modeling and satellite-based tracking systems, an advancement that should greatly enhance efforts to warn people of impending natural disasters and mitigate their impact. Timely and effective responses to these warnings can significantly reduce losses of lives and property, an issue that has been of considerable interest in post-Katrina assessments. Impressive too are the advances in "preventive" civil engineering, including improvement in the strength of materials and the design and construction of floodwater management equipment and facilities. Evidently these engineering advances were not effectively applied to the design and construction of levees (water containment/control devices) protecting New Orleans. This was corroborated by several teams of civil engineers who told a U.S Senate panel in 2005 that poor design and construction bears much of the blame for the flood in New Orleans. Speaking of this failure, Senator Susan Collins (R-ME), the chair of the Senate committee on Homeland Security and Governmental Affairs, which conducted a hearing in November of 2005, said "Many of the widespread failures throughout the levee system were not solely the result of Mother Nature. Rather they were the results, it appears, of human error in the form of design and construction flaws."[17–19]

Consequences

It is in this setting that John McLachlan, director of the Tulane/Xavier Center for Bio-environmental Research, a New Orleans based academic center, referred to the environmental and health consequences of Katrina as the "mother of all multidisciplinary problems." Prominent among these problems was environmental contamination, including contamination from arsenic, lead, volatile and semi-volatile organic compounds (untreated sewage, with a bacterial and viral load, over-flowed into housing and streets, and standing water was a breeding site for mosquitoes and other insect vectors of disease). There were also tons of spoiled food in warehouses along the docks and mold growth in houses damaged by Katrina. This is not the place to belabor these risk factors for disease because they have been widely enumerated in volumes of governmental and non-governmental reports and professional journals and elaborated in Congressional testimony and in a huge number of workshops and seminars.[17,20–25]

One of the most striking assessments of Katrina's impact on the New Orleans health care system—one of the community's main avenues of advance in its broad societal attack on disease problems—was offered by Tyler Curial, MD, MPH, who along with his wife, Ruth Berggren, MD, an infectious disease specialist at Tulane and Charity Hospitals, were physicians on duty at the Medical Center of Louisiana at New Orleans (Charity) as Katrina bore down. His assessment is instructive and worth quoting at length:

> Katrina's floodwaters crippled emergency power generators, transforming hospitals into dark, fetid dangerous shells. Extremely high temperatures killed some people. We were under tremendous strain: in addition to the dire medical circumstances of many of our patients, we confronted uncertainty about our own evacuation, exacerbated by tensions, threatened by violence by snipers and frazzled soldiers and guards. I saw competent professionals reduced to utter incoherence and uselessness as the crises unfolded. I saw others perform heroic deeds that surprised me. Clearly a better personnel selection process was needed.[26]

Plainly, many of the determinants of the health consequences and conditions of Katrina were part of a broad economic, social, and political construct, and thus, beyond the direct control of health service professionals in either the public or the private sector. What is more, many of the environmental components, here broadly defined, were socially conditioned, relating to poverty, racism, overcrowding, substandard housing, and a broad spectrum of social ills that require political solutions rather than repeated or expanded answers from health sciences and biomedical research. Concerning political solutions to public health problems, Laurie Garrett gave voice to a side of the problem that is very relevant here. Writing about the politics of preparing for an influenza pandemic, she opined, "There may be some who lost parents, aunts, or uncles, to the 1918–19 pandemic, and perhaps even more heard the horror stories that were passed down. But politics breeds shortsightedness and for decades the threats of an influenza pandemic has been easily forgotten, and therefore ignored at budget time."[27] Public health departments and medical care institutions do not have an easy handle with which to grab hold of and shape priorities of state or municipal budgets, or to manage such health-related services as transportation, public works, and land-use planning. Action in these areas at the state and local levels requires an alignment of public policy in transportation, land use, and infrastructure maintenance in ways that promote health.

Finally, as we write, there are many other lessons still being learned from Katrina, the most evident of which include the frequently cited need for a comprehensive but dynamic and flexible disaster-preparedness plan that involves all key components of society. The blueprint should be designed to force leaders to rehearse their response to crises, preparing emotionally and intellectually so that when the disaster strikes the community can face it. For environmental health, specifically, Hurricane Katrina made it clear that there is an unmet need for a national coordinated response plan to assess environmental and biological exposures to hazardous agents, and to understand the relationship of exposures to adverse health outcomes through appropriate surveillance.

Such a plan, according to the National Institute of Environmental Sciences, would facilitate prevention and early intervention strategies designed to identify at-risk individuals and reduce morbidity and mortality.[28]

Conclusions

In Hurricane Katrina, risk factors for disease, disability, and premature death due to environmental hazards took root and became rampant in New Orleans. It would be encouraging if we could report that the multiple and complex issues arising from Katrina's impact have been effectively addressed. But our recent visit to the area forces us to conclude that the situation in New Orleans continues to require long-term sustained commitment and the administrative, scientific and technical skills of both the private and public sectors. Perhaps a *New York Times* (February 16, 2007) page one headline said it best: "New Orleans's New Setback: Fed-Up Residents Giving Up."[29] It is clear that post-Katrina health problems, physical and mental, cannot be solved by short-term strategies in the form of a few new laws, rearrangement of the bureaucracy, and a few dollars thrown in the direction of the problem, in hopes that it will go away. To be sure, the public health archives are replete with evidence of long-term adverse effects resulting from efforts to apply short-term solutions to problems that require long-term sustained commitments. So, we are cheating the entire nation if we in the private and public sectors attempt to cover up the consequences of Katrina with short-term solutions. Undoubtedly, Katrina's aftermath poses diverse challenges—a bewildering array of environmental hazards and social and economic disruption—for us all. For the sake of future generations, we must take them up.

Notes

1. Institute of Medicine, Committee on Environmental Justice. Toward environmental justice: research, education, and health policy needs. Washington, DC: National Academies Press, 1999.
2. U.S. General Accounting Office. Siting of hazardous waste landfills and their correlation with racial and economic status of surrounding communities. (GAO/RCED-83-168.) Washington, DC: U.S. Government Printing Office 1983.
3. Olden K, White SL. Health-related disparities: influence of environmental factors. Med Clin North Am. 2005 Jul;89(4):721–38.
4. United Church of Christ, Commission for Racial Justice. Toxic wastes and race in the United States: a national report on the racial and socioeconomic characteristics of communities with hazardous waste sites. New York: United Church of Christ, 1987.
5. Johnson BL, Coulberson SL. Environmental epidemiological issues and minority health. Ann Epidemiol. 1993 Mar;3(2):175–80.
6. Cook RR, Calabrese EJ. Hormesis is biology, not religion. Environ Health Perspect. 2006 Dec;114(12):A688.
7. Cook R, Calabrese EJ. The importance of hormesis to public health. Environ Health Perspect. 2006 Nov;114(11):1631–5.
8. Rietjens IM, Alink GM. Future of toxicology—low-dose toxicology and risk—benefit analysis. Chem Res Toxicol. 2006 Aug;19(8):977–81.

9. U.S. Council on Environmental Quality. Environmental justice: highlights of Executive Order 12898. In: U.S. Council on Environmental Quality. Environmental quality: twenty-fifth anniversary report. Washington, DC: Executive Office of the President, 1994–1995; p. 113.

10. Wolf SH, Johnson RE, Geiger HJ. The prevalence of severe poverty in America: a growing threat to public health. Am J Prev Med. 2006 Oct;31(4):332–41.

11. Walker B, Mays VM, Warren R. The changing landscape for the elimination of racial/ethnic health status. J Health Care Poor Underserved. 2004 Nov;15(4):506–21.

12. Institute of Medicine, Board on Global Health. Microbial threats to health: emergence, detection, and response. Washington, DC: National Academies Press, 2003.

13. National Center for Health Statistics (NCHS). Health, United States, 2004 with chartbook on trends in the health of Americans. Hyattsville, MD: NCHS, 2004.

14. Institute of Medicine. Committee on Assuring the Health of the Public. The future of public health in the 21st century. Washington, DC: National Academies Press, 2002.

15. Trust for America's Health. Ready or not? 2003. Protecting the public health in the age of bioterrorism. Washington, DC: Trust for America's Health, 2003.

16. U.S. Conference of Mayors, Homeland Security Monitoring Center. First mayors' report to the nation: tracking federal Homeland Security funds sent to the 50 state governments. Washington, DC: U.S. Conference of Mayors, 2003 Sep 17.

17. Manuel J. In Katrina's wake. Environ Health Perspect. 2006 Jan;114(1):A33–9.

18. Travis J. Hurricane Katrina. Scientists' fears come true as hurricane floods New Orleans. Science. 2005 Sep 9;309(5741):1656–9.

19. Bohannon J. Katrina leaves behind a pile of scientific questions. Science. 2005 Sep 23;309(5743):1981.

20. Berggren RE, Curiel TJ. After the storm—health care infrastructure in post-Katrina New Orleans. N Eng J Med. 2006 Apr 13;354(15):1549–52.

21. Institute of Medicine. Roundtable on Environmental Health Sciences Research and Medicine. Environmental health impacts of disasters: Hurricane Katrina. (unpublished) Washington, DC: National Academy of Sciences, 2006.

22. Lambrew JM, Shalala DE. Federal policy response to hurricane Kartina: what it was and what it could have been. JAMA. 2006 Sep;296(11):1394–7.

23. Greenough PG, Kirsch TD. Hurricane Katrina. Public health response—assessing needs. N Engl J Med. 2005 Oct 13;353(15):1544–6.

24. Voelker R. Katrina's impact on mental health likely to last years. JAMA. 2005 Oct 5;294(13):1599–600.

25. Kinitisch E. Hurricane Katrina. Levees came up short, researchers tell Congress. Science. 2005 Nov 11;310(5750):953–5.

26. Curiel TJ. Murder or mercy? Hurricane Katrina and the need for disaster training. N Engl J Med. 2006 Nov 16;355(20):2067–9.

27. Garrett L. The next pandemic? Foreign Aff. 2005 Jul/Aug;84(4):3–23.

28. Schwartz DA. The NIEHS responds to hurricane Katrina. Environ Health Perspect. 2005 Nov;113(11):A722.

29. Pareles J. New Orleans's new setback: fed up residents giving up. The New York Times. 2007 Feb 16:1.

PART I: What It Was Like and What Happened

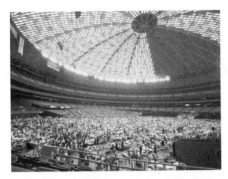

Figure 1. Evacuees from New Orleans filling the Houston Astrodome. Photograph courtesy of Baylor College of Medicine Office of Public Affairs.

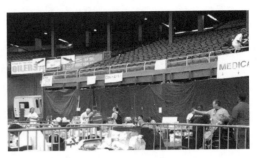

Figure 2. Post-Katrina triage in the Astrodome. Photograph courtesy of Baylor College of Medicine Office of Public Affairs.

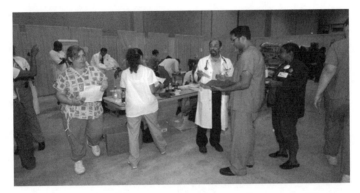

Figure 3. Clinicians in the Astrodome. Photograph courtesy of Baylor College of Medicine Office of Public Affairs.

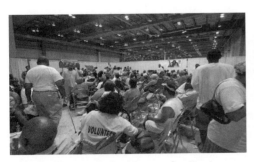

Figure 4. Waiting for health care after Katrina. Photograph courtesy of Baylor College of Medicine Office of Public Affairs.

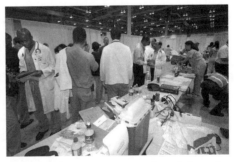

Figure 5. Clinicians took marathon shifts at the Astrodome. Photograph courtesy of the Baylor College of Medicine Office of Public Affairs.

Chapter 3
Persevering through the Storm: Educating Nursing Seniors in the Aftermath of Katrina

Sharon W. Hutchinson, PhD, MN, RN
Charlotte Hurst, PhD, CNM, RN
Sheila C. Haynes, MN, CNS, RN
Betty P. Dennis, DrPH, RN
Sheila J. Webb, PhD, CNS, RN

If I had to summarize my experience in two words, I would say heart ache. Heartache because I could not help each and every one or rewind time . . . I could not do either and that broke my heart.

—Dillard University Senior Nursing Student (DUSNS)

On August 29, 2005, native New Orleanians and the world watched as water surging from Hurricane Katrina began to breach levees and the rushing waters flooded homes of over a half a million people.[1] The nation glued its eyes to radios and television sets, listened and watched and wept as stranded neighbors, family members, friends, and fellow citizens struggled to obtain the necessities of life. The media depicted a fallen city with residents of all social levels asking for guidance and assistance in finding temporary shelter. Being stranded without the necessities of life and not knowing where to go, or when you would be able to return home left many confused, bewildered, and searching for a temporary home. Doubly traumatic was also seeing friends and family members go through the same experience. Senate hearings with Homeland Security produced cost projections for rebuilding in excess of the already allocated 62 billion dollars.[2]

More than 300 thousand former New Orleanians evacuated to Baton Rouge, Louisiana, the state capital.[3] Among the evacuees were Dillard University Nursing faculty, nursing students and staff. Unable to return to the Dillard University's campus, which was located directly next to the London Avenue Canal, one of several levee breaches, the University's administration had to respond to the overwhelming crisis.[4]

Dillard University had long been admired for the classic beauty of its campus, where white-columned Georgian buildings stood among spacious green lawns. The expansive branches of many huge, old live oak trees shaded the buildings and walkways of the campus. Following Hurricane Katrina and the failure of the levees, water surged onto

SHARON HUTCHINSON is an Associate Professor at Southern University School of Nursing in Baton Rouge. During the aftermath of Katrina, Dr. Hutchinson was the Assistant Dean of Nursing for Dillard University. CHARLOTTE HURST and SHEILA HAYNES are Assistant Professors at Dillard University, Division of Nursing, where BETTY DENNIS is a Professor and Dean. SHEILA WEBB is the Associate Director of Clinical Services at EXCELth, Inc. in New Orleans.

the campus and into the surrounding community. For almost two weeks, the lawns, buildings, and trees sat submerged or partially submerged under about 10 feet of water. In the immediate aftermath, the campus could only be accessed from the air. Aerial views showed that the most extensive water damage had occurred in the rear of the campus, its lowest point. One building was a total loss, and others would need to be gutted and extensively repaired. In the front of the campus, although there was less water from the levees, the roaring winds and heavy rain of the hurricanes had ripped shingles from the roofs and left water in classroom buildings, computer labs, the library, the chapel, and administrative offices. Two dormitories caught fire and burned to the ground because fire service could not respond until the waters receded. Of the several universities in the New Orleans area, Dillard University sustained the greatest damage to its physical facilities. It was not possible to return to campus until September 2006.

Like other universities and nursing schools closed by Katrina, Dillard was left with the task of educating future nurses in the aftermath of a major disaster.[5] The account given here reports the efforts of faculty and administration of the Division of Nursing at Dillard University to enable senior-level baccalaureate students to complete their coursework. The students' reflections concerning their unique learning experience are interwoven throughout the chapter.

Educating in Unfamiliar, Distant Environments

There were times of sorrow, but for the most part the spirit of New Orleans was alive.
—DUSNS

After Hurricane Katrina, Dillard University's administrators, including the Dean of the School of Nursing, relocated to Atlanta, Georgia. It was from this temporary head-quarters that school officials continued to conduct the business of the University and make plans for future recovery. All classes had been cancelled for the fall semester and students in majors other than nursing had been admitted to other universities for the semester. The Division of Nursing and the Dillard administration acknowledged that it would be difficult for students to realize fully a senior experience in a nursing program at another university. It was also understood that the demand for nurses in the greater New Orleans area would increase as the City's health care infrastructure was abruptly dismantled.[6-7] Therefore, the administration granted permission for the Division of Nursing to continue nursing classes for its seniors at an alternate site.

In the midst of the chaos of being displaced and creating a post-disaster future, for which there was no model, Dillard's Dean of Nursing located the Assistant Dean and two senior faculty members who had relocated to Baton Rouge. Students and faculty communicated by cell phone and text messages regarding plans for senior nursing students to continue their studies in Baton Rouge. The students were told their classes would resume on October 6, 2005 in Baton Rouge and that they would receive details as soon as arrangements had been finalized.

Creating and Finding Resources for Nursing Students

When I first saw the living area . . . I thought a shelter, but I grew to love that place. We all did.

—DUSNS

At no time in our lives did Maslow's hierarchy of needs seem so applicable.[4] Having found our students scattered across Louisiana and Texas, faculty had to locate centralized housing for the students very quickly. Dillard University is associated with the United Methodist Church (UMC) and sought the assistance of the Wesley Foundation (which is a ministerial affiliate of the UMC) at Southern University in Baton Rouge. The Wesley Foundation was able to provide housing for our nursing students at their facilities directly across from Southern University's main campus. The former director, Reverend Rodney Wooten, readily responded to the University's request for assistance with the housing of 14 nursing students. He met with the nursing faculty to plan the transformation of the Foundation's facility into a temporary, safe, female dormitory. Word of the University's and the Foundation's efforts traveled fast and charitable contributions for the students poured into the Foundation's office. Contributions of beds, linen, towels, water, snack foods, clothing, personal items, electronic textbooks, provisions for daily meals, and computers arrived almost immediately. The procurement and installation of a shower trailer from the Federal Emergency Management Agency (FEMA) completed the supply of daily necessities and Southern University School of Nursing provided classroom space. The Wesley Foundation conference room served as a study area. Prior to the students' arrival, Dillard University hired 6 residential coordinators from the Baton Rouge area to assist in the provision of 24-hour security and assistance with immediate student needs. Every effort to provide a stress-reduced learning environment was made prior to the students' arrival.

On October 6, 2005, 14 senior nursing students from Dillard arrived at the Wesley Foundation to continue their nursing studies, leaving behind their families and loved ones in parts of Texas and Louisiana to which they had either evacuated or returned home.

Getting Creative—Continuing the Curriculum with a Limited Number of Faculty

A lot of changes took place within the class, but we were able to adapt and make it through.

—DUSNS

Having solved the problem of housing and classroom availability, the focus changed to acquiring sites for clinical experiences and continuation of the curriculum. The senior nursing courses taught immediately after Katrina were *Community Health Nursing I (Community Health)*, *Nursing Leadership and Management (Leadership and Management)*, and *Nursing Research*. The curriculum had previously called for *Adult Health Nursing III*, but this was not available due to the unavailability of some faculty after the disaster. Fortunately, some faculty members evacuated with their USB computer keys and had access to course syllabi for *Community Health* and *Leadership and Management*. Faculty reviewed the course objectives and agreed that they could be accomplished in the remaining time period. Dillard nursing faculty taught *Community Health* and *Leadership and Management*. With the assistance of the Southern University nursing faculty, students cross-enrolled to study *Nursing Research* at Southern's School of Nursing. Dillard's Dean of Nursing notified the Louisiana State Board of Nursing regarding its plans to continue the curriculum for senior nursing students only and that classes would resume for all other baccalaureate students in the Spring of 2006.

Faculty agreed that Katrina presented a learning opportunity unlike any other that faculty and students had encountered before and they began to identify agencies that could provide the students with learning experiences related to the hurricane, its aftermath, and health care. To do this, faculty reached out to other health care personnel. A home health agency and a federally qualified health center were identified as possible clinical affiliates for the *Community Health* and *Leadership and Management* courses. Both health care organizations were originally located in New Orleans and had re-established themselves in the Greater Baton Rouge area. The Division of Nursing entered into a clinical affiliation agreement with EXCELth, Inc. to permit the students to engage in a community-based learning experience for *Leadership and Management* at the FEMA trailer site known as *Renaissance Village*, located in Baker, Louisiana. An affiliate agreement with a home health agency was already in place prior to the storm. Faculty also arranged for other clinical activities, including health promotion presentations at middle schools, and planning and implementation of a health fair at a church in the Greater Baton Rouge area. Students were required to write reflections regarding their on-site educational experiences and their association with other Katrina evacuees.

A Unique Learning Opportunity: Establishing a Leadership and Management Clinical at a FEMA Site

The first time I went to Renaissance Village, I was overwhelmed. Some people were really receptive and some were not because they believed they were being mistreated. The biggest problem was the gap between them and receiving health care. It was a learning experience for all of us. I also learned to cope with a lot of my own personal Katrina issues.

—DUSNS

Traditionally, Dillard's senior nursing students' *Leadership and Management* clinical experiences were held in acute care settings. However, given the impact of Katrina and the obvious presence of nurse leaders and managers operating outside of the acute care setting,[8] the faculty felt that the health center's Mobile Health Clinic would provide a valuable learning opportunity. Senior nursing students enrolled in the nursing *Leadership and Management* course had the opportunity, through lecture and selected clinical sites, to analyze the role of a nurse leader and nurse manager during the recovery phase of a disaster; the role of nurse manager in the establishment of community-based health care post-disaster; and the need for continued professional development and self-management.

Weekly clinical rotations were developed along with the nurse managers at the health center to provide students with learning experiences in leadership development. The initial clinical experiences allowed students to work as case managers and to develop strategies to meet the needs of clients at the FEMA site. This proved to be challenging because, not only were there adults at the site, there were children of various ages who had a variety of health care as well as social needs. An open system MODEL approach was used.[9] This approach allowed Dillard nursing students, members of the health center, and other community-based organizations to come together to meet the needs of adults, families, and children. It was imperative that the students understood they would be required to make house calls with the registered nurse or physician on duty to determine if an individual needed assistance in keeping his or her appointment with the mobile unit. One student saw the learning experience this way:

> It was a different experience. We had limited resources that were utilized the best we could to provide the best care. I learned how to adjust to situations and make the most out of what you have, to get the work done. It was an eye-opening and compelling experience.

The Dillard nursing student was also involved in the development of a land-based clinical site. This part of the clinical experience focused on disaster health care management, economics and finance, public policy, human resources, quality improvement, and marketing. Coursework was also carried out through hands-on activities at EXCELth's land-based facility in North Baton Rouge.

Reflecting: More on What They Thought

I found myself holding back tears in front of the person I was registering. It really opened my eyes to how blessed I am.

—DUSNS

Living and learning in this non-traditional setting was a life-changing experience for all involved. Everything that was once familiar no longer existed for the students and faculty living at the Wesley Foundation. Life as they knew it, and the lives of the individuals they encountered during their clinical experiences, had been forever changed. Individuals affected by Katrina experienced (and continue to experience) a myriad of mental health conditions as a result of the storm; they needed opportunities to explore their feelings concerning the disaster caused by the hurricane.[10] Faculty therefore took up the reflective tool as an opportunity for students to critically think about their learning experiences and as a venue for them to explore their own feelings regarding Katrina.[11] Both the *Community Health* and *Leadership and Management* clinical experiences included a reflective component. Additional excerpts from the DUSNS reflective papers follow.

I realized some people just needed to talk . . . to talk about their feelings . . . we were able to come together to help others, despite the circumstances.

At the school I interacted with students that were displaced. Most students talked about the difficulty of trying to adapt to a new school when you were suppose to be at your own school. This was an eye-opening experience.

These experiences have made me appreciate a lot of things in life and I am grateful to have been able to experience them. Despite the bad things that have happened, I learned a lot.

A Paradigm for the Future

Two words that I would use to summarize this experience would be life changing.
—DUSNS

Prior to Katrina, no paradigm existed for establishing a learning experience for nursing students in a post-disaster setting. What worked for Dillard University Division of Nursing can serve as an effective guide for re-establishing health care learning experiences in the aftermath of disasters. The steps taken by Dillard University Division of Nursing and the University's administration were: (1) reestablish an operational base with key administrators, (2) establish lines of communication to locate faculty and students, (3) assess the damage and remaining resources, (4) take stock of the diminished health care infrastructure, (5) grant permission for the continuation of educating nursing students to meet impending health care demands, (6) identify external resources, (7) review curriculum and course offerings, (8) establish shelter and daily necessities of life for continued educational experience, (9) notify boards of nursing regarding planned educational experience, (10) establish clinical sites, (11) evaluate in an ongoing manner. While the steps are listed in a linear sequence, by no means did they occur in such a fashion, or without the collaboration of appropriate authorizing agencies. The majority of the steps occurred simultaneously as tasks were delegated to administrators and faculty to be executed in a timely manner.

We can only echo the students' words: the experience was *life changing* and *overwhelming*. An event such as Katrina affects everyone. The on-site faculty administrator with the Dillard nursing students found that prayer, communication, organization, prioritization, delegation, support systems, and constant assessment and evaluation were essential to mental and physical survival during those difficult months. The community of Baton Rouge, the nursing community, and our families helped all the authors endure when at times we could only see the past and immediate present. We are forever appreciative of everyone's contribution to our efforts to overcome the challenges posed by the hurricanes of 2005.

In July 2006, Dillard University Division of Nursing held its Annual Pinning Ceremony, a rite of passage commencement activity for future nurses. The 14 young women who were seniors in 2005–6 chose *Persevering through the Storm* as their class theme. Like so many Katrina survivors, the students and faculty of the Dillard University Division of Nursing continue to move forward both professionally and emotionally, changed and gradually stronger.

Acknowledgments

The authors wish to acknowledge the efforts of Dr. Marvelene Hughes, President, Dillard University; Dean Janet Rami and the faculty and staff of Southern University School of Nursing; Mike Andry and the staff of EXCELth, Inc. (a federally qualified health center); Lisa Crinel and the staff of Abide Home Health, Inc.; Scottlandville Magnet High School; Elsevier Publishing Co.; San Buras of MIRT; Louisiana Conference United Methodist Churches—Baton Rouge District and the Wesley Foundation at Southern University; Adrianne Lebean of Dr. Bryan Lebean's, Lafayette, LA; Louisiana Sen. Michael J. Michot; Residential Coordinators—Elmira Beal, Nell Johnson, Marquitta Gill, Jeffery Parker, Angelica Peterson, Hallique L. Dawson, Angela Pittman, and Joseph Cole; Southern University Credit Union; Chapters of Alpha Kappa Alpha, Inc. and Delta Sigma Theta, Inc., and Community Partners at Work.

Notes

1. Knabb RD, Rhome JR, Brown DP, et al. Tropical cyclone report: Hurricane Katrina, 23–30 August 2005. Miami, FL: National Oceanic and Atmospheric Administration, National Weather Service, National Hurricane Center, 2005 Dec.

2. United States Senate. Recovering from Hurricane Katrina: the next phase—hearing before the Committee on Homeland Security and Governmental Affairs. Washington, DC: United States Senate, 2005 Sep 14.

3. Appleseed. A continuing storm the on-going struggles of Katrina evacuees: a review of needs, best practices and recommendations. Washington, DC: Appleseed, 2006 Aug.

4. Varcarolis EM, Carson VB, Shoemaker NC. Foundations of psychiatric mental health nursing: a clinical approach. 5th edition. Philadelphia, PA: W. B. Saunders, 2006.

5. Sumner J. Struggling to regain normalcy: LSUHSC after Hurricane Katrina. J Nurs Educ. 2005 Dec;44(12):531–2.

6. Sofer D. Will Katrina and Rita change the nursing landscape? Thousands of nurses and nursing students have evacuated damaged regions. Will they return? AJN. 2005 Dec;105(12):19.

7. Kleinpeter MA. Rebuilding New Orleans and the Gulf Coast—lessons learned to strengthen nation's healthcare. Response to Ferdinand's "public health and Hurricane Katrina." J Natl Med Assoc. 2006 May;98(5):814–5.

8. Spurlock WR, Hill JJ. The role of an academic nurse managed center in the provision and coordination of healthcare services to hurricane evacuees. Pelican News. 2006 Sep;62(3):9.

9. Gillies DA. Nursing management: a systems approach. Philadelphia, PA: W. B. Saunders, 1982 Feb;56–74.

10. Saenger E. The psychological aftermath of Hurricane Katrina: an expert interview with Edna B. Foa, PhD. Medscape Psychiatric & Mental Health. 2005;10(2).

11. Billings DM, Halstead JA. Teaching in nursing: a guide for faculty. 2nd edition. Philadelphia, PA: W. B. Saunders, 2005.

Chapter 4
A Diabetes Pharmaceutical Care Clinic in an Underserved Community

Adrienne Allen, PharmD
Wayne Harris, PhD
Kathleen Kennedy, PharmD

Background

Xavier University of Louisiana is an historically Black University (HBCU) located in New Orleans. Xavier's reputation for graduating students in the scientific disciplines is well known. It is the leading producer of African American students graduating in the fields of biology and the life sciences and number one in placing African Americans in medical schools. Additionally, as one of five HBCUs with a pharmacy school, Xavier has been a leader in producing African American pharmacists. Xavier's College of Pharmacy is dedicated to developing pharmacists who are experienced and competent in delivering pharmaceutical care, especially to those individuals in the community served by Xavier University. Its vision is to prepare pharmacy practitioners who demonstrate leadership and dedication to the medically underserved populations in our society, while striving to eliminate health care disparities. As a result, the College has developed partnerships with several ambulatory care clinics in medically underserved neighborhoods. These clinics serve as sites for clinical service and experiential education, and represent excellent resources for development of ongoing projects in disease state management, health outcomes and disparities research, and prevention research. One such clinic was the Diabetes Pharmaceutical Care Clinic (DPCC). The objectives of this report are to provide a description of the DPCC; to discuss the ongoing DPCC activities involving faculty and students prior to Hurricane Katrina in August 2005; and to discuss the impact of the abrupt discontinuation of its operation.

Overview

In 2002, Xavier University of Louisiana established the Minority Health and Health Disparities Research and Education Program (MHDREP), funded by research endowment

ADRIENNE ALLEN was the Director of the Diabetes Pharmaceutical Care Clinic of Xavier University of Louisiana prior to Hurricane Katrina. She is Associate Professor of Clinical Pharmacy and, most currently, the Director of the Center for Diabetes Prevention and Research at Xavier. WAYNE HARRIS is Professor and Dean of the College of Pharmacy at Xavier. KATHLEEN KENNEDY is Malcolm Ellington Professor of Pharmacy, Associate Dean and Director of the Center for Minority Health and Health Disparities Research and Education at Xavier.

grants from the National Center on Minority Health and Health Disparities of the National Institutes of Health, in order to contribute to the national goal of eliminating health disparities. An important goal of the MHDREP, now renamed the Center for Minority Health and Health Disparities Research and Education (CMHDRE), is to develop and test the effectiveness of models of diabetes management characterized by pharmacist-directed diabetes patient education in medically underserved communities. Pursuant to this goal, Xavier University of Louisiana's College of Pharmacy (XULACOP) established the Diabetes Pharmaceutical Care Clinic (DPCC), which was also partially supported through Xavier's Center of Excellence grant funded by the Health Resources and Services Administration of the United States Department of Health and Human Resources, in October 2003. The purpose of the DPCC was to provide a site for clinical education of Doctor of Pharmacy students, to engage community residents more actively in diabetes management, to increase the level of self-monitoring of blood glucose by patients, and ultimately to lead to better glucose control and decreased diabetes complications. This model of practice would later be expanded, based on outcomes, to include management of other chronic diseases that contribute to the problem of health disparities, including asthma and hypertension.

Description of a University-Based Diabetes Pharmaceutical Care Clinic

The College of Pharmacy acquired space through a partnership with the City of New Orleans in a city-operated clinic known as the Mandeville-Detiege Health Center, which was located in the Gert Town (GT) community less than half a mile away from Xavier's campus. Established as a residential neighborhood in the late nineteenth century, GT has historically been a predominately African American community and the home to many musicians, the hard working poor, and some small industries. In those early years, GT was recognized as a viable neighborhood in New Orleans, but more recently has seen a drastic decline in population. Xavier University has taken an active role in the community advocacy group called the Gert Town Revitalization Initiative. This group strives to improve the future outlook of the neighborhood through various channels including health care, education, housing, safety, and economics. Pre-Katrina, the GT community had a population of approximately 4,748 people, nearly 95% of whom were African American. It was estimated that earners in 40% of the households in this community brought home an annual salary of less than $10,000.[1]

With the availability of office and clinic space and funding support, the XULACOP prepared and equipped the DPCC soon after the appointment of the clinic director. The purpose of the DPCC was to provide pharmacist-directed diabetes education to patients with Type 2 Diabetes, particularly African American patients residing in underserved neighborhoods. The director of the clinic was a clinical pharmacist (PharmD) and a full-time faculty member who had 6.5 years of experience counseling and educating adult patients in an ambulatory care clinic. The director had also completed 2 years of pharmacy residency training with one of those years specializing in ambulatory care.

To ensure best practices in diabetes, a diabetes internal advisory committee was identified and a Certified Diabetes Educator and Registered Dietician were brought in as consultants. The internal advisory committee included six XULACOP faculty members with experience in diabetes care/diabetes research. As early as January 2004, the clinic started enrolling patients. Patient participation in the clinic was voluntary and diabetes education, medication counseling, and point of care testing were provided to patients at no cost. Since extramural grant support, as described previously, was obtained to demonstrate improvement in patient outcomes by pharmacist intervention and to provide the DPCC's infrastructure (e.g., equipment, reference material, office furniture, faculty salary support), we were able to perform point of care testing for baseline and follow-up laboratory tests at no cost to patients.

Informed consent was obtained from patients prior to clinic enrollment and this was considered the patient's first visit. The first visit involved the administration of a basic diabetes knowledge test and a 50-minute interview by the pharmacist or a trained senior pharmacy student (i.e., a pharmacy student completing a clinical experiential rotation). The primary purpose of the interview was to obtain information on prior diabetes education and knowledge of the disease and preventing its complications. This information was compiled in a 10-page document and was retained as a primary component of the patient's chart. In addition, a baseline HbA1c and lipid profile [low-density-lipoprotein (LDL) cholesterol, high-density-lipoprotein (HDL) cholesterol, total cholesterol, triglycerides], glucose, blood pressure (BP), weight, and body mass index (BMI) were also obtained during this visit. The lipid profile was obtained only for those patients who reported to the clinic in a fasting state. If a patient did not own a glucometer, a starter kit and a 7-day supply of glucose strips were provided with 20–30 minutes of instruction to ensure appropriate use.

After enrollment, the patient was scheduled for a diabetes class before leaving the DPCC. Patients were given a choice between attending a class of 10 patients or a one-on-one education class. The pharmacist or a trained senior pharmacy student under the pharmacist's supervision provided the classes.

The Education Component

A curriculum for the DPCC was developed using a series of diabetes teaching outlines developed by the Michigan Diabetes Research and Training Center for patients and health professionals.[2] The outlines were modified based on the needs of patients and updated with the most current diabetes standards of care.[3] Upon completion of the curriculum, patients will have received 10 hours of instruction. Class scheduling was arranged for patients to complete the program in one month, with the incentive of patients receiving a month's supply of glucose test strips upon completion.

The curriculum was organized into four classes: 1) *Diabetes Process, Monitoring and Acute Complications, and Medications*; 2) *Long Term Complications and Monitoring*; 3) *Nutritional Management and Monitoring and Acute Complications*; and 4) *Nutritional Management*. Patients were encouraged to begin with the class that included the Diabetes Process since the remaining classes required a basic understanding of the disease. After completion of the first class, patients could attend the remaining classes in any order. The *Nutritional Management* teaching outline was one of the most extensive outlines, having 10 subtopics (of which we used 5).[2] The nutrition class was divided into 2 separate classes due to the extensive content and extensive patient participation required to demonstrate learning (e.g., understanding how food affects glucose levels, reading food labels, understanding the difference between a serving and a portion, practicing good nutrition by making plates using NASCO Life/form® food replicas). Each week the DPCC offered a different class twice a day (e.g., first week: *Diabetes Process, Monitoring and Acute Complications, and Medications* at 9:00 a.m. and 1:00 p.m. on Thursday; second week: *Long Term Complications and Monitoring* at 9:00 a.m. and 1:00 p.m. on Thursday). The basic knowledge test was administered a second time after completion of all courses and anytime a patient missed a class or anytime a patient was not seen in the clinic for more than a week. The test questions were formulated from objectives taken from the teaching outlines and used to determine if patients required an overview of content from classes previously completed. The test was also used as a method to help determine the effectiveness of the education provided.

Patients were allowed to repeat classes anytime they were offered. The DPCC mailed monthly class schedules 1–2 weeks in advance to allow for advanced planning. Patients enrolled in the clinic were encouraged to attend these classes or to schedule an independent class. The intent of the DPCC was to see patients once a week until the entire curriculum was completed. Patients with an HbA1c greater than 7% were encouraged to work one-on-one with the pharmacist or senior pharmacy student to devise an individualized meal plan. After the patient's enrollment date, follow-up appointments were scheduled 2–3 months later to obtain an HbA1c and 4–6 months later to obtain a lipid profile. Glucose, BP, weight, and BMI were obtained at every visit.

DPCC Hours of Operation

The clinic's hours of operation were selected to provide patients with a greater opportunity to participate in the clinic services. Usual days and hours of operation were Monday through Friday from 8:00 a.m. until 5:00 p.m.; however, at times, the clinic opened as early as 7:00 a.m. and closed as late as 6:00 p.m. to obtain fasting lipids and glucose for patients who were non-fasting on the day of enrollment or to accommodate patients who could not attend a class during the scheduled class times.

Overall, the clinic director spent about 40 hours at the clinic during the week preparing for diabetes classes, providing patient education and counseling, coordinating class scheduling, enrolling patients, serving as preceptor to senior pharmacy students, and handling other administrative responsibilities (e.g., clinic advertising, diabetes research).

DPCC Activities and Accomplishments

The existence of the DPCC afforded the opportunity for patient education in the clinic as well as in off-site community centers. The DPCC also fostered scholarly activities among faculty and students and served as a training site for pharmacy students to complete their advanced experiential program.

Patients

Community outreach was an integral service of the DPCC that allowed for the provision of diabetes education for patients who could not travel to the clinic for various reasons. By August 2005, 230 patients were provided with diabetes education off-site at various community centers and health fairs (e.g., senior living centers, a women's shelter, and local churches) as an extension of the DPCC services. On site, nearly 30 diabetes classes had been provided to approximately 34 patients actively enrolled in the clinic (i.e., patients participating in some type of DPCC service) by the time of Hurricane Katrina. Due to the extent of our interactions with the patients we served, we can say without hesitation that over 90% of the patients educated were African American women with Type 2 Diabetes. At the time of this writing, we are unable to provide other patient characteristics because it has been impossible to retrieve patient records from the clinic, which was deluged by 4–6 feet of flood water on the first floor. Although the DPCC offices were located on the second floor, the devastating effects of stagnant water (e.g., mold and rodent infestation) made entering the building by anyone other than experienced clean-up workers a major health-hazard.

Scholarly Activities

The DPCC provided opportunity for scholarly activities for both faculty and students. Two XULACOP faculty projects were funded, one by the Department of Health and Human Services Office of Women's Health and the second by the National Library of Medicine (NLM). The goal of the first project, *Pharmacy Peer-Partners to Enhance Diabetes Education and Prevention in African American Women*, was to empower women as lay health educators (called *Pharmacy Peer Partners*) to deliver information regarding healthy lifestyles and diabetes management and prevention to a medically underserved community, specifically African Americans in the GT neighborhood. The project was to be completed in three phases by October 2006. When Katrina struck, the investigators were in the third phase of the project, which entailed determining the clinical improvement of the Peer Partners (i.e., improvement in HbA1c and lipid panel) and the level of satisfaction of community participants through focus group participation. The DPCC served as the education site, the training site, and the focus group site.

The NLM project was to begin in September 2005. The goal of this project, *A Diabetes Community Outreach Project*, was to increase the use of the NLM's patient health web site, Medline Plus®, by installing a kiosk and computer software at the DPCC site. Due to the loss of the DPCC, this project could not be completed.

Two XULACOP senior pharmacy students paired up while on rotation at the DPCC in July 2004 and initiated a community project, *A Pilot Study: Taking Diabetes Education on the Road*. The project's primary goal was to determine patient barriers to participating in diabetes education provided on-site (e.g., education provided at a senior living center). The students' preliminary work was presented as a poster at the American Society of Health System Pharmacists meeting in Orlando, Florida in December 2004 but the completion of the study was interrupted due to the unknown status of the patients after the hurricane.

Collaboration Agreement

A collaborative effort between the DPCC and a nephrologist from a local hospital began in June 2005. The physician agreed to participate in the DPCC's effort to prevent diabetic nephropathy by holding a clinic at the DPCC every other week to conduct patient screenings for diabetic nephropathy. This agreement also included serving as a link to primary care physicians for patients without a primary care practitioner (PCP).

Advanced Professional Experience Practice Rotation Clerkship Site

As a Centers of Excellence institution, XULACOP counts among its objectives motivating underrepresented minority students to pursue research or academic positions by completing fellowships or pharmacy residencies. The DPCC was an ideal setting to fulfill this objective because it served as an ambulatory care rotation site for senior pharmacy students in the XULACOP's advanced professional experience program.

Before Katrina, 40 senior pharmacy students rotated through the DPCC. Of those 40, 53% (21) of the students were African American and of those 21 students, 14% (3) pursued pharmacy residency programs after graduation.

Impact of Hurricane Katrina

The university could not assess the damages caused to the DPCC by the hurricane since the DPCC was housed in a non-Xavier building. Because of the impossibility of taking an inventory of equipment and retrieving patient files and records of patients enrolled at the DPCC or patients involved in ongoing faculty or student projects, we believe the impact sustained to be enormous. Although projects were not completed, the need for diabetes education to improve diabetes management and to increase diabetes awareness was clearly evident based on some clinical interventions (i.e., patients with baseline HbA1cs greater than 9%, newly diagnosed patients not advised about the importance of obtaining a glucometer, insulin user with frequent bouts of hypoglycemia unfamiliar with the glucagon kit).

Continued Efforts to Eliminate Health Disparities

Efforts to locate working space in a community to resume the DPCC services are ongoing. Although the services of the DPCC were abruptly disrupted, the need for diabetes education continues, but in different communities. In Louisiana, diabetes remains the fifth leading cause of death in the adult population. African Americans, women, and those with household income of less than $15,000 annually are at increased risk for diabetes.[4]

Future endeavors to continue our quest to eliminate diabetes health disparities in minority populations are ongoing as residents continue to return to New Orleans and as demographic changes in the city occur. The future plans of the XULACOP include a mobile diabetes unit to provide diabetes education and awareness in communities across the city and the redevelopment of a college-directed diabetes pharmaceutical care clinic. Currently, clinical faculty members are providing diabetes education to patients at federally qualified community health centers throughout Orleans Parish and are involved in collaborative initiatives in diabetes and hypertension management.

Notes

1. Greater New Orleans Community Data Center. Census 2000 Data Tables. New Orleans, LA: GNOCDC, 2007. Available at http://www.gnocdc.org/orleans/4/62/index.html.
2. Funnell MM, Arnold MS, Barr PA, et al. Life with diabetes: a series of teaching outlines by the Michigan diabetes research and training center. 2nd ed. Alexandria, VA: American Diabetes Association, 2003 Jun.
3. American Diabetes Association. Standards of medical care in diabetes. Diabetes Care. 2005 Jan;28 Suppl 1:S4–S36.
4. Centers for Disease Control and Prevention (CDC). Behavior Risk Factor Surveillance System, Prevalence Data: Louisiana—2004, Diabetes. Atlanta, GA: CDC, 2006. Available at http://apps.nccd.cdc.gov/brfss/displayasp?yr=2004&cat=DB&qkey=13 63&state=LA.

Chapter 5
Dental Care as a Vital Service Response for Disaster Victims

Nicholas G. Mosca, DDS
Emanuel Finn, DDS, MS
Renée Joskow, DDS, MPH

Introduction

On August 29, 2005, Hurricane Katrina ravaged the southeastern United States, causing extensive and severe damage to the socioeconomic infrastructure in Louisiana and Mississippi and displacing over 750,000 citizens.[1] With top winds exceeding 130 miles per hour and a storm surge topping 30 feet as the storm made landfall, Hurricane Katrina battered nearly 93,000 square miles across 138 parishes and counties, killing well over 1,300 people (deceased identified through December 2005).[2]* The states where communities were destroyed were among the poorest in the nation, with one-fifth of those displaced by the storm living in poverty and 30% having incomes below the federal poverty level.[1]

Katrina damaged all fourteen hospitals and three federal medical facilities in the lower six counties of Mississippi, and made eleven hospitals in the New Orleans area flood-bound. Early reports estimated that 1,292 primary care physicians were affected by storm-related damage in affected Louisiana and Mississippi counties.[3] In Mississippi, 85 dental providers experienced office damage in the affected areas. Additionally, 44 dentists lost their homes.[4]

In the immediate aftermath, rapid needs assessments (health and medical) were performed by the U.S. Department of Health and Human Services (DHHS) Secretary's Emergency Response Teams as part of the process of supporting local requests for federal assistance. Emergent medical care was provided in Mississippi by the remaining open hospitals, DHHS's federal medical shelters staffed by U.S. Public Health Service (USPHS) Commissioned Corp officers and federalized civilian volunteers, and nine FEMA Disaster Medical Assistance Teams (DMAT). However, no dental treatment or dental

---

* Later estimates of the number of deaths from Hurricane Katrina are considerably higher. The Earth Institute at Columbia University has kept tabs on vital statistics associated with Katrina. See their website (http://www.katrinalist.columbia.edu/index.php) for more information.

NICHOLAS MOSCA is the Dental Director of the Mississippi Department of Health, **EMANUEL FINN** is the Dental Director of the District of Columbia Department of Health, and **RENÉE JOSKOW** is a Biosecurity Senior Medical Epidemiologist with the U.S. Public Health Service, Department of Homeland Security.

personnel were part of the DMAT or DHHS medical response and, thus, no definitive emergency dental services were available from these medical response teams.

To estimate the needs of Katrina evacuees and survivors early on, several organizations, such as the Kaiser Foundation and the *Washington Post*, conducted survey assessments.[5] However, few surveys asked questions about dental health needs. Public health personnel living in Mississippi's special needs shelters reported a need for toothbrushes and toothpaste among shelter residents. Some shelter residents also asked for denture adhesive so they could eat, and some evacuees reported having lost their dentures while trying to evade the high winds and storm surge. A telephone survey of 47 shelter directors in Mississippi conducted during the second, third, and fourth weeks after the storm by researchers at Mississippi State University's Family and Children Research Unit found that the single greatest unmet need reported was oral health care, at 17%. In comparison, 9% of shelter directors reported children with unmet needs for health care and mental health care, and 4% reported a need for toiletries.[6]

To assess the impact of destruction on the dental care infrastructure of the affected regions, Mississippi's state dental director worked closely with the Mississippi Dental Association (MDA), the American Dental Association (ADA), and the Centers for Disease Control and Prevention (CDC) to obtain information. Initially, land-based communication was impossible due to downing of power and telephone lines. Mississippi Dental Association (MDA) staff members were able to reach some dental providers through personal cell phones to determine the status of their homes and practices. Some dentist's offices that could not be reached by telephone were visually inspected for damage by search and recovery teams with the cooperation of local emergency operations incident commands. Within days, the ADA was able to provide mapping with the location of dentist homes and offices in the affected areas, mapping that was then used to estimate the impact of damage based on severe wind and storm surge effects.

Oral Health Care at Hurricane Katrina Ground Zero

The eye of Hurricane Katrina made landfall in Hancock County in Mississippi, which had a pre-storm population of about 45,000 people. Hancock's population centers were the cities of Bay St. Louis and Waveland, both located south of Interstate 10 near the Gulf waters. On September 7, we determined that 5 of 8 dental offices (62%) located in Hancock County were closed due to storm damage. The county's only hospital, Hancock Medical Center, was also closed due to damage. The state incident command made arrangements for the State of North Carolina to send its state medical assistance team and mobile hospital. It was the first time that North Carolina's mobile hospital (Carolina MED-1) was deployed in an actual disaster response. This mobile hospital was developed by Carolinas Medical Center with funding from the U.S. Department of Homeland Security and featured 14 intensive-care beds, 100 acute-care beds, and an operating room. However, no dental treatment or dental personnel was included as part of this deployment. The mobile hospital arrived after September 2 and was positioned in the parking lot of a damaged strip mall in the city of Waveland. In its first week of operation, Carolina MED-1 (pictured in Photograph 1) reported seeing about 200 patients a day.

In response to the media's humanitarian coverage, many out-of-state dental professionals contacted Mississippi's health department to offer support. On September 8, a general dentist in Birmingham, Alabama agreed to send a two-chair mobile dental van to Mississippi. The dental director decided that the mobile dental van should be positioned next to the mobile hospital's emergency triage tent in order to be accessible to those seeking emergency care. On September 12, the state dental director began providing emergent dental care to locals using the mobile dental van. The local incident command arranged to provide the gas and potable water required to operate the dental equipment. Dental care was limited to urgent procedures, such as extractions and temporary fillings, using dental supplies that were donated by dental corporations and private dentists (Photograph 2). The Mississippi Department of Health stationed an immunization van next to the dental clinic to provide tetanus vaccinations. Additionally, there was a need to provide local community and regional shelters with oral health care supplies. As the population seeking dental care grew larger, a tent and portable dental equipment were stationed next to the van.

Private volunteer dentists from Illinois and Georgia joined the dental mission after they obtained temporary dental licensure through the state's Emergency Management Agreement Compact (EMAC). The EMAC, established by federal law in 1996, is an agreement among member states that outlines the legal agreements and procedures for providing assistance to other member states in the event of an emergency or disaster. Additionally, in coordination with the Office of Force Readiness and Deployment, Office of the Surgeon General, and the USPHS Chief Dental Officer, USPHS dental officers were deployed to provide dental treatment to hurricane victims and response personnel. Dental services were provided on the mobile dental van at Carolina MED-1 from September 12 to September 20.

On September 20, the Sullivan-Schein Corporation's *Tomorrow's Dental Office of Today* (TDOT), a fully-functional dental convention exhibit van, arrived and was used

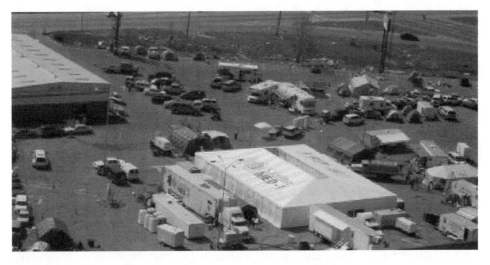

Photograph 1. Aerial photo of Carolina MED-1 in Waveland, Mississippi.

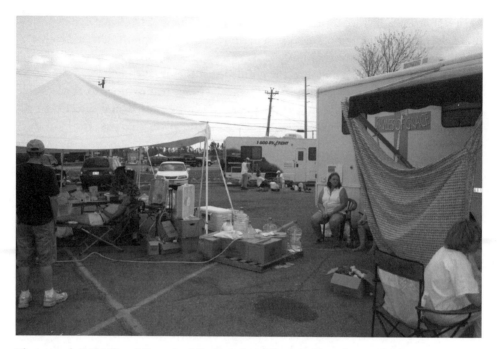

Photograph 2. *Smiles of Grace* mobile dental van from Birmingham, Alabama.

to provide dental care until October 29. After establishing a facility, the next objective was to ensure that the facility had an adequate and sustainable dental workforce to meet the demand for treatment. This was achieved through the DHHS's deployment of the USPHS Commission Corps dentists and dental hygienists to staff the TDOT in Waveland (Photograph 3).

The city of Gulfport, Mississippi, located in Harrison County, had a pre-storm population of over 190,000 people. On September 28, through coordination with DHHS, FEMA, and the Nevada Hospital Association, Nevada-One, an in/out patient, hospital tent compound was established on a vacant lot in Gulfport (Photograph 4). At Nevada-One, USPHS dental officers and hygienists provided dental services using a mobile dental van provided by the State of Virginia and portable dental equipment that was housed in one of the medical treatment tents. Dental care was provided to civilians at Nevada-One until October 26. Nearly half of the total patient visits from September 21 through October 29 at the previously mentioned Waveland and Gulfport medical sites were dental patient encounters.

Oral Health Care for Displaced Victims 1,000 Miles Away

On September 4th, the Mayor of the District of Columbia announced plans to broaden the District's Katrina relief efforts to include an airlift of several hundred Hurricane Katrina evacuees from Louisiana who had been evacuated to Alabama. The Mayor agreed to use the D.C. National Guard Headquarters (D.C. Amory) as a temporary shelter because it could hold up to 400 Hurricane Katrina evacuees. Multiple agencies

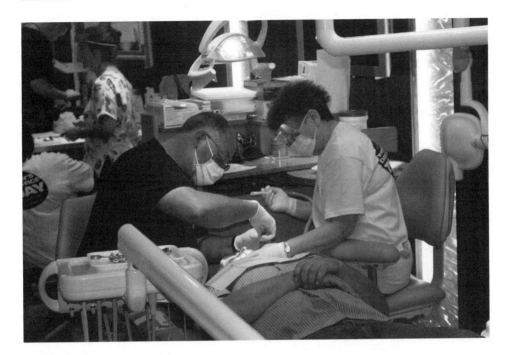

Photograph 3. Dental care provided by Commission Corps Officers on TDOT.

convened to develop an evacuation plan, including the D.C. Department of Health, Metropolitan Police and Fire Departments, Washington Metropolitan Area Transit Authority, and D.C. Public Schools. The dental director for the District of Columbia was invited to join the planning team and prepare a dental services plan before the first wave of evacuees arrived. The dental plan included positioning the Colgate Mobile Bright Smiles Dental Van; the Mary's Center for Maternal and Child Health Mom Baby Bus; Howard University College of Dentistry staff, residents and students; local dentists; and staff with the St. Elizabeth's Hospital Dental Program at the Armory. They all answered the Mayor's call to make the plan for the evacuees an unprecedented reality.

On September 5th, nearly 300 evacuees who were airlifted from Louisiana and other Gulf States arrived at the Armory. This facility had turned instantly into a welcoming

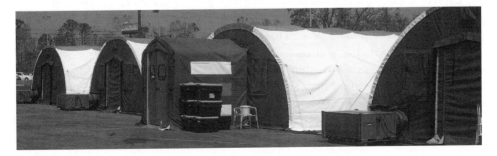

Photograph 4. Nevada-One hospital unit.

and comfortable but emotional shelter for unfortunate victims of one of the worst hurricanes to hit the United States mainland in modern times. The dental team was on hand to welcome, comfort, and treat evacuees when the first buses rolled through the security gates of the D.C. Armory.

In just days after the first buses arrived at the Armory with evacuees, the population dropped from nearly three hundred to fewer than one hundred and fifty as dozens of individuals and families found living arrangements with relatives and friends. Two hundred evacuees were immediately enrolled in the D.C. Medicaid Program and 100 in the City's Health Care Safety Net Program. The District passed emergency legislation to provide evacuees with access to health care and other services. The Relocation and Recovery Assistant Emergency Act of 2005 authorized the Mayor, upon declaration of a state of emergency or disaster relief, to provide disaster services, relocation, and recovery assistance to disaster evacuees. The legislation ensured that there would be no impact on existing services for D.C.-based homeless or low-income individuals and families. The legislation also permitted the District of Columbia to waive documentation requirements such as for a Social Security card, birth certificate, or photographic identification, all of which might have been lost or destroyed due to disaster, and instead to seek third party verification.

Outcomes

In Mississippi, over 1,250 people received dental care and more than 1,400 patient visits were recorded with 75% of visits (n=975) occurring in Waveland and 25% (n=276) in Gulfport. About 968 people reported that they lived in Mississippi and 41 people reported being displaced from Louisiana. Among the 1,020 people who recorded their sex, 537 were female and 483 were male. Among the 1,026 people who provided their date of birth, 73 were younger than 18 years of age, and 953 were older. Some patients were disaster relief workers who developed acute dental problems while assisting in the relief efforts.

Seven patients reported having tuberculosis (TB) but it is unclear whether they had received treatment for active TB or had experienced an exposure. Ten of the women who received dental care were pregnant. About 147 patients reported that their health situation had changed over the last 12 months. The recorded health history findings for people treated in Mississippi are listed in Table 1. Dental extractions and temporary or sedative dental fillings were the most commonly performed dental procedures.

In the District of Columbia, clinical dental services were provided to 51 adults and 9 children. Initial care was provided to the evacuees with the greatest dental need and those who suffered injuries during the hurricane. The last of the evacuees moved out of the D.C. Armory 5 weeks after they were airlifted to Washington. This brought an end to a rescue and shelter effort that helped hundreds of victims get back on their feet. The city had mobilized dozens of agencies and hundreds of Washington area residents and volunteers in an unprecedented effort to offer assistance and assurance to the people of the Gulf Coast region devastated by Hurricane Katrina.

Discussion

The Mississippi Department of Health's primary responsibility under the state's emergency plan was to ensure medical support for survivors. Prior to Hurricane Katrina, Mississippi's state dental director was not familiar with the operational and planning needs associated with disaster response. Furthermore, the state oral health program did not include any action steps tied to the state emergency response plan. Through our experiences in providing dental care after Katrina, we realize the importance of participating in disaster preparedness education and training to ensure that all health personnel can respond effectively in disasters.

For many weeks after Hurricane Katrina, two-thirds of the dental treatment infrastructure in the affected areas remained closed. People seeking relief from dental pain and infection had one option: locate medical assistance quickly or leave for unaffected areas. Emergent health care delivery in the aftermath of a wide-scale emergency must include support for all types of anticipated emergencies, including dental; have a competent, properly trained workforce; and ensure the appropriate mobile technological infrastructure to meet these needs.

It is recommended that all state oral health program personnel understand their state emergency response plans, as well as the national response plan, and complete the appropriate Incident Command Training, available through FEMA. This would help to ensure that oral health leaders have the knowledge and information necessary to respond and to request available resources from local, state, and federal governments, and private and corporate sources after a disaster.

It is also recommended that state oral health programs have an emergency prepared-

Table 1.

HEALTH FINDINGS FOR KATRINA SURVIVORS SEEKING DENTAL CARE IN MISSISSIPPI (N=1,250)

Reported medical history	Number reported
Rheumatic fever or rheumatic heart disease	7
Congenital heart disease	8
Cardiovascular disease (including high blood pressure)	193
Asthma or hay fever	139
Liver disease	28
Abnormal bleeding problem	15
Diabetes	83
Tuberculosis	7
Taking prescription medication	589
Reported drug allergies	345
Active pregnancy	10

ness plan that ensures the appropriate planning for the delivery of emergent dental services to disaster victims. Having a plan allows the state oral health program to develop written mutual aid agreements with other state programs and with non-government entities so that critical resources, such as mobile dental facilities, supplies, and properly trained personnel will be available during the initial response to a disaster. The Secretary of the DHHS and the Surgeon General were instrumental in setting up a system to solicit, enroll, and credential civilian health care volunteers, allowing them to become temporary, non-paid federal employees in order to ensure the proper protection against liabilities. State participation in the Emergency Management Assistance Compact is also very important for health workforce volunteers because of the liability and workman's compensation arrangements that are included in the agreement.

Many of the oral health injuries that required treatment in Mississippi were associated with pre-existing disease, such as untreated tooth decay or chronic periodontal disease. Our experiences show that a pre-existing disease condition can and will make people acutely ill when left untreated. In fact, at the Waveland and Gulfport sites, the dental clinicians treated several life-threatening infections of dental origin. This is especially true for victims who lack clean water or antiseptic rinses, which can help to minimize the pathogenic impact of bacterial infections in the oral cavity. Finally, with so many elders who lost their homes and possessions due to the high winds, tornadoes, and storm surge, there was a great demand for replacement dentures.

Conclusion

In our communities, oral health's involvement was small compared with the other medical services rendered. In spite of that, oral health had a vital role in disaster relief to help the people of New Orleans and the Gulf Coast heal and recover. Valuable experience was gained in coordinating the dental efforts during this disaster crisis in these communities and there is strong motivation to ensure a greater role for oral health care providers in disaster relief, emergency preparedness, and management, no matter the magnitude or nature of the catastrophe.

We believe that these experiences will have a tremendous impact on dental education and the dental profession for the foreseeable future. To prepare for a wide-scale disaster, we must have a well-defined preparedness plan that considers the contributions of all types of health professionals, the appropriate mobile technology to respond to emergent health risks, and a competent workforce ready and able to respond. Such preparation will require our dental education programs to develop disaster preparedness competencies to achieve the desired level of understanding.

Notes

1. Gabe T, Falk G, McCarty M, et al. Hurricane Katrina: social-demographic characteristics of impacted areas. Washington, DC: Congressional Research Service, Library of Congress, 2005 Nov.
2. White House Staff, Katrina Lessons Learned Review Group. The federal response to

Hurricane Katrina: lessons learned. Washington, DC: The White House, 2006 Feb. Available at http://www.whitehouse.gov/reports/katrina-lessons-learned.pdf.

3. Williamson D. Study shows Hurricane Katrina affected 20,000 physicians, up to 6,000 may have been displaced. (No. 444.) Chapel Hill, NC: University of North Carolina, Chapel Hill News Services, 2005 Sep. Available at http://www.unc.edu/news/archives/sep05/ricketts092605.htm.

4. U.S. Department of Health and Human Services (HHS), Mississippi Department of Health (MDH). Hurricane Katrina: Medical Support/Demobilization/Transition Plan for the State of Mississippi. Washington, DC: HHS, MDH, 2006 Jan.

5. Brodie M, Weltzien E, Altman D, et al. Experiences of hurricane Katrina evacuees in Houston shelters: implications for future planning. Am J Public Health. 2006 Aug; 96(8):1402–8.

6. Family and Children Research Unit, Mississippi State University Social Science Research Center. Shelter survey provides insight into services, children's needs. Starkville, MS: Mississippi State University Social Science Research Center, Family and Children Research Unit, 2005. Available at http://www.ssrc.msstate.edu/Divisions/fcru/pdf/fcru_ka_pr_0905c.pdf.

Chapter 6
Mental Health Interventions by Telephone with Katrina Survivors

Don C. Combs, EdD

Much has been written about the delivery of face-to-face mental health crisis intervention services to both disaster survivors and first responders to those disasters.[1-15] In fact, an intense national debate as to the most effective ways to intervene immediately following a traumatic or disaster-related event remains unresolved.[1] In question is the efficacy of a long-standing psychological debriefing procedure, Critical Incident Stress Debriefing. This approach, developed by Mitchell and Everly,[2-4,5] has yielded somewhat disappointing results according to McNally, Bryant, and Ehlers, who indicate that, "Although the majority of debriefed survivors describe the experience as helpful, there is no convincing evidence that debriefing reduces the incidence of post-traumatic stress disorder (PTSD) and some controlled studies suggest that its use may impede natural recovery from trauma" (p. 45).[1] As an alternative, crisis intervention specialists currently recommend a relatively new approach, Psychological First Aid.[1,6-8] The principles of this approach, which focuses on meeting each individual's crisis-related psycho-bio-social needs in a practical manner, through developing an action plan for recovery, among other things, are outlined in significant detail at the National Center for PTSD and the National Child Traumatic Stress Network website.[9] The effectiveness of this approach requires continued empirical analysis.[1,6]

Although telephone hot-lines have been considered integral to crisis-oriented mental health services[6,10,11] since the mid-1950s,[11] only one research study[6] has investigated their use as part of early intervention disaster-oriented mental health services.[6] Interestingly, the national debate noted earlier has focused primarily on face-to-face contact rather than contact via telephone. Notably, the delivery of mental health interventions by telephone was widely used by the American Red Cross in the aftermath of Hurricane Katrina.

Description of Telephone Services Model

Several years ago, the American Red Cross established a National Call Center in Falls Church, Virginia whose on-going purpose is to act as a 24-hour a day, 7 days a week information clearinghouse for callers needing emergency assistance and services as a result of disaster-related losses. The role of the call agent answering incoming calls

DON COMBS *is an Associate Professor in the College of Education at the University of Texas at El Paso (UT-El Paso).*

is to connect the caller with local resources and services near the caller's home area. A unique characteristic of the call center approach is the provision of psychological assistance on an as-needed basis to those callers experiencing mental, emotional, and/or behavioral distress. When a call agent identifies a caller in need of such assistance, a licensed mental health professional is asked to plug in to the agent's phone system to assist with the call. The assistance rendered by the mental health professional is based on the caller's needs and thus, follows an individualized plan as suggested by the Psychological First Aid model.[1,6–8]

The National Call Center became a major hub for Gulf Coast callers after Katrina. What was unique about Katrina calls was that all callers were using cell phones, since landlines were not functional. Call responders worked eight-hour shifts (7 am–3 pm; 3 pm–11 pm; or 11 pm–7 am) each day. A high volume of incoming calls daily (approximately 100 to 150) was the norm, occasionally resulting in a distressed caller having to talk to a call agent until a mental health worker was available. More mental health volunteers were needed than were available, especially on the night shift, which only had two or three workers (compared with the three to five workers on the day and evening shifts).

My Experience

As a licensed professional mental health counselor and certified American Red Cross Disaster Mental Health worker, I volunteered to assist with the Katrina relief effort and was deployed to the National Call Center in mid-September 2005 for a 12-day period. I attended a mandatory general orientation session the day after my arrival and began working the phones the following day. I worked the 11 pm–7 am shift each night. I was not given specific instructions concerning how to respond to clients but, instead, was expected to do what licensed mental health professionals do during times of disaster. It was emphasized that I should focus on the caller's current crisis-related distress and refer callers needing more in-depth and/or on-going interventions to local counseling agencies. Although prior to Katrina I had participated in the 2-day American Red Cross Disaster Mental Health (DMH) course, this training program, which incorporated components of Psychological First Aid, involved face-to-face contact only and did not include telephonic crisis intervention support as an early intervention after disasters. As a mental health professional, I was ultimately responsible to decide my own course of action as a telephone responder. As described below, the track I took was mapped out using Psychological First Aid. In retrospect, I would have benefited had the American Red Cross included simulated telephonic role-playing exercises as part of its DMH course.

My individualized approach to callers was to engage in active listening as long as the client needed to talk and then to assist the caller in formulating an action plan designed to structure the next few hours or days. Both of these (active listening and formulating a plan) are widely accepted components of the Psychological First Aid approach.[1,6–8] I used these techniques in an attempt to help the caller acquire a greater sense of control over his/her immediate environment. Most calls lasted approximately 30 minutes, though a few lasted an hour or more. Except for two obscene phone calls,

I always stayed on the line until the caller indicated a desire to terminate. Occasionally, termination seemed premature, and I asked callers to continue talking. By my assessment, callers were, for the most part, shocked, overwhelmed, somewhat detached from reality, and experiencing some degree of hopelessness due to the deteriorated conditions they were forced to endure. Overall, they were experiencing significant emotional distress and cognitive impairment to the extent that they were unable to think clearly or make timely decisions. Many were calling out of deep frustration at not being able to reach Federal Emergency Management Agency (FEMA) Financial Assistance Centers, hoping that I could connect them. (I could not.) Occasionally, I needed to ask for medical assistance and advice for a caller. At such times, I asked nursing staff working with me to assess a caller's pre-existing medical condition(s) and to provide information concerning how to replace lost medications and obtain emergency medical care. Primarily, callers were experiencing significant, but expected, coping difficulties due to the gravity of the disaster. I stressed to them that their fears, anxieties, and depressive reactions, including sleeping and eating difficulties, were, for most of them, very normal reactions to highly abnormal and unusual circumstances. (Those providing disaster-related mental health services generally stress the importance of a normalizing approach.[2,6,10–13])

The calls I received were uniformly and without question from the poor, the disadvantaged, and those with pre-existing mental and/or physical disabilities. Many callers had experienced difficulty, for a variety of reasons, leaving their immediate environments. Some callers did not have access to transportation and indicated that they were simply forgotten or ignored during evacuation prior to the storm. Some were too frightened to leave and decided to remain in their homes. Others related that shelters near them had closed, that they had no way to get to a shelter, and/or that they had had a bad experience at a shelter and, as a result, decided to return to their damaged homes. A noticeable number indicated that they were afraid to go to a shelter based on media as well as first-hand reports of violence at places such as the Superdome. Some had moved in with other families and were now living in crowded, very cramped spaces with no personal privacy. By their reports, most callers had no one else to turn to at the time of their call, whether they were displaced or still in their own homes.

Telephone interventions appear to have been helpful as callers indicated experiencing a significant sense of relief just knowing that someone cared enough to listen. During the relatively short time I spent with callers, I observed them move from a place of despair and despondency to one where they again felt hope. After talking through the difficult and trying situations they were facing, most callers began to think more clearly and were able to develop an action plan regarding needed changes in their living conditions. The sense of relief in their voices after having the opportunity to discuss their fears, anxieties, and concerns openly was unmistakable. Toward the middle of my 12-day assignment, I began making follow-up calls to check on those people who had seemed exceptionally distraught when they called. In most cases, those I called back had followed through with the recommended course of action and appeared to be coping more effectively. Callers were very appreciative when re-contacted and stated how validating it was to them that they had not been forgotten. I usually waited at least 24 hours before making follow-up calls.

I found that the time spent in listening and interacting with callers was very meaningful to them. They indicated feeling more confident and stronger after talking with someone, as if they had found a renewed sense of self. Nearly every caller thanked me for being available, while knowing that I had no magic answers. Callers did not expect immediate resolution of their problems; instead, they were seeking some time and attention from someone who cared at a time when their world had been destroyed. The callers I spoke with were very humble and appreciative. It was a distinct pleasure and privilege to be on the phone with them, and their strength and courage is something I will always remember. I doubt I could have coped as effectively as they had with the horrors they had faced and were continuing to face in Katrina's aftermath. I left the National Call Center deeply enriched by the experience.

Examples of Calls Received

Perhaps the most effective way to illustrate my experiences is to describe three of the calls received, and to summarize the action plan formulated during the call. All names have been changed and some basic identifying information altered to ensure confidentiality and anonymity.

Margaret, 73, called from New Orleans to ask if we could assist her in reaching FEMA so that she could schedule repairs to her damaged house. The call agent asked for a mental health intervention as she sounded confused and somewhat disoriented. Margaret told me that she was on a walker and did not leave her home either before or after Katrina as she was frightened that she might fall. In talking with Margaret, she indicated that there was water in her bedroom that she had to wade through in order to reach her bathroom. As Margaret continued talking, she seemed more tired and sleepy than confused or disoriented. **Action plan**: I talked with Margaret about the importance of going to sleep as soon as possible (it was the middle of the night) and to postpone attempting to reach FEMA until the next day. She agreed to this. The call agent had given her several emergency numbers to call to secure assistance in leaving her home if necessary. This information seemed to give her peace of mind. Margaret's 14-year old grandson was staying with her, and I spoke with him prior to the end of the call. He indicated that he would see that she made the calls the following day. I believe that Margaret needed permission to let go of her worries for the night, and that receiving it from the Red Cross call center along with the housing information we had given her made doing so easier.

Patty, 25, called from Slidell, Louisiana saying that she was alone and living in her car due to the damage to her home that made it uninhabitable. She said that her car was not operational and, as a result, that she could not leave the area. She indicated that she was nearly out of her prescribed antidepressant medication. She also reported that, although she had had suicidal thoughts several years ago, she was not currently suicidal. I concurred based on my assessment during our conversation. (Her thinking was clear, logical, and goal-directed with no evidence of suicidal ideation or emotional instability at the time of the call.) I was concerned that, without her medication, she might become suicidal. Her current inadequate living conditions also needed immediate attention. **Action plan**: Patty agreed to contact emergency personnel in her area to transport her to a local emergency room for continued evaluation and a refill of her prescription. She indicated that she had an emergency contact number for her local area but had not followed through as she had been preoccupied with the aftermath of Katrina. She also agreed to call the American Red Cross for corporate housing. In my professional opinion, Patty was capable of taking these steps, as she did not appear to be mentally or emotionally impaired to the extent that I needed to make the calls at time of our conversation. Triage decisions[10] such as this were a routine part of my assessment procedures. Patty needed a focused plan for the immediate future, which is what I helped her lay out.

John, 45, called from the area of Biloxi, Mississippi to say that he was disabled and had lost his artificial leg and foot in the storm. He was very frightened and worried that he would not be able to replace them as he had no money. He stated that he would not leave the area until he received replacements. He also needed to talk about numerous pre-existing medical problems that continued to worry him. As we spoke, the call agent located a number that he could call to obtain a set of replacement prostheses. This information created a definite calming effect for him. He stated to me how much it meant to talk with someone who seemed to take his concerns seriously. He was very appreciative of my time. **Action plan**: John was more than eager to make the necessary call to replace his lost prostheses.

Conclusion

As noted, the use of the telephone as an early intervention tool after disasters has apparently not yet surfaced in the debate regarding the merit of various approaches to disaster work. The incorporation of Psychological First Aid components in telephonic work is thought to be an important observation in the discussion, however, and depending on research outcomes, may serve to reinforce the use of Psychological First Aid as a routine part of disaster-related early intervention efforts.[1,6–8]

There is little or no current literature regarding the empirical effectiveness of disaster-related telephonic interventions, which means that there is a need for systematic outcomes assessment. As mentioned earlier, telephone interventions and Psychological First Aid approaches appear to mesh well. Assessment instruments measuring the impact of Psychological First Aid are still being developed.[1,6] These instruments, when available, may be of great assistance in determining the efficacy of telephonic interventions. Until such time as this occurs, however, the field may have to continue to rely on both call responder assessment and caller self-report regarding both symptom reduction and perceived satisfaction with service delivery as the basis for determining effectiveness. Callbacks, as described earlier, could be an important resource in this connection.

Notes

1. McNally RJ, Bryant RA, Ehlers A. Does early psychological intervention promote recovery from posttraumatic stress? Psychological Science in the Public Interest. 2004;4(2):45–79.
2. Mitchell JT, Everly GS Jr. Critical incident stress debriefing: an operations manual for CISD, defusing and other group crisis intervention services. Ellicott City, MD: Chevron Publishing Corporation, 1997.

3. Mitchell JT. Characteristics of successful early intervention programs. Int J Emerg Ment Health. 2004 Fall;6(4):175–84.

4. Jacobs J, Horne-Moyer L, Jones R. The effectiveness of critical incident stress debriefing with primary and secondary trauma victims. Int J Emerg Ment Health. 2004 Winter;6(1):5–14.

5. Mitchell JT. Major misconceptions in crisis intervention. Int J Emerg Ment Health. 2003 Fall;5(4):185–97.

6. Halpern J, Tramontin M. Disaster mental health: theory and practice. Belmont, CA: Brooks/Cole—Thomson Learning, 2007.

7. Parker CL, Everly GS Jr, Barnett DJ, et al. Establishing evidence-informed core intervention competencies in psychological first aid for public health personnel. Int J Emerg Ment Health. 2006 Spring;8(2):83–92.

8. Everly GS Jr, Flynn BW. Principles and practical procedures for acute psychological first aid training for personnel without mental health experience. Int J Emerg Ment Health. 2006 Spring;8(2):93–100.

9. National Child Traumatic Stress Network, National Center for PTSD. Psychological first aid: field operations guide, 2nd Ed. Los Angeles, CA: National Center for Child Traumatic Stress. 2006 Jul. Available at http://www.nctsn.org.

10. Greenstone JL, Leviton SC. Elements of crisis intervention: crises and how to respond to them. Pacific Grove, CA: Brooks/Cole—Thomson Learning, 2002.

11. James RK, Gilliland BE. Crisis intervention strategies. Belmont, CA: Brooks/Cole—Thomson Learning, 2005.

12. Walz GR, Kirkman CJ, eds. Helping people cope with tragedy and grief: information, resources, and linkages. Greensboro, NC: CAPS Publications, 2002.

13. Kanel K. A guide to crisis intervention. Belmont, CA: Brooks/Cole—Thomson Learning, 2007.

14. Everly GS Jr, Langlieb A. The evolving nature of disaster mental health services. Int J Emerg Ment Health. 2003 Summer;5(3):113–19.

15. Everly GS Jr. Early psychological intervention: a word of caution. Int J Emerg Ment Health. 2003 Fall;5(4):179–84.

Chapter 7
"They Blew the Levee": Distrust of Authorities among Hurricane Katrina Evacuees

Kristina M. Cordasco, MD, MPH

David P. Eisenman, MD, MHS

Deborah C. Glik, ScD

Joya F. Golden, BA

Steven M. Asch, MD, MPH

On August 29th, 2005, Hurricane Katrina made landfall just east of New Orleans, Louisiana. That night and the next day, levees in New Orleans collapsed, resulting in flooding of 80% of the city, with water levels reaching to the rooftops in many areas.[1] Despite strong evacuation warnings, followed by a mandatory evacuation order,[2] over 100,000 greater New Orleans residents failed to evacuate prior to the hurricane's landfall.[3]

Distrust of authorities, among numerous other factors,[4–5] seems likely to have played a role in New Orleans residents' reactions to evacuation warnings and public health authorities' advice. Prior to the hurricane, 72% of New Orleans residents were of minority race or ethnicity[6] and there is a long history of minority groups in the United States distrusting the medical and public health leadership.[7–9] Furthermore, distrust of authorities among New Orleans' impoverished residents is rooted in local history. In 1927, The Great Mississippi Flood was threatening to destroy New Orleans, including its crucial downtown regional financial institutions. To avert the threat, and in part to stabilize the financial markets, it was decided to perform a controlled break of the New Orleans levees, thereby selectively flooding poor areas and saving financial institutions.[10] This event lives on in the memories and oral history of the residents of the deliberately flooded areas.[11]

Faced with the knowledge that distrust hampers the success of recommended evacuations and other disaster responses, disaster and public health officials must learn how to build trust,[12–13] a complex and multidimensional phenomenon.[14] Research centered in health care settings has identified several components of trust, defined as the expectation that others will act in one's interests, including fiduciary responsibility,

KRISTINA CORDASCO is a Clinical Scholar in the UCLA/Robert Wood Johnson Clinical Scholars Program. DAVID EISENMAN is an Assistant Professor in the Department of General Internal Medicine and Health Services Research and DEBORAH GLIK is a Professor in the Department of Community Health Science, School of Public Health, both at UCLA. JOYA GOLDEN is a Health Research Specialist at the VA Greater Los Angeles Health Care System, with which STEVEN ASCH is also affiliated. Dr. Asch, additionally, is an Associate Professor at UCLA and is affiliated with RAND Health.

honesty, competency, confidentiality, and equity.[15] Residents' planning and response to Hurricane Katrina illustrate many elements of trust and distrust as they relate to disaster response and may provide lessons with policy implications.

The salience of trust and distrust was vividly demonstrated in interviews we performed from September 9th through 12th, 2005, days 11 through 14 after Louisiana landfall of Hurricane Katrina. As part of a study of the facilitators and barriers to evacuation,[4] we interviewed 58 English-speaking adults who were living in Louisiana prior to landfall of Hurricane Katrina and currently receiving shelter in one of three Houston, Texas, evacuation centers (The Reliant Center, The Astrodome, and The George R. Brown Convention Center). Because our semi-qualitative interviews did not include specific queries about trust and distrust, we were struck by the frequency and depth of distrust reflected in the spontaneous statements of the evacuees we interviewed. This report is intended to describe and contextualize those statements.

Not surprisingly, *competency*, the belief in another's qualifications to perform a specific act, was the category of distrust that was mentioned most frequently by interviewees. All levels of authority, from the federal and local government officials, to the emergency workers, were the subjects of these statements. The perceived incompetence was summed up in the statement of one participant who said, "They could of did a lot better than what they did." Another said "the whole deal was a total letdown."

Several people went further when discussing their distrust by addressing a second element of trust, perceived equity. The equity component of trust is the belief that one is being treated fairly, without consideration of class, race, gender, or other characteristics.[9,16] Seven people told us that they believed that the preparations or response were performed ineffectively or slowly because of the race or socioeconomic composition of their neighborhood. One person stated:

> If the President would have stepped in when they give that evacuation just like they were going to send six million dollars to save a whale, send all our men to Iraq, and send food and shelter and money over there, why couldn't he do it for the poor neighborhoods?

Distrust was expressed not only for government leaders but also for the people working on the evacuation. One person said that her family's signals for help were ignored by rescuers; instead of responding to their signals, "the helicopters were going back and forth getting people from the richer neighborhoods." Another perceived that he was discriminated against once he did receive help, recalling:

> I got in one of the military trucks and it dropped us off in the middle of the interstate because Jefferson Parish, which is the neighboring parish, they made it clear they didn't have any water, they didn't have any shelter, they didn't have any food. So what they're saying is they didn't want any of Orleans Parish residents in their parish. See, Orleans Parish is 87% Black and Jefferson Parish is predominately White, so they didn't want that there.

The fiduciary component of trust, in which people trust others to act with their best interests and well being in mind, was an element of many evacuees' distrust.[15-16]

Those who commented on this generally linked it to economic issues, and not race. For instance, the common belief that the rich are privileged over the poor in disaster response is illustrated by one man's comment:

> I've seen it on floods. We had some floods a few years back and you either take out this whole bunch of factories and the whole state's economy or 25 starving families . . . So what do they do? They knock a hole in the levy over here and knock these people out of pocket, destroy them, and they keep the big money in.

Another interviewee expressed doubt that the officials had acted in the best interests of the public with the statement "they could have saved people if they really wanted to save people."

A striking element of distrust expressed by interviewees was perceived dishonesty, or a lack of truthfulness and sincerity. Eight people we interviewed did not believe the reports in the media and claims of the authorities that the flooding in their neighborhoods came from the levees being overwhelmed by storm waters. Two people stated that they believed that the water was diverted into the poor neighborhoods to save the rich neighborhoods. Explaining how "the politicians broke the pump," one individual said: "They let the waters go in the poor neighborhoods and kept it out of the rich neighborhoods, like that French Quarter where tourists go at." Six people went further and stated that they believed that the levees were intentionally broken. One person stated:

> He sacrificed New Orleans. He cut that 17th bridge, because you've got to sacrifice something. Donald Trump is putting the tower on Canal Street downtown and they saved the French Quarter and the Garden District, the historical areas, the rich people, where the money is coming from, casinos and all that. And they drowned out all the poor people and the lower-middle class working people . . . And they do that all over the country, not just in New Orleans . . . they do stuff and then they lie, lie, lie.

Another person connected what he perceived as the breaking of the levees to issues of race, saying:

> I believe they do these things intentionally . . . so they can flood out those Black neighborhoods . . . because every time they have a hurricane, it always be that way. You know?

Honesty and dishonesty encompass what is not said as well as what is said. Some evacuees felt useful information had been withheld from them. "I heard from some people who watched the CNN news that these people knew about this hurricane a month ago."

These statements must be viewed in light of the participants having just experienced a horrific trauma, which clearly influenced their interpretations of events. In situations of fear and uncertainty people give more credence to negative perceptions.[17] Furthermore, as participants were living collectively and exchanging information and perspectives, some individuals' distrust may have been amplified by conversations with other people living in the shelter. It is not possible from our interviews to separate this element of blame as stemming from a coping mechanism versus a reflection of underlying distrust.

Despite these limitations, the evacuees' interpretations of events after Hurricane Katrina reflect an underlying, profound distrust of authorities. Evacuation and post-evacuation experiences heightened this distrust for some individuals. Given the importance of trust in disaster preparedness and communications,[18-19] addressing existing distrust is critical to mounting effective responses in the future.

Each of these elements has specific implications for disaster planning and risk communication. The level of a community's distrust will be partially buffered based on the extent to which authorities display competency, fairness, empathy, honesty, and openness prior to a disaster.[20] The historical depth of fiduciary concerns highlights the necessity of improving trust now between public officials and vulnerable communities where distrust may be long-standing and chronic.[7,13,21] For instance, public health and emergency response officials charged with planning for disasters, from natural disasters (e.g., hurricanes, pandemic flu) to terrorist events should include community representatives—drawn from churches, social clubs, schools, or labor unions—at all levels of disaster planning and response. The success of involving churches in African American communities in other public health endeavors buttresses this recommendation.[22-23] Ensuring that authorities are viewed as honest requires addressing both the completeness of information as well as its accuracy.[24] People are more likely to trust authorities whom they view as genuinely concerned about the welfare of others.[25]

As has been previously proposed,[9, 25] the issue of disaster planning and communications is especially amenable to the methods of community-based participatory research (CBPR), in which partnerships between researchers and communities are formed. Capacity-building, exchange of information, and enhancement of trust are central to the process.[26] Community advisory boards are formed to impart cultural knowledge, provide transparency, and strategize and assist in implementation and dissemination of results.[25] Community-based participatory research differs from traditional research methods in that it fosters social change as part of the research method and has been shown to be particularly effective in addressing public health issues in historically disenfranchised populations.[27-28] In conclusion, public health authorities must attend to matters of distrust when crafting policy and direct outreach for disaster preparedness and communications.

Acknowledgments

We thank the evacuees who generously volunteered their time and responses during the most difficult of experiences. In addition, this project was made possible through funds awarded to D. Eisenman by the Natural Hazards Research and Applications Information Center from the National Science Foundation (CMS 0408499), an award to Dr. Eisenman from the Centers for Disease Control and Prevention (K01-CD000049-02), and an award to Dr. Cordasco from The Robert Wood Johnson Clinical Scholars Program. The authors have no financial conflicts of interest with this project.

Notes

1.   The Brookings Institute. Hurricane Katrina Timeline. Washington, DC: The Brookings Institute, 2005 Oct. Available at http://www.brookings.edu/fp/projects/homeland/katrinatimeline.pdf.

2.   Murphy B, Rad S, Bryant S, et al. Houston: buses bring thousands from Superdome to Astrodome. The Houston Chronicle. 2005 Sep 1:A1.

3.   Nigg JM, Barnshaw J, Torres MR. Hurricane Katrina and the flooding of New Orleans: emergent issues in sheltering and temporary housing. Ann Am Acad Polit Soc Sci. 2006;604(1):113–28.

4.   Eisenman DP, Cordasco KM, Asch SM, et al. Disaster planning and risk communication with vulnerable communities: lessons from Hurricane Katrina. Am J Public Health. (In press.)

5.   Brodie M, Weltzien E, Altman D, et al. Experiences of Hurricane Katrina evacuees in Houston shelters: implications for future planning. Am J Public Health. 2006 Aug: 96(8):1402–8.

6.   U.S. Census Bureau. State & County QuickFacts: New Orleans (city), Louisiana. Washington, DC: U.S. Census Burea, 2007. Available at http://quickfacts.census.gov/qfd/states/22/2255000.html.

7.   Jacobs EA, Rolle I, Ferrans CE, et al. Understanding African Americans' views of the trustworthiness of physicians. J Gen Intern Med. 2006 Jun;21(6):642–7.

8.   Corbie-Smith G, Thomas SB, Williams MV, et al. Attitudes and beliefs of African Americans toward participation in medical research. J Gen Intern Med. 1999 Sep; 14(9):537–46.

9.   Eisenman DP, Wold C, Setodji C, et al. Will public health's response to terrorism be fair? Racial/ethnic variations in perceived fairness during a bioterrorist event. Biosecur Bioterror. 2004;2(3):146–56.

10. Barry JM. Rising tide: the great Mississippi flood of 1927 and how it changed America. New York: Simon & Schuster, 1997.

11. Brinkley D. The great deluge: Hurricane Katrina, New Orleans, and the Mississippi Gulf Coast. New York: William Morrow & Co., 2006; p. 8.

12. O'Toole T, Mair M, Inglesby TV. Shining light on "Dark Winter." Clin Infect Dis. 2002 Apr 1;34(7):972–83.

13. Blanchard JC, Haywood Y, Stein BD, et al. In their own words: lessons learned from those exposed to anthrax. Am J Public Health. 2005 Mar;95(3):489–95.

14. Goold SD. Trust, distrust and trustworthiness. J Gen Int Med. 2002 Jan;17(1): 79–81.

15. Thomas CW. Maintaining and restoring public trust in government agencies and their employees. Administration and Society. 1998;30(2):166–93.

16. Hall MA, Dugan E, Zheng B, et al. Trust in physicians and medical institutions: what is it, can it be measured, and does it matter? Milbank Q. 2001;79(4):613–39.

17. Covello VT, Peters RG, Wojtecki JG, et al. Risk communication, the West Nile virus epidemic and bioterrorism: responding to the communication challenges posed by the intentional and unintentional release of a pathogen in an urban setting. J Urban Health. 2001 Jun;78(2):382–91.

18. Quinn SC. Hurricane Katrina: a social and public health disaster. Am J Public Health. 2006 Feb;96(2):204.

19. Quinn SC, Thomas T, McAllister C. Postal workers' perspectives on communication during the anthrax attack. Biosecur Bioterror. 2005;3(3):207–15.

20. Wray R, Rivers J, Whitworth A, et al. Public perceptions about trust in emergency risk communication: qualitative research findings. Int J Mass Emerg Disasters. 2006 Mar;24(1):45–75.

21. Boulware LE, Cooper LA, Ratner LE, et al. Race and trust in the health care system. Public Health Rep. 2003 Jul–Aug;118(4):358–65.

22. Davis DT, Bustamante A, Brown CP, et al. The urban church and cancer control: a source of social influence in minority communities. Public Health Rep. 1994 Jul–Aug;109(4):500–6.

23. Yanek LR, Becker DM, Moy TF, et al. Project Joy: faith based cardiovascular health promotion for African-American women. Public Health Rep. 2001;116 Suppl 1:68–81.

24. Glass TA, Schoch-Spana M. Bioterrorism and the people: how to vaccinate a city against panic. Clin Infect Dis. 2002 Jan;34(2)217–23.

25. Peters RG, Covello VT, McCallum DB. The determinants of trust and credibility in environmental risk communication: an empirical study. Risk Anal. 1997 Feb;17(1):43–54.

26. Israel BA, Eng E, Schulz AJ, et al. Introduction to methods in community-based participatory research for health. In: Israel BA, Eng E, Schulz AJ, et al., eds. Methods in community-based participatory research for health. San Francisco: Jossey-Bass, 2005.

27. Themba MN, Minkler M. Influencing policy through community based participatory research. In: Minkler M, Wallerstein N, eds. Community-based participatory research for health. San Francisco: Jossey-Bass, 2003.

28. O'Toole TP, Aaron KF, Chin MH, et al. Community-based participatory research: opportunities, challenges, and the need for a common language. J Gen Int Med. 2003 Jul;18(7):592–4.

Chapter 8
Hospitals in Hurricane Katrina: Challenges Facing Custodial Institutions in a Disaster

Bradford H. Gray, PhD
Kathy Hebert, MD, MMM, MPH

The evacuation order contained exemptions for certain people, including city, state and federal officials, inmates of the parish prison, those in hospitals, tourists staying in hotels, and members of the media.

New Orleans Times-Picayune, Sunday, August 28, 2005

Hospitals were part of the problem and part of the solution during the Hurricane Katrina crisis. In a city characterized by high rates of poverty and poor health,[1,2] hospitals cared for some of the most vulnerable people. These institutions also presented some of the most difficult challenges once flooding made evacuation necessary.

In the days after Hurricane Katrina struck and New Orleans's infrastructure failed, hospitals and other organizations that have custodial responsibility for human beings (such as nursing homes and jails) faced special difficulties. In some two dozen hospitals,[3] patients had to be evacuated because of the loss of power, water, and sewage service, and many of these hospitals required external assistance that was slow to arrive. Meanwhile, patients' needs for care continued unabated. Some hospitals evacuated all patients successfully, but by the end of that long week, some had become places of death.

This chapter explores what happened in New Orleans-area hospitals during and after Hurricane Katrina and why hospitals had such varied experiences. We conclude with lessons based on the Katrina experience.

A Note on Methods

This chapter is based on interviews with a dozen hospital executives, public officials, leaders of trade associations, and others who had firsthand experience of the flooding in New Orleans. We also use accounts published during and after the events of that terrible week.

At the time of our interviews, the Louisiana attorney general's office had opened criminal investigations into the deaths of hospital and nursing home patients, once the scale of the tragedy became clear. Some hospital officials were not willing to speak with

BRADFORD GRAY *is a Principal Research Associate in the Urban Institute's Health Policy Center and the Editor of The Milbank Quarterly.* **KATHY HEBERT** *is Medical Director of the Jay Weiss Center for Social Medicine and Health Equity and Associate Professor of Medicine, Division of Cardiology, University of Miami School of Medicine.*

us, and some spoke only off the record. Some information we obtained in interviews is thus unattributed. Also, one hospital responded to our questions in writing rather than in an interview. We are grateful to all who shared their experiences with us.

The institutional review board at the Urban Institute, a nonprofit policy research organization in Washington, D.C., approved this project. At its suggestion, we obtained a Confidentiality Certificate from the National Institutes of Health to assure that we could not be compelled in any legal proceedings to identify anyone who gave us information.

The Problem

Hurricane Katrina presented New Orleans and its hospitals with the effects of two related but distinct events. The first was the hurricane itself, which arrived on Monday morning, August 29, 2005, with heavy rain and sustained winds of 120–130 mph, with gusts up to 160 mph. Electrical and communications services were disrupted by the destruction of landlines and the toppling of cell phone and radio repeater towers, but hospitals and other large buildings suffered only superficial damage.

For hospitals, the problems created by the storm would have been minor were it not for the second event—the failure Monday night of the levees protecting New Orleans from Lake Pontchartrain and the Mississippi River. By Tuesday morning, large sections of the city were under as much as 15–20 feet of water, far exceeding the capacity of the city's pumping system (which was designed to pump water into the very canals whose walls had been breached). Evacuation became essential in the flooded areas.

The situation was particularly urgent for the hospitals that lost power, communications, and water/sewer service, and that couldn't re-supply such essentials as drugs, blood, linens, and food. According to figures assembled by the Louisiana Hospital Association (LHA) during the storm, 1,749 patients occupied the 11 hospitals surrounded by floodwaters.[3] Many of these beleaguered hospitals received much publicity during the crisis—Charity Hospital, University Hospital, Tulane University Hospital, Veterans' Affairs Medical Center, Lindy Boggs Medical Center, and Memorial Medical Center.

The LHA's compilation also showed more than 7,600 people in these 11 hospitals in addition to the patients. Some, but by no means all, were staff members. Hospitals, like the Superdome and convention center, became refuges for patients' families and for thousands of others who left their homes. Hospitals also housed pets. Personnel at Lindy Boggs Medical Center dealt with 45 dogs, 15 cats, and a pair of guinea pigs brought in by staff and patients to ride out the storm.[4]

Conventional modes of transportation were used to evacuate a dozen or so hospitals that were not isolated by water. But evacuation from the 11 flood-bound hospitals posed particularly difficult problems, requiring boats or helicopters.

Why Didn't Hospitals Evacuate in Advance?

Hospitals threatened by the approach of Hurricane Katrina faced a dilemma. It was certainly understood that Katrina was an unusually powerful storm with the potential to do terrible damage, but its course was uncertain, and hospitals had survived numerous previous storms. Officials at Charity Hospital said they did not consider evacuation in advance because Charity had always been where nursing homes and other facilities sent patients in major storms.

In advance of the hurricane, many hospitals in the New Orleans area discharged ambulatory and stable patients. One hospital told us that its psychiatric patients were bused to Tennessee on Saturday. Officials at another hospital wanted to evacuate patients in the intensive care unit in advance of the storm, but were unable to find a hospital that would accept them. These hapless patients were then transferred to another local hospital that was subsequently surrounded by floodwater.

But many patients could not simply be discharged in advance of the storm. Some were recovering from surgery or debilitated by disease. Some depended on mechanical assistance to breathe. Demented patients, newborn babies, and others also couldn't be released. Some patients had even come to hospitals in anticipation of the storm, including those requiring dialysis and those transferred from nursing homes.

Once the mayor gave the evacuation order for the population at large on Saturday—an order that excluded hospitals—exit routes from the city became heavily congested. Moreover, there was no city or state plan for moving hundreds of patients from multiple institutions. Nor were enough vehicles available once it became apparent that New Orleans would be struck. Hospitals did have contractual arrangements for ambulance services in an evacuation, but one hospital official said that when he called on Sunday to move 12 ventilator patients to Lake Charles, he was told that the mayor had taken control of all ambulances and that, in any case, the traffic was so bad that they would not likely get back and forth before the storm hit.

An additional practical problem was the need for a destination for the patients. Critically ill patients could not simply be transported north or west. Some hospitals reported that in advance of the storm, they had been unable to find hospitals that were both reasonably close and willing to accept patients from New Orleans, in part because those hospitals did not know how they would be affected by the storm.

But even had advance evacuation been possible, it was not clearly the correct course of action. For patients who were disoriented or on respirators or in traction, for example, evacuation posed enormous logistical challenges, especially because external conditions were harsh. Hospital officials believed that many patients in critical condition would be put at undue risk in a hasty evacuation, particularly considering the expected traffic jams. The patients were thought to be safer where they were.

Moreover, before the storm, it was not clear that evacuation would be necessary; where Hurricane Katrina would make landfall and how New Orleans would be affected were both uncertain. The unpredictability of hurricanes was well understood by hospital and governmental officials. A year earlier, New Orleans was threatened by Hurricane Ivan, and what the *Times-Picayune* called "mind numbing-congestion" resulted, as more than 600,000 people tried to flee the city in a single day.[5] At its peak, traffic backed up for 30 miles. The hurricane then changed paths, turning east to strike the Alabama-Florida coast. New Orleans was spared. Had hospitals evacuated unnecessarily, any patient deaths would have been criticized harshly.

A Hospital That Evacuated before Katrina

Although none of the New Orleans hospitals evacuated in advance of Hurricane Katrina, St. Charles Parish Hospital in Luling, Louisiana, some twenty miles west of New Orleans, made a different decision. That hospital's patients were evacuated on Sunday afternoon in advance of the storm. (Personal communication, Guillot K., COO and North D., Director of Nursing, St. Charles Parish Hospital, 2006 Apr 17.)

Hospital officials began to consider advance evacuation on Saturday, even though the hospital had never before evacuated in advance of a hurricane. But the hospital was a single-story building, and Katrina seemed particularly threatening. On Saturday afternoon, the chief executive officer (CEO) called several hospitals; Desoto Hospital in Mansfield, Louisiana, some 300 miles away, agreed to accept the patients. After a night of planning, the decision was made on Sunday morning to evacuate the hospital's medical patients using three ambulances (for the six sickest patients) and two wheelchair-accessible school buses that had been outfitted for the parish's medically needy. Two additional school buses transported the psychiatric patients. The nursing and pharmacy staff assembled a week's worth of medicines and supplies, and patient care staff members (both physicians and nurses) were organized to accompany the patients.

The buses left at 1:00 p.m. on Sunday; the ambulances did not leave until after 4:00 p.m. because of the complexities in arranging a transfer in Baton Rouge to ambulances that would complete the trip to Mansfield. The buses soon encountered gridlock traffic. The first leg to Morgan City, normally a one-hour trip, took 6–7 hours. At 10:00 p.m. the buses stopped at a shelter for the medically needy in Lafayette, 120 miles from Luling. The patients rode out the hurricane there, and some were admitted to a hospital in Lafayette. Others were transported to Mansfield, as planned, after the hurricane passed.

Patients who were transported by ambulance had a different experience. With the assistance of an escort from the sheriff's department, the patients reached their destination in Mansfield (320 miles from Luling) at about the same time the bused patients reached Lafayette. The transferred patients remained there for the rest of the week, cared for by personnel transported with them from St. Charles Parish Hospital. That hospital's emergency room reopened late Monday afternoon on emergency power, with ancillary clinical department (e.g., lab, x-ray, respiratory) support, but the inpatient units did not admit new patients until full power was restored at the end of the week. At that time, most of the patients who had been evacuated were returned to the hospital. (The exceptions were those who had been admitted to the hospital in Lafayette and several who were transferred to a nursing home in Mansfield.) In retrospect, hospital officials believe that they made the right decision in evacuating before the storm.

Conditions inside Hospitals after Hurricane Katrina

Our interviews and press accounts provide a picture of the terrible conditions faced by medical staff and others trying to care for patients after Hurricane Katrina. Many hospitals were short-staffed because of personnel who did not come to work; those who made it in worked long shifts in adverse conditions. Patient care became exceedingly difficult as hospitals lost power to operate vital equipment such as lab and x-ray equipment, dialysis machines, and elevators. Temperatures rose to above 100 degrees in many institutions (fixed windows were smashed from the inside with furniture at some), toilets backed up, and essential supplies dwindled. Many hospitals reported struggling to care for ventilator-dependent patients after hospitals lost electricity. One hospital told us of emergency surgery being done by flashlight, with little or no anesthesia.

The most detailed descriptions of conditions during the crisis came from Charity Hospital, the venerable public hospital that was surrounded by waist-deep water. There were accounts of dozens of critically ill patients being carried up and down dark stairwells because the elevators were not working (the ICU was on the 12th floor), hospital personnel using "jerry-rigged ventilators" to "physically breathe" for patients, family members fanning patients for hours in sweltering rooms, workers using buckets or plastic bags as toilets, doctors making rounds by flashlight, personnel unable to check lab values or use electronic devices for IV medications, patients occupying stretchers in the halls, the emergency department moving from the first to the second floor to escape the floodwaters, personnel brushing teeth and feeding each other with IV fluid after food ran out on Wednesday, people sleeping on the roof to escape the heat and stench, bodies being stacked in a stairwell because the basement morgue was both full and inaccessible, and personnel feeling that the hospital had been forgotten after telephones and electronic communication failed.

By Tuesday morning, after flooding put Charity's generators (which were in the basement) out of commission, it became evident that patients in the ICU had to be evacuated. By Wednesday, *all* patients (from 250 to more than 350 by various accounts) clearly had to be evacuated. The process was not completed until the end of the week. Even so, and notwithstanding the terrible conditions described above, only 8 patients at Charity died during the ordeal, mostly ICU patients who, according to the CEO, were expected to die.

Many more deaths were reported at two hospitals owned by Tenet Healthcare Corporation: Memorial Medical Center and Lindy Boggs Medical Center. Nineteen bodies were found at Lindy Boggs and 45 at Memorial, though company officials indicated that 11 had died before the storm. Those deaths became the subject of separate criminal investigations by Louisiana's attorney general and the New Orleans district attorney,[6–7] so information is limited to contemporary press accounts and an interview given by George Saucier, the CEO of Lindy Boggs Medical Center, to Joseph Parker, the president of the Georgia Hospital Association.[8]

By Saucier's account, Lindy Boggs Medical Center suffered only superficial damage during the storm. But by that Monday evening, flooding had begun, the hospital's generators had stopped working, water pressure was gone, and all communications with the outside world were severed. When the hospital heard from no one on Tuesday, people began to get nervous.

The hospital lost power in the storm or soon thereafter. Saucier reported that a team of nurses alternated 30-minute shifts to hand operate the ventilators sustaining four ICU patients; then family members were trained to take over. Dr. Thiagarajan Ramcharan, a transplant surgeon working at Lindy Boggs during the crisis, said in a press account a few days later that patients in the hospice unit were already dying by

Tuesday from heat and dehydration.[4] He believed that hospice patients accounted for most of the deaths at Lindy Boggs.

A lack of supplies contributed to the crisis. The hospital ran out of blood for transfusion and had "very little medication besides morphine."[4] At some point the pharmacy was locked, which Dr. Ramcharan described as standard evacuation procedure. The water supply was also depleted.

The experience at Memorial Medical Center was even grimmer. Between 220 and 300 patients and 1,500 others were stranded.[9] Only fragmentary information is available on conditions in the hospital. The failure of generators and the resulting debilitating heat are undisputed, as is the loss of running water and sewage service.[10] But reports about, for instance, whether looters broke into the hospital and whether the hospital had to ration food and water, conflict with one another. Heroic efforts by hospital personnel were reported,[9] as were allegations that hospital personnel had ended the lives of some patients they believed would not survive the ordeal.[11-12]

Louisiana's attorney general opened an investigation of the deaths at Memorial by issuing 73 subpoenas in late October 2005 and calling for autopsies of all 45 bodies removed from the hospital after the storm.[13] There were conflicting reports about Tenet's cooperation in the investigation. The company claimed that it cooperated fully, but the attorney general charged that a letter from Tenet's assistant general counsel to advise staff members of their rights if "contacted by a representative of a state or federal agency [or] the media" had a "chilling effect," prompting subpoenas.[13] After an 11-month investigation, Attorney General Charles Foti announced the arrest of a physician and two nurses from Memorial on charges of second-degree murder for allegedly purposely administering fatal doses of morphine or other drugs to four patients in the days after the hurricane.[14] The case had not gone to trial when this article was written.

The two hospitals where so many died shared several characteristics. First, control of both hospitals had changed several times over the previous decade. Both had a long history as religiously affiliated (Baptist and Catholic) before merging in 1994 and being acquired by Tenet in 1995. Tenet had been operating them as separate institutions for little more than a year when Katrina struck.[15] Second, both hospitals contained entities other than traditional medical/surgical units: Lindy Boggs Medical Center had a hospice unit, and Memorial Medical Center had an 82-bed "long-term acute care" unit operated by LifeCare Holdings. Who was responsible for the seriously ill patients in the unit may have been unclear. Although the patients were in a Tenet hospital, the company quickly announced that 24 of the patients who had died were "under the care and supervision of LifeCare Holdings and its staff."[16]

On September 6, 2005, LifeCare Holdings issued a press release stating that all patients and staff had been evacuated from its units in three hospitals in the New Orleans area and that, although these hospitals had "contributed approximately 12.5% of [the company's] consolidated revenue in the previous six months," the financial impact on the company could not yet be estimated.[17] The statement did not mention the deaths of the 24 patients in LifeCare Holdings' unit at Memorial Hospital.

The Evacuation

Options are limited for evacuating patients from hospitals surrounded by floodwater. A few hospitals were accessible by helicopter. To leave other hospitals, patients had to be taken by boat to where ground transportation or a helicopter was available. From there, some patients were transferred directly to another hospital, but many went to triage points on a nearby highway overpass or the Louis Armstrong New Orleans International Airport. Some boats, the ambulances, and many of the helicopters could transport only one or two patients at a time, and the round trip could take an hour or more. This, combined with the inadequate number of boats and delays resulting from security fears after shooting was reported, made the pace of evacuation excruciatingly slow.

Some stories about the evacuation were almost as disturbing as the events inside the marooned hospitals. The Veterans Affairs Medical Center (VA) and the nearby Tulane University Hospital were relative success stories because they shared a common trait—access to an effective external source of help.

In a published account, critical care nurse Frank Millette described the experience at the VA hospital, which housed 150 patients and about 550 others.[18] By Tuesday morning, the hospital had no running water or air conditioning, the heat was stifling, and flood damage to the electrical wiring in the basement knocked out the elevators. A distress call to the Veterans Affairs Department in Washington prompted someone to contact the VA Law Enforcement Training Center in North Little Rock, Arkansas. The center's director, Ron Angel, who had recently returned from Iraq, called upon his colleagues from the Arkansas National Guard. Without getting higher authorization, 16 national guardsmen and 7 military trucks headed toward New Orleans, arriving at the VA Medical Center at 9:30 Tuesday evening. Putting patients on mattresses in the truck beds for the one-hour trip, the guardsmen began evacuating patients to the airport on Wednesday. Fifteen critically ill patients were reportedly transported to a heliport at the Superdome from where they were evacuated Tuesday. Another 55 people were evacuated by the same route on Thursday. The hospital was not completely evacuated until Friday afternoon. Although Millette felt that the hospital had been well taken care of by the federal government, saying "We were lucky in that we were under the wing of the federal government,"[19] elements of the evacuation were clearly *ad hoc*.

At Tulane University Hospital, officials told us that planning for evacuation began three days before the storm hit. The decision to evacuate was made mid-afternoon on Tuesday, prompted by the rising waters endangering the generators in the plant facilities area, and by advice from the Louisiana State Office of Emergency Preparedness. (This was the only hospital official we interviewed who mentioned this agency as part of the decision to evacuate.)

Helicopters that landed on the roof of its parking garage carried out the evacuation from Tulane University Hospital. Some helicopters were arranged by the hospital through the local company Acadian Ambulance, and some were secured from elsewhere by the hospital's parent organization, the Hospital Corporation of America (HCA, the nation's largest investor-owned hospital company). The company was also instrumental in finding places for patients at its other hospitals; the transfer of each patient to a specific hospital was arranged before evacuation. Many other hospitals were not able to make such arrangements.

The evacuation of Tulane University Hospital began on Tuesday and was completed on Friday. It included both 120 patients who had been hospitalized during the storm and another 58 who arrived Sunday evening from the Superdome. Some patients from nearby Charity Hospital were also evacuated from Tulane's roof after they were ferried over by boat. The evacuation of Tulane University Hospital was not without its challenges. Since elevators were not functioning, patients had to be carried down stairwells to the second floor of the garage, from where they were taken on the back of a truck to the roof for transport out. Some patients required larger helicopters. Two patients had to be moved with 500-pound heart pumps. Two others were bariatric surgery patients each weighing more than 600 pounds. (Officials at another hospital told of the staff using sheets to carry five patients who each weighed more than 500 pounds up stairs to their hospital's roof for evacuation by helicopter.) Some patients had to be accompanied by a nurse. According to Tulane's CEO, none of their patients died during the evacuation, although two patients who had been moved from Charity Hospital to Tulane died during the evacuation.

Notwithstanding this success, Tulane's management told us that its disaster plan, implemented a few days in advance of the storm, was not referred to during the event and was of little help, in part because the hospital's complete inability to communicate was not anticipated. (However, another flooded hospital's CEO told us that their disaster plan's provisions for food, water, medications, security, and physician care all worked.)

Two factors beyond the staff's hard work and competence seem particularly important in the successful evacuation of Tulane University Hospital. First, the hospital was accessible by helicopter. Second, the hospital had external assistance, from its parent company, HCA.

However, a parent company was not enough to ensure success in dealing with the crisis presented by Katrina. The two hospitals with the most deaths, Lindy Boggs Medical Center and Memorial Medical Center, were both owned by Tenet, the nation's second-largest hospital company.

The CEO at Lindy Boggs reported that the hospital lost communications systems early in the crisis. On Tuesday, Thomas Jordan, a neighbor who had waded to the hospital to check on conditions, volunteered to wade to the New Orleans Health Department (three hours through thigh-deep water) to carry news of the increasingly desperate situation in the hospital; on his return he expressed doubt that any response would result because the health department itself seemed to be helpless.[19]

Two boats operated by firemen from Shreveport, Louisiana, arrived at Lindy Boggs Medical Center on Wednesday morning, and the evacuation of the 120 patients began, with patients and families loaded into boats to be ferried one fourth mile to a dry berm where they could be airlifted by helicopter. Many patients had been carried down several flights of stairs. Before evacuating patients, doctors had prepared cards for each indicating whether they could walk out on their own ("A") or had medical problems that needed attention ("B"). "C" meant "condition critical"; "C" patients were told by the doctors they would be evacuated first, in accord with hospital policy. But the rescue team brought different priorities, insisting, according to the CEO, that the city was under martial law and women, children, and the most ambulatory patients had to be evacuated first.[8] By day's end, the rescue team was called elsewhere, leaving 30 patients and 80 employees and family members feeling abandoned and worrying that the rescuers might not return.

On Thursday, hospital employees borrowed a boat and siphoned gasoline from abandoned cars.[4] Late in the morning, the remaining patients and staff were transported to the berm, in hopes that a helicopter would come, and the evacuation of Lindy Boggs was complete, with at least some of the patients transported by helicopter to an overpass on Interstate 10 for triage and further transportation.[20]

Regarding Memorial Hospital, where so many patients died, the CEO and some health personnel provided details to the *New York Times* about the evacuation.[10] By this account, the CEO sought assistance from Tenet's Dallas offices by e-mail on Tuesday, after the telephones failed. Workers successfully cleared an abandoned helicopter pad on top of the hospital's parking garage, and extension cords from the still-functioning generator supplied light to guide pilots. Patients had to be passed to the hospital garage through a hole in a second-floor maintenance room, transported by vehicle up the parking garage, and then carried up three flights of steps to the landing pad. The first two helicopters that sought to land intended to deliver evacuees *to* the hospital. Some pilots wanted to transport only pregnant women or babies. Boats were also used to ferry patients and 1,800 residents who had taken shelter at the hospital to dry land for further evacuation.

Midday on Wednesday, Memorial's generators failed. On Wednesday evening, while 115 patients still awaited evacuation, the boats stopped coming. Patients who had been prepared to evacuate had to be brought back in, fed, given fluids, and put onto cots. On Thursday morning, 6 helicopters chartered by Tenet arrived and the remaining living patients were all evacuated.

At Charity, the most fragile patients, ICU patients, were evacuated first, but press accounts indicate that 28 babies (including 18 in intensive care) were among the last to be evacuated.[10] Among the critically ill patients who required evacuation were 2 from the hospital's prison ward. (Disagreement among staff members was reported, about whether these prisoners should be evacuated before other, critically ill patients.[21]) Many details of Charity's experience in trying to evacuate their patients plus some 1,200 other people come to light in interviews with senior officials, including these:

- Telephone communication was spotty.
- No single person or agency could be called for help. Hospital personnel said they had to beg agency by agency for help, since agencies were not coordinated.
- Evacuation plans were not useful because of the flooding, and no one had experience arranging for boats and staging areas.
- Personnel initially had difficulty finding places to send patients, though this was relieved by the availability of other public hospitals in the state.
- Hospital personnel did not know the landing coordinates that helicopter pilots requested.

- There were complications moving bedridden patients, as well as patients on oxygen and IV medications, up and down stairways and in boats.
- Spinal boards needed to move patients down stairwells had to be brought from storage in Baton Rouge.
- A truck high enough to deliver the spinal boards through the floodwaters was located but it would not fit on the ramp into the hospital, so personnel hot-wired another truck in the parking garage to complete the delivery.
- Personnel had to make arrangements with the state police to allow the truck through.
- Personnel had to figure out what kinds of buses could be used to move patients.
- Personnel had to triage patients by type, destination, and mode of transportation. For example, ICU patients were evacuated to the triage area at the airport. Ninety psychiatric patients were medicated and sent by bus to a psychiatric hospital in Alexandria, Louisiana.
- Reports of gunfire near several hospitals heightened the need for security and made obtaining help more difficult.

Evacuation was a completely different task at institutions that weren't flooded. Children's Hospital, for example, had to evacuate because the water pressure dropped to zero and the air conditioning failed. Patients were evacuated by ambulances, helicopters, and private cars. Children's Hospital reported no difficulty finding places to transfer patients. In fact, children's hospitals elsewhere offered more help than needed, according to the CEO. Patients were triaged to hospitals (mostly in Kansas and Miami) that had doctors trained to deal with their particular problems. (The Kansas Children's Hospital also flew doctors and nurses to New Orleans.)

Experiences with FEMA and Other Authorities

Several of our interviews with hospital officials, most of whom would talk only off the record, concerned negative experiences with the Federal Emergency Management Agency (FEMA) or the authorities controlling access to the city. One hospital successfully requested supplies from its corporate headquarters, only to have them confiscated by FEMA before they reached the hospital. Authorities turned back ambulances that had been arranged by another hospital. Another interviewee charged FEMA with diverting a shipment of fuel ordered by a hospital whose generators had run out. After one organization experienced difficulty getting supply trucks into the city, they downloaded a logo from the state police web site and fashioned authorization letters that got the trucks past the police barricades blocking the city. Methodist Hospital reported that supplies sent by its corporate parent were confiscated by FEMA at the airport; thereafter, the company sent food, water, and diesel fuel to Lafayette (130 miles from New Orleans) then had them transported to the hospital by helicopter, while also evacuating some of the most seriously ill patients.[22]

There were also other accounts of negative experiences with FEMA. One official we interviewed reported that FEMA replaced some patients' hospital bracelets with

FEMA ID bracelets, which made tracing transferred patients difficult. Another hospital reported that it had called the police, national guard, and FEMA when alarming rumors about gang looting had them feeling vulnerable; none of these agencies sent assistance for lengthy periods of time.

Lessons from Hospitals' Experiences in Katrina

Many of the most important lessons of Katrina are not peculiar to hospitals. The congressional and White House reports, for example, emphasize the need for better advance planning, better communications, more rapid deployment of resources, and better coordination.[23,24] The experiences of New Orleans's hospitals affirm these conclusions, and the failure of communication modes exacerbated all of the hospitals' other problems. But hospitals (and nursing homes) present distinctive and difficult challenges in a community-wide disaster. No other facilities house such large concentrations of people who cannot meet their own needs, who may require ongoing life support, and who cannot manage their own evacuation. Yet, officials at several hospitals spoke of feeling abandoned in the wake of Katrina.

Lessons from Hurricane Katrina

The Possibility of Advance Evacuation

In considering the human misery and tragedy in urban hospitals in the wake of Katrina, should hospitals be evacuated in advance of predicted disasters? Future circumstances may well warrant advance evacuation. Yet, the calculus for whether to evacuate is complex, involving the cost and risk of evacuation, the certainty and anticipated severity of the event, and the time available for action.

Certainly, calls for mandatory evacuation of a metropolitan area should not automatically exclude hospitals. (One hospital CEO told us that the mayor's exclusion of hospitals from his evacuation order created "emotional pressure" to stay behind as the city emptied.) At the same time, a general policy of moving hospitalized patients anytime the authorities recommend evacuating a metropolitan area seems unwise. Buildings such as hospitals can withstand events that would severely damage or destroy smaller buildings. Moreover, the evacuation of large numbers of severely ill patients will always be difficult, dangerous, and costly in both economic and human terms. When disaster threatens, its severity and location will be uncertain and, when a city's entire population seeks to evacuate, fierce competition will arise for such scarce resources as emergency personnel, vehicles, and highway space. The possibility of adverse consequences for an evacuation that proves unnecessary must also be considered, since transferring fragile patients is difficult and risky.

We described the experience of St. Charles Parish Hospital, which did evacuate in advance of the storm. Except for the handful of patients who were transported by ambulance with police escort, patients transported by bus (starting from 20 miles west of New Orleans) became ensnared in traffic and rode out the storm in an emergency shelter established for medically needy patients 120 miles from their hospital and adjacent to a full-service hospital. The St. Charles Parish Emergency Operations Center and the State Department of Emergency Medical Services coordinated use of this shelter. None of this hospital's patients died in the ordeal. In retrospect, hospital personnel believed that evacuation was the correct decision and regretted not leaving earlier.

Advance evacuation of patients involves complex tradeoffs between certainty about the location and severity of the disaster and the amount of time needed to transport people with challenging needs. Clearly, sirens and lights and police escorts facilitate the process once gridlock has set in. Gridlock will set in, it appears, even when multilane highways are converted to one-way arteries away from the city (the so-called contra-flow scheme used in the pre-Katrina evacuation). Dedicating a lane for people with special needs (e.g., hospital patients) is an idea that deserves consideration, although many practical difficulties would have to be solved.

Thus, even though it is difficult to imagine a more disorderly and dangerous under-taking than the evacuation of hospitals *after* Katrina, it should be assumed for planning purposes that many affected hospitals will not evacuate in advance of catastrophic events.

Improved Planning

Hurricane Katrina showed that hospitals' advance planning was inadequate in several respects. First, planning was left to individual hospitals, though the disaster was area-wide. Advance arrangements (e.g., contracting with an ambulance company) may be inadequate if multiple facilities must be evacuated simultaneously. Clearly, hospitals must be a major part of *area-wide* disaster and evacuation planning.

Second, disaster plans before Katrina implicitly assumed that hospitals (and other large buildings, such as hotels and office buildings) could withstand a hurricane. The New Orleans Emergency Preparedness plan, for example, included instructions for nursing homes, but nothing for hospitals. Although the assumption that hospitals would not be destroyed proved to be correct, their vulnerability to the secondary consequences of the storm was not anticipated by either governmental officials or by hospitals themselves. (One hospital CEO told us that its disaster plan was not helpful because it did not include evacuation procedures and had no provision for a com-mand center.) Katrina showed that hospitals depend heavily on citywide infrastruc-ture (electrical power, communications, water, security, and transportation) that can be disrupted by an area-wide disaster. As described here, it was the combined loss of essential infrastructure and utilities that put hospitals and their patients into such perilous circumstances. Disaster planning for hospitals must incorporate the possible loss of essential infrastructure.

More particularly, special attention must be devoted in disaster plans to the pos-sibility that hospitals (and other facilities with custodial responsibility for people) will need to evacuate their charges. In locales vulnerable to flooding, this possibility must be considered both in facility design and in contingency planning for evacuation. It is now obvious, for example, that generators should not be vulnerable to predictable contingencies and that plans for refueling should be in place. Indeed, the generators' failure, for reasons that seemed to vary from institution to institution, is one of the most striking and disheartening parts of the post-Katrina experience.

Even with better planning, however, under similar circumstances, some hospitals will likely have to care for at least some patients for several days. During Katrina, in hospitals that lacked power, surgery was performed, babies were born, and severely ill patients received care. But hospitals were generally unprepared for the loss of essential services and shortages of food, water, and supplies. Delivery of supplies stopped before the storm hit. Thereafter, ordinary deliveries were completely disrupted and in some instances, authorities diverted supplies *en route*. Hospitals are not ordinarily prepared to be self-sufficient for a week. Authorities assisting after a disaster must recognize and accord priority to hospitals' need for supplies.

The Challenges of Evacuating Patients

Hospitals' experiences with evacuation contained important lessons for the future. Among the lessons gleaned from firsthand experience with Katrina are these:

1. Evacuating a hospital is very different from evacuating a similar-sized hotel or apartment building. Many patients have special requirements for both transportation and an appropriate destination. Patients who require artificial life support or who are immobilized (e.g., in traction) pose particular problems. Officials at several hospitals mentioned challenges posed by bariatric surgery patients. (One patient was evacuated from a second story window into a boat.) In the future, advance evacuation efforts should focus on patients who pose especially difficult evacuation problems. Some patients panic or become agitated or disoriented, suggesting that qualified psychiatric personnel should be included in emergency response teams.

2. External coordination is essential, as hospital evacuation is logistically complex. Solutions to hospitals' problems cross agency lines and require assets for which there will be competing demands. After Katrina, some hospitals needed supplies or equipment to be able to evacuate patients. Destinations had to be identified and transportation arranged. Hospital officials had to make these complex arrangements themselves under the most adverse conditions. Some supplies or transportation arranged by hospitals were diverted by authorities for use elsewhere. Clearly, when large numbers of patients must be evacuated, particularly in chaotic situations in which communications have been disrupted, hospital personnel are not well situated to coordinate necessary services. The need for coordination is a vital topic for disaster planning.

3. Suitable destinations must be identified for patients who are to be evacuated, particularly those who have critical care needs. Such arrangements should be planned in advance, for example, by identifying partner hospitals outside the geographic area. (One hospital CEO suggested that undamaged hospitals in a disaster-hit region be required to accept evacuated patients.) Before Katrina struck, some hospitals could not find another hospital to accept their patients. At least one hospital stopped evacuating its patients after learning that they were being transported to a triage location with little capacity for patient care. Thereafter,

the hospital decided to release patients only on helicopters that would take them to a hospital on the other side of Lake Pontchartrain.

4. Their medical records must accompany evacuated patients. In the post-Katrina evacuation, even though hospitals such as Charity put summary records into ziplock bags attached to patients, some patients became separated from their records. As a result, the receiving hospitals did not have vitally important information about some patients' diagnoses, medical history, medications, and so on, and not all patients could supply it themselves. As use of electronic health records grows, similar circumstances (e.g., the need to evacuate patients from institutions that lost power) should be considered to ensure records are available after evacuation.

5. A system for tracking evacuees is essential, particularly since some patients, including newborns and Alzheimer's patients, were separated from their families. Some patients were transported more than once. Some hospital officials expressed concern that they did not know where their patients had been taken. One hospital CEO told us that three months after the storm, the staff still couldn't locate some patients who had been evacuated. Two things are clearly needed. One is making certain that identifying information is physically attached to patients and is not removed when they are rescued. The other would be the use of a clearinghouse to which post-evacuation information about the location of evacuation would be reported by telephone or email.

6. That many patients had family members with them was both a boon and a complication. Family members performed services ranging from fanning patients in the extreme heat to hand-pumping oxygen. But many family members wanted to be evacuated along with their relatives, which complicated the situation. At one hospital, a family member became extremely agitated when her mother was evacuated without her, leading the CEO to fear that a riot might break out. Policies concerning relatives should be part of planning for disasters that affect institutions with custodial responsibilities.

7. More generally, it must be recognized that in a crisis, hospitals become magnets for people who want to help or who are seeking refuge. The presence of hundreds of extra people created a significant management problem for hospital officials, exacerbated many of the difficulties faced by hospital staff, and added to the challenge of evacuation. These people, too, needed food, water, and plumbing facilities. The newcomers were disruptive in some cases and added to the evacuation challenge. Some hospital executives concluded that, if ever again faced with similar circumstances, they would refuse to shelter family and pets. In any event, decisions should be made in advance about how a possible influx will be handled.

8. Advance agreement is needed among key parties about which patients will be evacuated first. As we have recounted, several disputes developed over priorities in the days after Katrina. There was disagreement, for example, over whether the sickest patients or those more likely to survive should be evacuated first. There is also a need to decide on the circumstances under which patients (including

infants and demented elderly patients) will be separated from attendant family members.

9. A disaster creates special security problems for hospitals. Hospital personnel and patients need protection. In the wake of Katrina, hospital officials mentioned several security problems, including protecting hospital supplies (e.g., particular drugs), controlling refugees or patients' relatives, and even protecting space in the garage (many people saw hospital garages as places their automobiles might be safe from the storm). Security concerns delayed evacuation at some hospitals (e.g., Charity), particularly after gunfire was reported. At Touro Infirmary, where half of the 240 patients were evacuated by ground, buses, cars, and vans went in caravans under police guard for patients' safety.

From the interviews and the published accounts of hospitals' experience after Katrina, we want to draw one final lesson pertaining to institutions responsible for people who cannot take care of themselves. Notwithstanding the unresolved allegations of criminal neglect at several nursing homes and hospitals where multiple deaths occurred, there were countless accounts of staff members and volunteers doing extraordinary things under extremely difficult circumstances. It should be recognized, not taken for granted, that many staff members went to the hospital when the city was ordered evacuated, worked day after day until they were exhausted, and improvised with enormous creativity when equipment failed or supplies were depleted.

Conclusion

The story of New Orleans' hospitals in the days after Hurricane Katrina is a reminder of their vital importance and of the deep sense of responsibility shared by the people who work there. It is a story of both success and failure under unthinkably terrible conditions. Shortcomings in planning can be laid at the feet of almost all of the hospitals, but this was an experience without precedent and the goal now should be to learn, not to blame. In any case, such shortcomings pale in comparison with the failures of public authorities to understand what flooding would do to hospitals and to respond quickly and effectively to the conditions at hand. The way hospitals dealt with adversity is a part of the Katrina experience that must be remembered for the future.

Notes

1. Zedlewski SR. Building a better safety net for the New Orleans. Washington, DC: The Urban Institute, 2006.
2. Zuckerman S, Coughlin TA. Initial health policy responses to Hurricane Katrina and possible next steps. Washington, DC: The Urban Institute, 2006.
3. Louisiana Hospital Association (LHA). Hurricane Katrina evacuation report. Baton Rouge, LA: LHA, 2005 Aug 31–Sep 2. (Unpublished Excel worksheet.)
4. Davis R. Hope turns to anguish at intensive-care unit. USA Today. 2005 September 16.

5. Grisset S. Louisiana, Mississippi hurricane evacuation plan gets rerouted. New Orleans Times-Picayune. 2005 April 13:1.

6. Schuler M. State probes 13 nursing homes, 4 hospitals. The Advocate. 2005 September 29:2.B.S.

7. Johnson K. Grand jury to probe hospitals. USA Today. 2006 January 15.

8. Parker JA. A story you probably haven't heard. GHA Today. 2005 Nov;49(5):11.

9. Ritea S. Hospital staff fought to save dying patients: 45 bodies protected from water, looters. New Orleans Times-Picayune. 2005 Sep 13:A-06.

10. Chan S, Harris G. Hurricane and floods overwhelmed hospitals. New York Times. 2005 September 14.

11. Roig-Frazia M, Conolly C. La. investigates allegations of euthanasia at hospital. Washington Post. 2006 Oct 15:A03.

12. Kahn C. New Orleans hospital staff discussed mercy killings. National Public Radio. 2006 Feb 17. Available at http://www.npr.org/templates/story/story.php?storyId=5219917.

13. Griffin D, Johnson K. Dozens subpoenaed in hospital deaths. Atlanta: CNN.com, 2005 Oct 26.

14. Nolan B. Ethicists: any deliberate killing crosses the line. New Orleans Times-Picayune. 2006 Jul 9.

15. Tenet Healthcare. 2004. Tenet Louisiana announces split of Memorial Medical Center campuses. Dallas, TX: Tenet Healthcare, 2004 Jun 1.

16. Tenet Healthcare. Tenet comments on search of New Orleans hospital campus. Dallas, TX: Tenet Healthcare, 2005 Oct 2.

17. Lifecare Holdings, Inc. reports evacuation of three New Orleans hospitals. Plano, TX: Lifecare Holdings, Inc., 2005 Sep 6.

18. McClenny P. VA Medical Center 'was the lucky one.' Mobile (AL) Register. 2005 September 26.

19. MacCash D. No shoes, but lots of soul: bootless paramedic wades miles to give generator to hospital. New Orleans Times-Picayune. 2005 Sep 26:B1.

20. Plohetski T. Austin medics see 30 victims an hour. Austin (TX) American-Statesman. 2005 Sep 2:A1.

21. Anonymous. Mayhem hampering hospital evacuations. Atlanta: CNN.com, 2005 Aug 31.

22. Herbert B. Sick and abandoned. The New York Times. 2005 Sep 15.

23. Select Bipartisan Committee. 2006. A failure of initiative: final report of the Select Bipartisan Committee to investigate the preparation for and response to Hurricane Katrina. Washington, DC: U.S. Government Printing Office.

24. White House Staff, Katrina Lessons Learned Review Group. The federal response to Hurricane Katrina: lessons learned. Washington, DC: The White House, 2006.

Chapter 9
Hurricane Emergency Planning by Home Health Providers Serving the Poor

Dahlia V. Kirkpatrick, MD
Marguerite Bryan, PhD

The purpose of the study reported on here was to gather critical information to help improve official emergency response to impending disasters for underserved and indigent populations. A retrospective study that evaluated the emergency preparation for and response to Hurricane Katrina, this qualitative research project took a case study approach, focusing on the emergency planning that was in place among home health providers at the advent of Hurricane Katrina.

The research team conducted in-depth interviews of the two top administrative staff of five selected home health agencies operating in Orleans Parish (which comprises the City of New Orleans). Administrative and social work staff members of the agencies estimate that the average household income of their clients was $12,000.

Existing state and local emergency preparedness plans at the time of Hurricane Katrina. *The State of Louisiana emergency plan.* The state of Louisiana had an operating emergency plan for home health providers at the time of Hurricane Katrina, titled, "Southeast Louisiana Hurricane Evacuation And Sheltering Plan."[1] The plan prescribed a procedure for the parishes to follow in response to a catastrophic hurricane. It did not replace or supersede any local plans, nor did it usurp the authority of any local governing body. A *catastrophic hurricane* was defined as a slow-moving hurricane in Category 3, or any hurricane in Category 4 or 5. Hurricane Katrina peaked as a Category 5 hurricane; at the time of landfall on Louisiana it was a Category 3.[2]

The state's plan called for evacuation of the low-lying parishes (including Orleans Parish) to shelters in the northern part of Louisiana and adjacent states, as needed. Much discussion surrounds when to declare recommended and mandatory evacuations, the various evacuation routes, *contra* flow procedures, and estimated number of shelters accessible to southeast Louisiana evacuees.

City of New Orleans emergency planning. The City of New Orleans had an emergency plan at the time of Hurricane Katrina, titled "City of New Orleans Comprehensive Emergency Management Plan."[3] It addressed the various tasks of the Mayor, the police, the Regional Transit Authority and the Orleans Parish School Board.

Existing home health care agencies' emergency plans. At the time of Hurricane Katrina, the State of Louisiana, through the Department of Health and Hospitals

DAHLIA KIRKPATRICK is Medical Director at the Acute Care Clinic in Houma, Louisiana. MARGUE-RITE BRYAN is a Lecturer in the Department of Sociology at Xavier University in New Orleans.

(DHH), had a generic emergency preparedness plan for home health agencies. This plan was established in 2000 and was posted on the website of the Louisiana Department of Homeland Security (DHS), rather than the state's Department of Health and Hospitals. The plan comprised several boilerplate parts, allowing individual agencies to fill in the blanks, as it were. The parts included Purpose, Situation and Considerations, Concept of Operations, Organization and Responsibilities, Administration and Logistics, Authentication, Signatures, and Index of Tabs.[4]

The plan specified how patients were to be categorized in terms of their need for community assistance. The plan outlined what agency staff should do in preparing for emergencies and what they should do during and after the emergencies. The plan specifically stated that home health providers must file annually with relevant Offices of Emergency Preparedness in each parish in which they provided care to patients.[4]

Hurricane Katrina. Hurricane Katrina struck the New Orleans area in the early morning on August 29, 2005. The storm surge breached the city's levees at multiple points, leaving 80% of the city submerged, tens of thousands of victims clinging to rooftops, and hundreds of thousands scattered to shelters around the country.[2] Three weeks later, Hurricane Rita struck much of the same area. The devastation to the Gulf Coast caused by these two hurricanes may be the greatest disaster in U.S. history.

Katrina is estimated to be responsible for $100 billion (2005 U.S. dollars) in damages, making it the costliest natural disaster in the nation's history. The storm killed at least 1,300 people,[2] making it the deadliest U.S. hurricane since the 1928 Okeechobee Hurricane. Criticism of the federal, state, and local governments' reactions to the storm was widespread and resulted in an investigation by the United States Congress and the resignation of the Federal Emergency Management Agency (FEMA) head Michael Brown.[5]

Methods

Review of the literature. A great deal of attention has been given to the assessment of the disaster response.[6-8] Among others, components that have been assessed include emergent social organizations and groups that form after a disaster,[8] the decision to evacuate and the process of evacuation,[9] shelter,[10] disaster management/administration,[11] and coordination of activities.[12]

One of the vexing problems of community disasters has been coordination and management of the emergency situation by public service providers.[11-13] Some of the confusion has been attributed to lack of agency staff training,[12-15] while other factors, such as communication breakdown[12,13,15] and agency "turf" competition and conflict,[12-15] have been cited as reasons for coordination failure.

In this article, the focus is on allied health provider agencies and their management of the Hurricane Katrina disaster. This article integrates traditional community disaster research concerns about emergency planning and implementation of emergency plans with another set of concerns addressing results-based performance of public agencies. The latter literature, part of public administration, addresses the program management, performance, and outcome. The survival and success of organizations are determined in large measure by the style of management of the organization and its ability to understand and work within its external environment.[16-19]

Method of data collection and analysis. The home health agencies studied for this paper were selected because they served the poorer, primarily African American and elderly patients in Orleans Parish. Orleans Parish had the largest concentration of African Americans in the state of Louisiana. About 68% of Orleans Parish residents were African American.[20] The households of Orleans Parish were among the poorest in Louisiana.[20] The parish had about 19.2% uninsured people, a greater proportion than Louisiana as a whole (which was 15.6%) or the nation. About 31% of Orleans Parish residents received Medicaid, compared with 23% of the residents of state of Louisiana. Moreover, the health of parish residents based on several standard indicators such as death rates due to heart disease, accidents, stroke, and cancer and proportion of the population with HIV infection showed that Orleans Parish was among the neediest and unhealthiest parishes in the entire state of Louisiana.[20]

More directly to the point, the home health providers selected for this study provided service for households that were among the poorest of Orleans Parish. Whereas Orleans Parish median household income was $27,408 (much lower than the median household income for the state of Louisiana, which was $33,792, or the nation),[20] administrators and social work staff members of the agencies we studied estimated that that the average household income of their clients was $12,000.

This retrospective study evaluated the emergency preparation for and response to Hurricane Katrina by means of qualitative research, taking a case study approach focusing on Hurricane Katrina and the status of the emergency planning that was in place among home health providers at the advent of the hurricane. Researchers conducted in-depth interviews of the two top administrative staff members at five selected home health agencies that operated in Orleans Parish.

Evaluation questions. The questionnaire was adapted from a study done by North Carolina's Department Health and Human Services in assessing hurricane emergency preparedness of the state between Hurricane Floyd in 1999 and Hurricane Isabel in 2003.[21]

The study addresses how the various agencies implemented emergency plans, the nature of response activities, the agencies' own assessments of their emergency responses, suggested areas of improvement and recommendations, and the impact of the hurricane on staff, capacity, and patient population. The evaluative component of the study utilized procedures from program evaluation literature.[16,17]

Results

What planning for hurricane emergencies existed at home health agencies? *Agencies' own plans.* Preliminary research into the nature of planning for hurricane emergencies at the time Hurricane Katrina landed in the New Orleans area suggests that all the agencies had some form of written plan in place. Overall, the plans consisted of maintaining a list of all the agency's patients and their caregivers along with contact telephone numbers and addresses, indicating whom the agency should contact during an emergency. In most cases, the patients had to sign forms indicating that an agency representative, often the visiting nurse, had explained the agency's emergency protocol and that they understood it and agreed with it.

The agencies prepared and left folders at their patients' homes with information on evacuation procedures, how to prepare kits to take with them during evacuations, what shelters they should evacuate to, contact telephone numbers and addresses for emergency first responders, and how to contact the agency or agency staff, should they need assistance. Direct quotations from the interviews with home health agency staff on this topic follow.

[1] The policy was to have home care professionals to make sure that folders were to be kept in the patients' homes . . . [the folders were] . . . about shelters, telephone numbers of who to call, where to go, etc. at the time of disaster, such as a hurricane . . . [This is called] the Red Folder.

In addition to establishing written guidelines and protocol for hurricane emergencies, the agencies indicated that they filed copies of their lists of patients who needed transportation in case of evacuation with local emergency responder agencies, such as the sheriff's office or police department in the parish or city where these special-needs patients resided. The lists included all the patients and their addresses and telephone contact numbers, with the special-needs patients' names highlighted, with an indication of their special needs.

[2] We had written policies. The Plan . . . went into effect [which consisted of] 1) Identified patients who needed to be moved or evacuated. Anything over #2 (patient level of special need) would qualify. [These are] Bed-bound patients or patients who didn't have available care givers or transportation; 2) We had sent a list to Orleans Parish and Jefferson Parish officials because we had patients in both parishes.

The home health agencies appeared to use similar methods of putting together their emergency plans and protocols. Staff members worked together to draft and implement the agency's hurricane emergency policy and plans. The usual duo was the Administrator of the agency and the Director of Nursing. However, some agencies reported that board members contributed as well. No agency interviewed indicated that their hurricane emergency policy and protocol was put together and implemented by a single staff member.

Local governments' coordination with home health agencies. Although home health agencies had written protocols for their staff and patients, there did not seem to be much coordination concerning emergency planning between them and local or state public health entities. Even those agencies that filed their patient information with the City of New Orleans and adjacent parishes did so at their own initiative rather than as a result of a required and written policy of the City of New Orleans. The procedure of filing with the City was not uniformly carried out, varying both in how it was done and whether or not it was done.

Filing a plan with the State Department of Health and Hospitals (DHH) was mandatory, but only negative feedback was given. There was no specific emergency coordinator or person to contact for guidance in emergency situations.

[6] No one was available to talk to. No call came from the state to implement the plan. No one person's name was given as the emergency coordinator.

Informal advice from local governmental agencies regarding disaster planning. Local governmental authorities appeared to lack written policies for disaster planning. If such a policy did exist, it was poorly disseminated, because none of the agency representatives knew of a specific plan for communicating with local government. This was in contrast to the state, which through DHH had mandated coordination of emergency preparedness policies. Some home health agencies asserted that the state authorities provided consultation to the agencies. This consultation took the form of disseminating literature on hurricane preparedness, hosting a website, and arranging a hurricane awareness meeting. Most of the home health providers felt that the state did provide leadership, but also reported that when the hurricane hit, they were unable to contact the state's Department of Health. Cell phone communication broke down. Even though people outside of New Orleans had cell phones that were electrically charged, the communication towers that transmitted the telephone signals were damaged by the storm. There was no command center available to the providers through the state.

Communication between individual agencies and Department of Health offices. Although most of the providers knew that there were individuals in need of assistance, they were unable to communicate with DHH; in spite of having cell phone numbers of key staff members, they were unable to obtain any assistance. Those providers who did not evacuate their clients before mandatory evacuation calls were unable to get the cooperation of city or state officials.

The agency that reported successful management of communications was the agency that evacuated all of its clients more than seventy-two hours before hurricane landfall and forty-eight hours before local agencies called a mandatory evacuation. One informant response was:

[2] Basically, we were in contact with the state, DHH [not the City]. Part of our agency's plan was to back up our computer records of all agency records. And we took the computer server with us during the evacuation from Katrina . . . We keep a cell phone directory of all of our staff persons and we are able to access the state DHH by telephone and by their website.

Training provided to staff prior to hurricane Katrina. Staff training was unevenly provided by individual agencies prior to Hurricane Katrina. Some agencies provided routine and comprehensive staff training for hurricane emergencies and other agencies did not provide any training at all or if they did, only in a perfunctory manner. Some of the informants' responses were:

[2] Yes. The agency had a staff meeting on May 30th. Every year on May 30th, the agency has in-service training for staff on emergency preparedness. On May 30, 2005, the agency had the emergency preparedness review for the entire staff, including volunteers. This is mandatory and documented records are kept of this training in staff records. During the end of May, we sent out hurricane alert fliers to each patient. We have the nursing staff discuss with all the patients what their plans are for emergency

evacuations in May and this is documented in their records and notes . . . We tested the policy protocol [in a mock emergency drill] for Hurricane Ivan in [September 2004] and this served as our test for the 2005 hurricane season.

[1] No training was provided to the staff, per se. A cascade list [of steps to take in getting ready for approaching hurricanes] was distributed to staff and discussed. The agency reminded staff to notify their patients and to alert them to prepare for hurricanes . . .

Preparation activities carried out as Katrina approached. *Preparation activities by projected hours before hurricane landfall.* The home health agencies took similar steps in preparing for Hurricane Katrina as it approached from 72 hours to 12 hours before landing. Upon hearing of the hurricane, the agencies called their patients to ensure their safety, concentrating on the special-needs and bed-bound patients. As the projected time for landfall approached, agency staff began making transportation and shelter arrangements for many of their patients who did not want to evacuate or were not able to link up with their designated caregivers. Eventually as the hours dwindled, the agencies began making preparations to preserve agency records and arrange their staffs' own evacuation from the city. Eventually the agencies were shut down as everyone evacuated. It must be noted that the Mayor of New Orleans had declared mandatory evacuation approximately 24 hours before projected landfall. After then, monitoring of patients and even staff location was being handled by cell phones by the administering staff and staff assigned to certain patients. Sample informant responses are given below according to hours before projected hurricane landfall:

Within 96 hours

[7] We secured all records medical records. Backed up computer records and took the server out of the building . . . We gave water to the patients as needed. We called all the patients to see who was going to be with whom and [what were their plans] . . .

Within 72 hours

[3] [We] called the office and field staff and asked them to start getting in touch with their patients to find out what was going on with them . . . where they were going. First we [contacted] the bed-bound and then the ambulatory . . . [We] cancelled the Health Fair scheduled that Sunday.

[6] Checked to make sure patients had their medicine in their possession.

Within 48 hours

All but one agency had begun implementing emergency plans. Most administrators were leaving the city with the computer servers containing the contact information for their patients.

[7] Did payroll . . . closed the facility down . . .

[3] The administrators were leaving. I instructed the nurses and staff to leave and make plans for themselves. We put some of the patients in hotels and [some of them] in the personal houses of some of the nurses.

[5] Continue with contacting patients and follow up with the patients . . .

Within 24 hours

[5] We contacted the City [of New Orleans] for evacuation plans and drop-off sites for patients to get to shelters.

[3] We shut the agency down . . . We put some of the patients in hotels and some with nurses.

[2] [We spent time] verifying that policy and procedures are in full implementa-tion...checking by telephone with patients to see if [they were taken care of] . . .

[1] Evacuation of staff and their families.

[6] Everyone was gone and all the patients had evacuated.

Within 12 hours

[1] None. We left Sunday morning. The staff were on their own.

[2] Evacuating self and staff.

[3] The agency was shut down.

[5] Making sure the patients were ready to be transported.

Agencies' interface with special-needs shelters. The agencies took part to different extents in the opening of special-needs shelters. Some of the informants reported being actively involved with special-needs shelters, while others indicated very little if any involvement.

Communication with government agencies in preparing for hurricane response. Although the informants reported having communication with government agencies in preparing for hurricane response, the extent of the communication appeared to have been cursory and not part of a thorough, comprehensive plan.

[6] All of the state agencies were closed on Friday without implementing their state plan. The state agency, DHH, did not call my agency to inquire about the status of the patients until October 2005, when they were reviewing the status of licensing for home health agencies.

[7] No. We were waiting on directions from the City [New Orleans] when to return . . . we heard on television the Mayor telling what areas [of the city] could come back . . .

How did home health agencies respond to Katrina? *How soon was assessment made?* The home health providers began assessment as little as 4 days after Hurricane Katrina landed, while others began it as long as 45 days afterwards. Generally, the informants noted that the extended delay in conducting response activities was one of the most disappointing parts of the implementation of their emergency prepared-ness plans. Many factors were cited for this delay. One was the breakdown in the cell phone communication systems. Anticipating perhaps that landline telephones would be in danger of being down from the effects of the heavy wind and rain of a hurricane, the agencies all appeared to rely on cell phones to continue their contact with their patients. However, cell phones failed in agency-to-patient communication. The following response reflects this:

> [1] About one month to forty-five (45) days after the hurricane landed [staff began assessing health and illness effects in affected areas] . . . The Tuesday after the hurricane, I got in touch with the owners of the home health agency. Lack of telephone contact [hindered ability to carry out assessment] . . . We used online system to verify benefits for patients. We did a merge mail out to 300–400 patients around late October, early November . . .

The catastrophic failure of cell phone communication systems in the aftermath of Hurricane Katrina was well documented in the national and local news coverage. This factor is generally agreed to be one of the major contributors to the poor handling of Hurricane Katrina at all levels of government.

Informants reported other factors they felt impeded their agencies' ability to initiate responsive activities. One was the fact that many of the patients changed their plans, particularly as to which caregiver was to take care of them and transport them to shelters or other safe locations. Notably, those interviewed also cited the fact that many of the patients and even their designated caregivers did not have cell phones (although this appears somewhat inconsistent with their reports of records kept for emergencies).

There were two other major issues that the informants hinted at but did not elaborate on, perhaps because it was so obvious to all who lived and worked in New Orleans. One was that the real problem that affected New Orleans was not so much the usual hurricane impact of high wind and heavy rain, but the ensuing break of the levees in New Orleans that caused catastrophic flooding of about 80% of the city. This unusual circumstance impeded any activity in the city. Second, because the street flooding was so extensive, involved toxic material, and did not subside for several weeks, people were not allowed to enter the city for weeks after the storm. Just about all points of entry were cordoned off and officially blocked. Access to the city was limited to air, such as by helicopter, and water, such as transport of official first responders and emergent private volunteers who used small boats to rescue stranded individuals throughout the city.

Most of the residents of the city had evacuated to other places by the time the hurricane hit land. Many of the remaining residents were either stranded in the infamous Superdome and Convention Center emergency shelters, or stranded in their flooded homes. Electricity was down. Sewerage and water systems were inoperative. Law enforcement was fragile and ineffective. This chaotic condition did not lend itself to effective response on the part of even first responders, much less home health agencies.

How effective was the response? The informants expressed disappointment with the effectiveness of their agencies' assessment activities. The ineffectiveness was partly due to the delay in reaching their patients. Some rated their agency response activities as mediocre to unsatisfactory. They indicated that the assessment was not adequate to help them make better response decisions. The following quotations from the respondents illustrate this frustration:

[3] Not as well put together initially due to delay 2–3 weeks. Once it got started we were able to contact the patients. We stayed in touch with 14 out of 65 patients. . . . No. [It didn't provide appropriate data to make response decisions.] It took so long [to get in touch with them after the hurricane] . . . Pre-Katrina [we were] very ill-prepared. Not well put together. Then the staff were overburdened with their own needs.

[2] [I would rate the] *agency-patient communication as D minus.*

One area of assessment the agency representatives seemed to concur was effective was the assessment of staff capabilities. Again, their satisfaction with this component of their assessment endeavor seemed to be influenced by the speed with which they were able to link to their staffs and meet obligations to and communicate with them. In this case, relying on cell phones often proved successful.

[2] Staff-to-staff communication was B minus. . . . I was able to reach 95% of the staff. . . . For staff [we had appropriate data]. We were able to do payroll—August 30th payroll to staff. The agency had [relocated] to Austin, Texas. We did bank wiring and transfers and moneygrams. [It was important to try to maintain staff in order to carry out agency's goals and activities].

[1] . . . The agency was able to handle payroll to staff just being one week late . . . We were better able to keep in touch with staff through cell phone and email.

How effective was evacuation of special-needs patients? The informants had mixed responses concerning how effective they were in evacuating their special-needs patients. Their self-evaluation ranged from poor to excellent. Some agencies indicated that they experienced a lot of problems and chaos due to the short evacuation notice given by the city, while other agencies that did not wait for the Mayor's mandatory evacuation orders reported excellent responses and outcomes. The latter were able to evacuate 100% of their special-needs patients, because they were able to enlist the assistance of the police departments and sheriffs' offices 72 hours before landfall, when first responders were still on the job and not evacuating themselves.

[3] All the patients were evacuated by 48 hours prior to the storm. We did not wait for the mayor [to declare mandatory evacuation].

Internal policy changes by providers in response to their personal assessment. Internal policy changes made by providers based on their personal assessment include the following:

1. Having every patient and employee provide two alternate telephone numbers in addition to their main contact number, including one number outside of the metropolitan area;
2. Changing from private answering service to an 800 number answering service in order to have continuity of care and better communication with patients and with staff;

Other areas that are being examined are:

1. Improving the means of following up on patients during and after hurricanes;
2. Trying to better match patients with staff to improve monitoring during hurricane emergencies;
3. Increasing in-service training to staff on emergency preparedness plans, including having more practice drills and mock evacuations.

How were the agencies affected by Katrina? Most of the agencies reported significant loss of staff and patients. Only one agency reported an increase in patients. (This was due to the fact that most of their patients evacuated to rural Louisiana outside New Orleans and the agency was able to relocate to the same rural area.) Another agency that did return to New Orleans in a part of the city that was not heavily flooded was still having problems with its facility at the time of the interviews. The building insurance payment had been delayed and this had hindered its capacity to provide services. Provision of services had also been hindered by the lack of housing for the agency's patients and staff. Many of the patients, even those that are handicapped, reportedly were still waiting for FEMA trailers.

Discussion

What worked? *Early evacuation.* Early evacuation is the most effective solution for home health patients and agencies. The most successful agencies implemented their plans long before the City of New Orleans called for a mandatory evacuation. Waiting for local leadership to call mandatory evacuation proved to be a critical mistake. The three agencies with the most successful outcomes left 72 hours before projected hurricane landfall. By doing so, the agencies avoided long waits to evacuate the city and easily found hotel or shelter space for their patients. They also experienced less stress in finding sheltering facilities for their special-needs patients.

Finding shelters for special-needs patients outside the high-risk area. Waiting for local leadership to provide special-needs shelter clearly was a mistake. The agencies that experienced more successful outcomes identified special-needs shelters outside the high-risk area early on. These shelters were open to special-needs patients long before the Superdome and Convention Centers began accepting evacuees. The agencies were able to relocate their patients to these shelters with minimum stress.

Implementing a volunteer cascading communication system. One agency recruited a group of volunteers who were responsible for calling clients and their doctors for emergency prescriptions and family caretakers for transportation assistance. This proved to be a very effective and efficient means of preparing special-needs clients for evacuation. The volunteers greatly improved the success of the communication between clients and staff before, during, and after the hurricane.

Conducting mock evacuation practice drills. One agency found that conducting mock evacuation practice drills regularly every year helped them in having a more orderly emergency response. Its staff members were better prepared than those of other agencies and its patients were able to adapt more successfully to the emergency situation.

Incorporating volunteers in agency emergency preparedness. Some providers were able to make use of volunteer workers, which made their efforts more efficient.

Lessons Learned

There are many lessons learned from the study both from a pragmatic as well as a theoretical point of view. Among the more salient are:

- *Do not limit emergency preparedness to written documents.*

The results of this preliminary assessment of home health agency responders seems to support the concerns Quarantelli addresses regarding emergency planning and emergency response.[13] According to Quarantelli, "Communities sometimes think they are prepared just because they have a written plan. Even worse, focus on a document often leads officials and organizations to ignore other more critical activities that are absolutely necessary for developing good community disaster planning."[13,p.5] This erroneous thinking seems to have underlain the Louisiana DHH's failure to interface with home health agencies by giving sufficient useful feedback to them on their emergency plans. Many respondents felt that the state only provided cursory review of such plans.

- *Do not rely on government offices to implement and coordinate emergency response.*

The home health providers reported that in many ways they would have had better emergency response outcomes, if they had not relied on government offices to coordinate the implementation of hurricane emergency plans. During the hurricane, communication between the government and individual agencies broke down. The agencies had to scramble on their own to rescue and find shelter for their patients. There was no designated state emergency coordinator to direct emergency preparedness activities in the face of the real disaster.

The Louisiana Department of Health and Hospitals (DHH) appeared to take a leadership role in requiring that all home health agencies have an emergency disaster preparedness plan for each client. Many of the contingencies of the plan, however, depended on having local government cooperation, including cooperation from city officials, police officers, and sheriff deputies to provide transportation for those clients who refused early evacuations. When city government officials, sheriff deputies, and even state troopers were called upon, as a backup, to ensure the safety of the clients, city and local government officials were unable to provide any assistance.

Most agencies felt that they were on their own and could not count on backup from local, state, or federal governments. The feeling of most of the administrators of the home health agencies is that they would have been infinitely better off if they had taken full responsibility early on. In the end, they noted, they were the ones who had to bear the brunt of criticism if their patients were not taken to a safe place that could provide for their special needs. To take just one example, an agency had contracted with a bus company to provide transportation, but when they called the company they were told that the company needed 48-hour advance notice in order to provide service. Needless to say, the Mayor of New Orleans only gave 24-hour mandatory evacuation notice to the residents of the city.

Recommendations

- *Identify patients reluctant to evacuate.*

The authors strongly feel that a practice drill should be performed in order to identify those individuals who are not likely to follow the plan. Those patients who are unwilling to go through the motions of a drill, will probably be unwilling to follow the evacuation plan, in the event of a real impending disaster.

- *Provide adequate security at special-needs shelters.*

No one realized the true numbers of people with special needs. No one provided adequate security for the large number of people who had to go to the emergency shelters set up at the last minute by the city officials. The Superdome was one such last minute shelter. The medical author of this article personally experienced the anarchy prevailing at one of the last-minute special-needs shelters provided by the City of New Orleans. The presence of even one government worker—not necessarily a police officer—would have curtailed the chaos and violence that occurred in the Convention Center and many other makeshift shelters. Therefore, the authors recommend that the same ratio of security to crowd that is used in regular crowd control be implemented in future emergency shelters.

- *Conduct practice drills.*

The authors recommend that more training be given to the agency staff, especially using simulated emergency situations to prepare them adequately for real hurricane experiences (or a pandemic, such as bird flu).

- *Train other first responders to handle special-needs people.*

The authors recommend the training of other first responders, particularly law enforcement officials, to handle special-needs people.

- *The Louisiana Department of Health and Hospitals must develop better evaluation procedures.*

The authors recommend that the Louisiana DHH improve its measures of emergency preparedness focusing on the following key factors:

1) Infrastructure,
2) Training of staff and patients,
3) Communication,
4) Partnership, and
5) Implementation of policies and procedures.

- *Improve communication systems.*

None of the home health providers anticipated complete failure of cellular telephones. Officials with FEMA, however, did know that loss of cell phone systems was a real possibility, which enabled them to have their communication up and running continuously. Some first responders expressed the belief that FEMA did not share all their information about communication systems with state and city officials. Wide sharing of state-of-the-art communication systems across all government levels and main first responders is strongly recommended.

- *Agencies should provide their own transportation to shelters.*

Some of the administrators who were interviewed expressed the desire to purchase their own means of transportation in order to get the special-needs patients to a safe facility early on in the evacuation process. Evacuating special needs clients is not an easy proposition because their health conditions tend to be so fragile that a long evacuation time could result in needless morbidity and mortality.

- *Agencies should evacuate their patients at least 72 hours before hurricane landfall.*

One agency implemented evacuation for their patients 48 hours before projected Hurricane Katrina landfall, even before the City of New Orleans declared mandatory evacuation for all residents. The agency experienced no loss in patients and reportedly less stress among staff in implementing the emergency plan. This policy is recommended for all home health agencies, especially for those with special-needs patients.

- *Adopt strategic management (best) practices.*

The authors recommend that the government, at all levels, as well as the individual home health providers look into adopting strategic management practices to achieve desired outcomes for emergency preparedness. This includes seeking best practices models and strategies from other sources, such as other cities, other states, and other home health care providers. It is felt that a large part of the shortcomings and even failure in the government and nonprofit agencies' responses to Hurricane Katrina was due to mismanagement. Certainly, the poverty of the patients and residents of New Orleans presented a daunting challenge. Yet other agencies and other state, local, and even federal government departments have addressed similarly tough challenges with more success. One such strategic management technique is what has been referred to in some circles as the *balanced score card* technique. Although this comprehensive approach to management originated in a commercial setting, it has since been widely applied to public agencies with reported success.[22-23] It has proven effectiveness in translating multiple points of view into shared goals aimed at achieving an agency's mission, vision, and measurable objectives. It prioritizes meeting the needs and wants of the customers/clients that are being served and establishes ongoing measurement and monitoring of agency objectives.

Conclusion

In the face of a major emergency or disaster the best laid plans of medical and public health planners failed for simple reasons such as lack of communication. No matter how detailed a plan or how well prepared the community seemed to be, the failure of the communication system ultimately led to chaos in the aftermath of Hurricane Katrina. The second most important factor in the failure of agencies and government to respond effectively to the disaster was a failure in management of human resources across all government levels. Although plans seemed to work well in theory, in practice implementation was difficult, if the agency waited for government response. The most successful agencies implemented their plans long before the City of New Orleans called for a mandatory evacuation. Early evacuation is the most effective solution. Waiting for local leadership to provide special needs shelter clearly was a mistake. That is why both local and state governments have now declared that no shelter will be set up within New Orleans city limits. Further studies of how to design and implement effective emergency plans are badly needed in this area.

Much knowledge must be shared among health care providers. There are hundreds of emergency plans that have not been shared. In interviewing the different health care providers for this study, it became apparent that some of the providers had skills and organizational plans that were so effective that they should be shared with others. Some providers were able to make effective use of volunteer workers, which made their efforts more efficient, for example.

This is a very limited study of some of the health care providers to the critically ill and special-needs patients of New Orleans. More studies are needed in this area. Major disasters tend to affect the poor and disadvantaged population disproportionately. Hurricane Katrina followed this pattern in a dramatic fashion. Better use of community resources (such as churches and service organizations) must to be factored into any major emergency plan in order to offset this disproportionate impact, in order to mobilize assistance for those who have no family resources.

Notes

1. State of Louisiana, Office of Emergency Preparedness. State of Louisiana emergency operations plan supplement 1A: southeast Louisiana hurricane and evacuation plan. Baton Rouge, LA: State of Louisiana, Office of Emergency Preparedness, 2000.
2. Grauman A, Houston T, Lawrimore J, et al. Hurricane Katrina: a climatological perspective: a preliminary report. Ashville, NC: National Oceanic and Atmospheric Administration, National Environmental Satellite, Data and Information Service, 2005 Oct. Available at http://repository.wrclib.noaa.gov/cgi/viewcontent.cgi?article=1000&context=nesdis_tech_reports.
3. City of New Orleans. City of New Orleans comprehensive emergency management plan: annex I hurricanes. (Date not available).
4. State of Louisiana, Office of Emergency Preparedness. Louisiana model home health emergency plan. Baton Rouge, LA: 2000 Jun.
5. Select Bipartisan Committee to Investigate the Preparation for and Response to Hurricane Katrina. A Failure of Initiative: Final Report of the Select Bipartisan Committee to Investigate the Preparation for and Response to Hurricane Katrina. Washington, DC: U.S. Government Printing Office, 2006 Feb 15.
6. Mileti DS. Disasters by design: a reassessment of natural hazards in the United States. Washington, DC: Joseph Henry Press, 1999.
7. Tierney KJ, Lindell MK, Perry RW. Facing the unexpected: disaster preparedness and response in the United States. Washington, DC: Joseph Henry Press, 2001.
8. Drabek TE, McEntire DA. Emergent phenomena and the sociology of disaster: lessons, trends and opportunities from the research literature. Disaster Prevention and Management. 2003;12(2):97–112.
9. Sorensen JH, Mileti DS. Warning and evacuation: answering some basic questions. Industrial Crisis Quarterly. 1988;2(2):1–15.
10. Quarantelli EL. Sheltering and housing after major community disasters: case studies and general observations. Washington, DC: Federal Emergency Management Agency, 1982 Jan.

11. Quarantelli EL. Ten criteria for evaluating the management of community disasters. Disasters. 1997;21(2):39–56.

12. McEntire DA. Coordinating multi-organizational responses to disaster: lessons from the March 28, 2000, Fort Worth tornado. Disaster Prevention and Management. 2002;11(5):369–79.

13. Quarentelli EL. Research based criteria for evaluating disaster planning and managing. (Preliminary Paper #247.) Newark, DE: Disaster Research Center, University of Delaware, 1997.

14. Farmer JC, Carlton PK Jr. Providing critical care during a disaster: the interface between disaster response agencies and hospitals. Crit Care Med. 2006 Mar;34(3 Suppl):S56–9.

15. Martchenke J, Rusteen J, Pointer JE. Prehospital communications during the Loma Prieta earthquake. Prehospital Disaster Med. 1995 Oct–Dec;10(4):225–31.

16. Hatry HP. Performance measurement: getting results. Washington, DC: Urban Institute, 1999.

17. Weiss CH. Evaluation. 2nd Ed. New Jersey: Prentice-Hall, 1998.

18. Kaplan RS, Norton DP. Using the balanced scorecard as a strategic management system. Harv Bus Rev. 1996 Jan–Feb:75–85.

19. Kaplan RS, Norton DP. The balanced scorecard—measures that drive performance. Harv Bus Rev. 1992 Jan–Feb:71–9.

20. Louisiana Healthcare Redesign Collaborative. Region 1 health care profile. Baton Rouge, LA: Louisiana Department of Health and Hospitals, 2006 Aug 17.

21. Davis MV, Temby JR, MacDonald PD, et al. Evaluation of improvements in North Carolina public health capacity to plan, prepare, and respond to public health emergencies. Chapel Hill, NC: UNC School of Public Health, The North Carolina Institute for Public Health, 2004 Sep.

22. National Partnership for Reinventing Government. Serving the American public: best practices in customer-driven strategic planning. Federal Benchmarking Consortium Report. Washington, DC: National Performance Review, 1997 Feb.

23. Syfert P, Elliot N, Schumacher L. Charlotte adapts the 'balanced scorecard.' American City & Country. 1998 Oct;113(11):32.

Chapter 10
Katrina and Vulnerability:
The Geography of Stress

Andrew Curtis, PhD
Jacqueline Warren Mills, PhD
Michael Leitner, PhD

Hurricane Katrina was a catastrophe in terms of structural damage, loss of life, and disaster-related morbidities, both at the time of landfall and for months afterwards. This chapter focuses on the links between morbidity, stress, and social vulnerability. The authors will draw from their experiences during the response and recovery to the catastrophe to show how geography and the mapping of stress-related phenomena might be used to understand and predict areas of elevated post-Katrina stress morbidity in New Orleans. The authors in no way suggest that they have achieved such a complex mapping, as many of the needed data sets are not readily available. We will show, however, how researchers can begin to move towards such a geographic prediction of stress-related risks with existing information.

The authors of this chapter were part of the Louisiana State University (LSU) team providing geospatial support to the Louisiana Office of Homeland Security and Emergency Preparedness Emergency Operations Center (EOC) during Hurricanes Katrina and Rita. Two of the authors (AC, JM) were a constant presence in the EOC, as part of a larger LSU-based volunteer team, performing tasks that included creating navigation maps for search and rescue teams, providing larger maps for briefing sessions and media releases, mapping the daily inflow of data (such as 911 calls or the latest flood imagery) and using online geospatial software such as *Google Earth* to provide coordinates for Public Health Service helicopter and ground missions. These tasks were performed under immense pressure. Stress arose from the importance of requests, often originating from high-ranking officials, including the President of the United States, and from the need for immediate results. We worked in a noisy and highly charged atmosphere, with official and unofficial reports about New Orleans diffusing through the EOC, while occasionally a misplaced phone call would be routed to the desk from someone attempting to find a missing relative.[1-2] One of the authors (AC), in addition to performing these tasks, played a more supervisory role coordinating the EOC, the Office of Public

ANDREW CURTIS *is an Assistant Professor of Geography and Anthropology at Louisiana State University (LSU) in Baton Rouge and the Director of the World Health Organizing Collaborating Center for Remote Sensing and GIS for Public Health.* ***JACQUELINE MILLS*** *is an Assistant Professor for Research in Disaster Science and Management and* ***MICHAEL LEITNER*** *an Assistant Professor of Geography and Anthropology, both at LSU.*

Health EOC, and LSU. This coordination included brainstorming sessions designed continually to improve geospatial response. Finally, all authors have been involved in the post-response phase of the catastrophe through the *LSU Geographic Information System Clearinghouse Cooperative* (www.katrina.lsu.edu), the world's largest geospatial data clearinghouse associated with a disaster. This clearinghouse has been widely used by local and national researchers, non-profit organizations, government contractors, state agencies and FEMA. The projects using the *LSU GIS Clearinghouse Cooperative* include both physical and social vulnerability investigations, ranging from how best to educate rural coastal communities about disaster mitigation and preparedness, to understanding the resilience of neighborhoods affected by Katrina and Rita.

Vulnerability to a disaster, or even to day-to-day societal risks, encompasses a great many characteristics worthy of analysis, and far more than can be addressed here. The authors draw from all their experiences with Katrina, and especially their understanding of the spatial aspects of the catastrophe, to focus on the geography of stress as experienced by Katrina-affected cohorts.

The Geography of Vulnerability, the Geography of Stress

Vulnerability to the effects of a disaster arises from a combination of factors, including physical proximity to a threat (e.g., living in a floodplain), the characteristics of the home (including construction and ownership), lack of a political voice, financial constraints, and choices made by an individual.[3-4] It is widely accepted that high-risk groups vulnerable to a disaster include those with lower incomes, the very young and the elderly, the disabled, women living alone, and female-headed households. Therefore, the social and economic cost of a disaster usually falls unevenly on different populations.[3,5-8] Such vulnerability can be expressed geographically in terms of *site* (proximity of a neighborhood to the hazard) and *situation* (the social context of that neighborhood). During Katrina, the site of many indigent neighborhoods made them vulnerable to flooding due to their proximity to a flooding source (such as a levee break), and the elevation of their homes (Figure 1).

The *situation* of a Katrina neighborhood is a construct encompassing the ability of residents to cope with the disaster. In an analysis of traditional socioeconomic vulnerability indicators and flood depth in Orleans Parish, conducted by LSU researchers, it was found that both heavily White and non-White neighborhoods were severely flooded. (See Curtis A, Pine J, Marx B, Li B. A multiple additive regression tree analysis of social vulnerability and Hurricane Katrina: implications for psychopathology and a disproportionate impediment to recovery; paper under review.) However, non-White residents were more likely to have remained behind, resulting in increased stresses from actually experiencing the hurricane.[8] In addition, non-White residents of New Orleans had a greater likelihood of having existing chronic health conditions.[9-10] These chronic health conditions, in addition to other poverty-related impediments resulted in people from these neighborhoods having the least ability to rebound and these communities having the worst prospects for recovery. In these fundamental ways, Katrina disproportionately affected non-White populations. The combination of site and situation can be used to estimate future patterns of stress-related morbidities and mortalities.

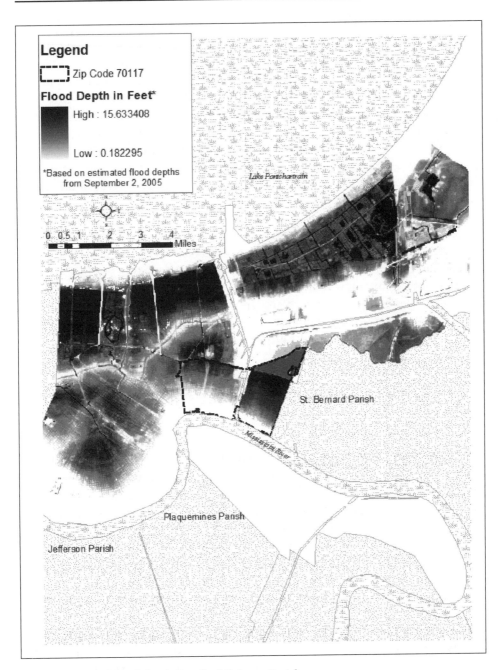

Figure 1. Map of flood depth for all of Orleans Parish.

Multiple stressors accumulated as a result of Katrina, especially during the first few days in New Orleans and the evacuation.[11] Several experiential papers provide insights into the stresses faced by those in the storm.[12–18] It is not surprising that these experiences have translated into health problems. Berggren and Curiel use the crude indicator of death notices reported in the *Times-Picayune* to show a 25% increase in deaths during

January 2006 (compared with the previous year), an increase they partly attribute to stress.[19] Post-traumatic stress has also resulted in increases in suicidal thoughts as well as suicidal attempts among children.[11] All of these stresses have a geography (residential address, pre-Katrina neighborhood characteristics, evacuation and relocation routes) whose parts can be mapped and overlaid on each other to estimate total stress load. Unfortunately such data are not readily available and we are left to piece together information from disparate sources as we build a geographic stress surface.

In a formal analysis of the geography of Katrina-related stress, the *site* is where the greatest damage occurred. It has previously been shown that post-traumatic stress is related to the degree of the disaster. Looking at things this way, Figure 1 (other things being equal) can be used as a proxy for neighborhood stress levels. As previously discussed, the situation of some communities made them more vulnerable because their residents were more likely to have experienced hurricane landfall, and to have other characteristics that magnify post-disaster stresses. In order to create a geographic stress surface, the geography of situation must be added to the geography of site. By combining these surfaces, community-level post-Katrina strategies can be prioritized. The maps that appear later in the paper, which are used to illustrate these geographies, focus on the Lower 9th Ward, by highlighting the ZIP Code that encompasses that section of the city. These maps can be broadly grouped into five categories of geographic stress:

1. The geography of experiencing the storm
2. The geography of evacuation and relocation stress
3. The geography of pre-Katrina stress
4. The geography of pre-Katrina health outcomes
5. The geography of rebound and recovery potential

The geography of experiencing the storm. There are many reasons why a segment of the population of New Orleans did not heed either the evacuation advisory or the subsequent mandatory evacuation order. In a survey of evacuees in a Texas shelter, 61% did not originally evacuate, with 29% not leaving because they underestimated the storm.[20] Hurricanes threatening Louisiana not long before Katrina led to evacuation advisories for residents of New Orleans even though no disaster ensued. Considering evacuation from New Orleans to Baton Rouge, a journey that usually takes between 1 and 1.5 hours, but took approximately 8 hours during the evacuation, many would have balanced the uncertain risk of the storm based on previous experience against a certain evacuation discomfort. Of course these are not the only reasons that people stayed behind; others included not wishing to leave their animals and having faith in the city's levee defense system.[20] All these reasons, however, can be viewed as choices. For indigent populations, however, there are reasons not to evacuate that cannot be overridden, such as the lack of any practical means of leaving the city. According to the 2000 U.S. Census, approximately 250,000 people in New Orleans did not have access to a private vehicle; of these 250,000, city buses could have evacuated only 10% (a means that was not, in any case, offered by the bus system).[21] In the Texas shelter survey mentioned above, the largest portion who did not evacuate (36% of all those interviewed) did not leave because they had no means to evacuate.[21] Even for those from poor neighborhoods with vehicles, the costs of evacuation (gas and motel stays) may have been prohibitive. These stranded residents have been likened to the underclass on the Titanic for whom there were not enough lifeboats.[22] Given all of this, it seems clear that people living close to or below the poverty line are forced to rely on the competence of evacuation planners,[23–24] who, if effective, must take such poverty-based traps into account in order to craft effective evacuations. Importantly, the understanding that a sizeable portion of the city's residents would not evacuate had been documented before Katrina by the Center for the Study of Public Health Impacts of Hurricanes at Louisiana State University.[25]

Although having individual level data showing who stayed behind is preferable, neighborhood-level maps can be created showing the lack of the ability to evacuate. For example, Figure 2 displays the spatial pattern of housing units wherein the occupant is without access to a vehicle. It has previously been shown that surviving or suffering through a human-created rather than a natural disaster exaggerates post-event mental health problems.[26] For many victims of Katrina this feeling of being left behind, as they didn't have the ability to evacuate, in combination with the length of time waiting for rescue, either from the floods or from the shelters in New Orleans, may have shifted their understanding of the disaster away from being a natural event to being humanly, even politically, caused. Therefore, maps such as the one presented in Figure 2, in combination with Figure 1, might help in estimating the geography of elevated stress from experiencing the storm. Two further maps (Figures 3a and b) represent census block groups of the population in poverty, and where residents are predominantly African American; these can be used to further develop our understanding of the geographic surface.

The geography of evacuation and relocation stress. Volunteers at one Texas shelter were struck by the smell when evacuees disembarked after their multiple hour journey from New Orleans, the smell having developed after several days spent inside the Superdome, standing for several hours in the Louisiana sun waiting for pick-up, and finally riding the bus to Texas.[27] This reflects something of the trauma of experiencing the storm, awaiting rescue, and being evacuated. The geography of this stress is best illustrated by a spider map, with the origin and destinations being portrayed as points, and the victims' journey between these locations being linked by lines. Figure 4 shows a sample of paths taken by people from the Lower 9th Ward. This information was extracted from a dataset provided by the Louisiana Department of Social Services (DSS) and represents a post-Katrina change in address for child support payments wherein the original address of the custodial or non-custodial parent is in the Lower 9th Ward. Each line represents the initial evacuation away from New Orleans. Stresses could be attached to these lines and nodes based on the known conditions of the evacuation route, combined with descriptions of the shelters; the more points and lines for each evacuee, the greater the stress loads irrespective of the conditions. Although more comprehensive representations of this information exist, most notably FEMA Individual Assistant (IA) application data, they have so far proved difficult to acquire.

Stress associated with disaster-caused relocation was well documented prior to Katrina.[11,28] Evacuees from Katrina-affected areas, like other disaster evacuees before them, were confronted with the uncertainty of when they would be able to return home, the loss of their communities, and even the loss of known and trusted caregivers (and

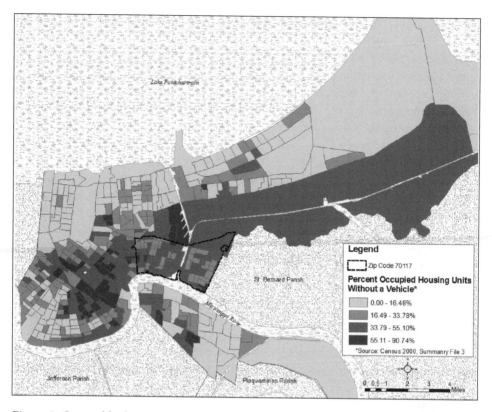

Figure 2. Census block groups displaying housing units without access to a vehicle.

medical facilities) for those suffering from a chronic illness.[29] Such evacuation stress can be either moderated or intensified by the official handling of the disaster.[11,30]

Children, like adults, can suffer posttraumatic stress. Previous disasters have shown that children have the ability to rebound more quickly than adults if they are quickly returned to normalcy.[31] However, an insensitive handling of the relocation process, with children being moved repeatedly without information, can intensify their distress.[11]

The final destination, or rather the last temporary residence before the return home, is another layer in stress geography. After Katrina, problems emerged in temporary FEMA villages, the individual not only facing the stress of being in a strange city, and being separated from the support structure of his or her home community, but also facing increased risk from crime.[32]

The geography of pre-Katrina stress. Disaster-related vulnerability is complex, comprising both community-level response and individual decisions.[33–34] Many of these vulnerabilities also extend into normal living conditions and are manifest in neighborhoods with limited employment opportunities, high crime rates, low educational attainment, and poor health outcomes. Problematic outcomes include elevated stress levels, which in turn can predispose a disaster victim to mental health problems such as posttraumatic stress, chronic health problems, which will be discussed in the next section, and a general inability to recover and rebound. Mapping vulnerable

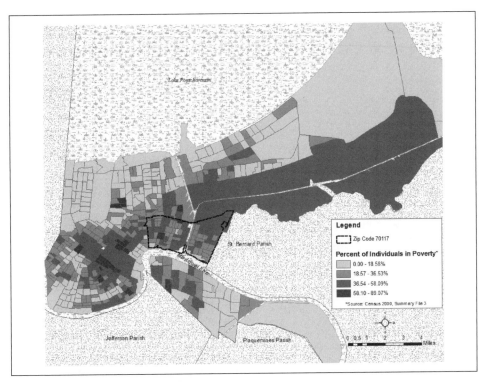

Figure 3a. Census block groups displaying population below the poverty level.

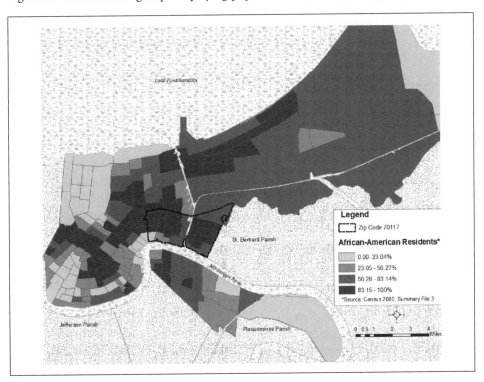

Figure 3b. Census block groups displaying African American population.

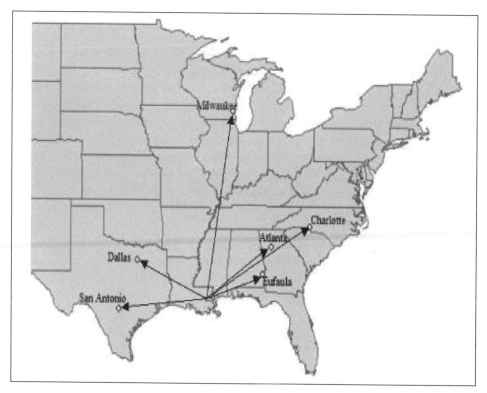

Figure 4. Sample evacuation routes away from the Lower 9th Ward.

neighborhoods prior to a disaster (for example by drug arrests) can indicate where people, with all other things being equal, will experience the effects of the disaster to a disproportionate extent.

Further geographic detail can be added to these surfaces by considering the sub-populations most at risk. For example, women often suffer post-disaster stresses disproportionately as they often have to spend more time in the (contaminated) home.[35-36] Furthermore, a major upheaval can cause irreparable damage to a marriage,[37] with the loss of normalcy and the memories associated with the relationship (in combination with stress) resulting in conflict and even abuse.[38]

Of particular importance to low-income African American women in New Orleans is the loss of a neighborhood support structure, which often extends beyond females in the household (mother and grandmother) to include immediate neighbors and community elders.[39] Louisiana, and especially New Orleans, is renowned for its culture and community, with many neighborhoods having distinct character. Within these neighborhoods, community ties, often based around churches, are especially strong. In the Lower 9th Ward, for example, there are two or three churches on every road. The thought of leaving the safety of this community could act as a deterrent to leaving New Orleans, and would be a source of depression once evacuated, especially with no known point of return. Neighborhood social structure is often viewed as being more important than losing personal possessions, including one's house.[38]

One female subpopulation that can be mapped is female as head of the household with young children in the home.[3] In this case, the woman might be without family other than her children, relying on close neighbors for support. She might not have the ability to evacuate with her children. All the previously described stresses will apply to her situation, though in addition she might have to face the physical needs of evacuation, or the stresses of caring for her children through the storm by herself. Figure 5 displays the surface of women as head of household with young children in the home. By comparing this pattern with maps of poverty, race/ethnicity, and neighborhood stressors such as crime, a pre-Katrina stress surface can be generated. All that is needed is to add the actual Katrina damage map (Figure 1).

The geography of pre-Katrina health outcomes. Approximately 11% of the residents of Orleans and Jefferson parish had diabetes,[29] a number skewed higher in poorer cohorts. Furthermore, approximately 7,000 residents of New Orleans were HIV-infected prior to Katrina.[19] According to the daily surveillance system initiated by the Louisiana Department of Health and Hospitals Office of Public Health (LAOPH), the American Red Cross and the U.S. Public Health Service, 31% of medical interactions between shelter workers and evacuees was for chronic illness, most of these contacts being to replace medications or resume treatment.[40] In one shelter, over half the evacuees had chronic health problems.[22] It has been estimated that some diabetics went as long as six months without insulin.[19] Diabetic concerns also extended to the diet provided at the shelters and limited opportunities for appropriate exercise. Hyperglycemia could

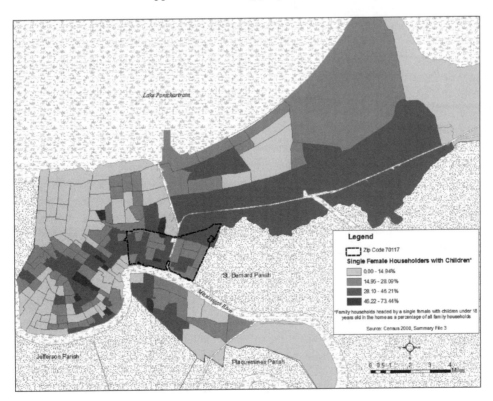

Figure 5. Women as head of household with young children in the home.

make the evacuee susceptible to other medical conditions, including severe depression, which in turn might affect diabetes, and skin infections, the later showing up regularly in shelter surveillance tools.[29,40] Other chronic illnesses common among evacuees were hypertension and gout.[27]

Additional stressful situations were caused by the loss of an evacuee's medical records. This resulted in doctors having to rely on a patient's memory in order to refill prescriptions.[29] As children began to attend school in their new locations, school care-givers were faced with a similar situation regarding vaccination status; in some cases, this was compounded by a lack of a guardian to recount the child's history.[11]

The geography of these chronic illnesses can be mapped as neighborhood rates. For example, Figures 6a and b display the infant mortality and low birth weight delivery surfaces for Orleans Parish for the period 2002 to 2004. New Orleans had severe prob-lems with poor pregnancy outcomes in African American neighborhoods, where a large number of births were to single mothers. After Katrina, this population is most likely to have experienced and to continue to experience the greatest stress load. Although other health conditions can be triggered by elevated stress,[41-42] poor birth outcomes, especially low birth weight deliveries (less than 2500 grams), have been strongly linked to anxiety and poor mental health.[43] In addition, many coping mechanisms associated with stress are also harmful to pregnant women and their fetuses, including smok-ing,[44-45] alcohol,[46] and drug use.[47-50] Unfortunately, this is one area where the legacy of Katrina will likely be felt by vulnerable populations for, literally, a lifetime to come. An increased chance of a low birth weight will persist as long as the mother continues to experience stress.

As previous poor birth outcomes can be used to predict similar future outcomes, the maps in Figure 6 can be used to give an indication of where the greatest risks will be faced in post-Katrina New Orleans. In addition, by combining these maps with the evacuation spider map in Figure 4, the diffusion of these pre-Katrina risks to other neighborhoods outside of New Orleans, and even outside of Louisiana, can be predicted.

The geography of rebound and recovery potential. The first set of stresses associ-ated with the return home arise from confronting the devastation: a destroyed home, removing possessions from inside the house and leaving them on the street outside, taping the refrigerator shut to keep the decaying food inside, possibly having a spray painted marking from animal rescue on the exterior of the house stating that the pet inside had died, the corpse left to be found and removed by the owner. The second set arises during rebuilding, amidst uncertainty about whether the damaged house can still serve as a safe living environment. In a joint survey by the Centers for Disease Control and Prevention (CDC) and the Louisiana Department of Health and Hos-pitals during October 22–28, 2005, 45.5% of properties had visible mold, while 17% had heavy mold, which is defined as one interior wall having at least 50% coverage.[51] In a second survey, 96.2% of returning residents believed that there was a health risk associated with mold growth, even though 42.1% had already cleaned mold, with 68.7% not always using respirators because of either discomfort or unavailability.[51] The returnee would also be uncertain about several other environmental hazards and health risks reported in the media. For example, continued exposure to damp interior spaces can lead to both upper and lower respiratory problems, and may result in the fabled

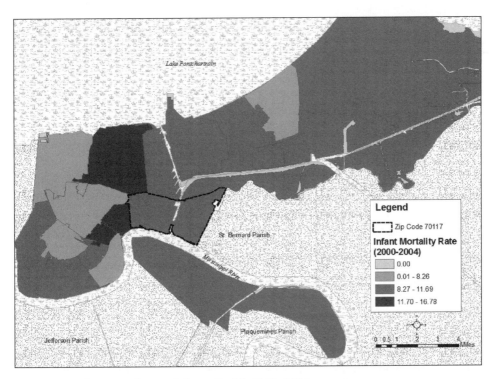

Figure 6a. Infant mortality in Orleans Parish 2002–2004.

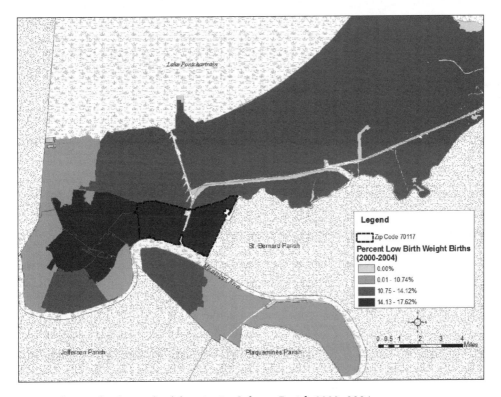

Figure 6b. Low birth weight deliveries in Orleans Parish 2002–2004.

Katrina cough.[51-52] Further uncertainties involved the neighborhood interdependence of cleaning: if there was no rebuilding next door, was there a developing toxicity in the neighborhood? The third series of stresses arises from the perceived futility of rebuilding, as returnees ask such questions as what the point of rebuilding the home is if the rest of the neighborhood, or even just a large proportion of the neighborhood, remains devastated; and whether the state of the entire neighborhood would result in the home eventually being compulsorily torn down anyway. According to one theory connected with disaster mitigation, the theory of interdependency, the actions of neighbors are almost as important as one's own actions.[19]

The stressors associated with first return and rebuilding are likely to affect all classes and races to some degree but, as previously discussed, socioeconomic groups differ in their ability to cope with these stresses in a post-disaster environment.[26,53] The geography of the environmental health risks can be displayed as neighborhood toxicity survey maps. For example, at the New Orleans Area Healthy Disparities meeting (held at the Hilton New Orleans Riverside on June 12, 2006), organized by the Poverty and Race Research Action Council (PRRAC), the Alliance for Health Homes, and the Health Policy Institute of the Joint Center for Political and Economic Studies, maps were displayed on the wall showing the spatial distribution of different environmental sensors and their toxicity readings.

Maps can also display the state of neighborhood return by showing the proportion of inhabited houses or locations of FEMA trailers. These data can come from door-to-door surveys, or even be extracted from high-resolution aerial photography. A cheaper and more dynamic data collection system is a video camera linked to a global positioning system (GPS). A car can drive the neighborhood (one GPS route is seen on the left side of the display in Figure 7), recording neighborhood activity. A second team can view the video and extract information from it, such as the level of rebuilding activity. These maps can be used to gauge neighborhood stress if we assume it is a function of returning residents to abandoned houses.

Finally, post-Katrina stress is developing in New Orleans, which had its roots in the problems of the city prior to the storm. A map displaying the location of murders was printed in the *Times Picayune* as part of an article entitled, "Murders so far," published on June 20, 2006. This not only shows neighborhoods where stress is likely to be elevated because of the fear of the emerging crime threat, but the map itself may actually create stress by revealing to returning residents where these new problems were emerging.

Discussion

Vulnerability is closely linked to poverty, which is compounded in New Orleans by race. Members of racial and ethnic minorities often feel left behind by society, sometimes literally so, as during the Katrina disaster.[54] An estimated 84,000 African Americans die per year because of health care deficiencies, the net result of which is widespread community distrust of "the system."[22,55] In a shelter survey of hurricane evacuees in Texas, 79% believed the official response was too slow, 68% feeling this was because the people stranded were both poor and minority group members, and 61% thought the government did not care.[21]

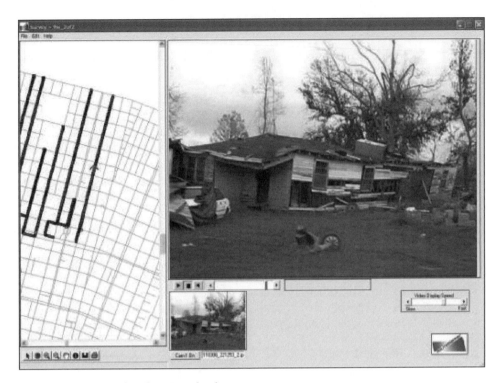

Figure 7. The Digital Video/GPS display.

If we are to learn something from Katrina, it is that—in their circumstances and their resources—all people are not equal in the United States, and that there is both a geography and a social character to vulnerability. Living in New Orleans, living in certain neighborhoods of New Orleans, being African American, having limited income, being female, being a head of household, having young children in the home, suffering from chronic illnesses, and being pregnant can all contribute to vulnerability. As we drill down through these risks, it is easy to see how spatially and socially complex vulnerability is. It is not enough to map poverty; we have to understand the social dimensions within our maps.

The maps presented in this chapter can all be used to predict where post-Katrina stress load, and stress-related health outcomes, are likely to be worst in New Orleans. These surfaces can be supplemented by individual information (which is preferred on a case-by-case basis). However, in the absence of individual counseling, and in the knowledge that poor and minority populations often do not seek help for disaster-related depression, the approach presented in this paper can be used to prioritize community level outreach. This is especially appealing as most of these datasets are either publicly available, or can be obtained with minimal effort as they do not contain confidential information.

Acknowledgment

The authors would like to acknowledge John Pine for his valuable comments on a first draft of this paper.

Notes

1. Curtis A, Mills JW, Blackburn JK, et al. University and government collaboration in Hurricane Katrina: geospatial decision support in the EOC. Int J Mass Emerg Disasters. (In press).

2. Curtis A, Mills JW, Blackburn JK, et al. Hurricane Katrina: GIS response for a major metropolitan area. (Quick Response Research Report 180). Boulder, CO: University of Colorado Natural Hazards Center, 2006.

3. Morrow BH. Identifying and mapping community vulnerability. Disasters. 1999 Mar; 23(1):1–18.

4. Jaspers S, Shoham J. Targeting the vulnerable: a review of the necessity and feasibility of targeting vulnerable households. Disasters. 1999 Dec; 23(4):359–72.

5. Mileti D. Disasters by design: a reassessment of natural hazards in the United States. Washington, DC: Joseph Henry Press, 1999.

6. Blaikie P, Brookfield H. Land degradation and society. New York: Metheun & Company, Ltd., 1987.

7. Cutter SL, Boruff B, Shirley WL. Social vulnerability to environmental hazards. Soc Sci Q. 2003 Jun;84(2):242–61.

8. Cutter SL, Mitchell JT, Scott MS. Handbook for conducting a GIS-based hazards assessment at the county level. Columbia, SC: University of South Carolina, 1997.

9. Bourque LB, Siegel JM, Kano M, et al. Weathering the storm: the impact of hurricanes on physical and mental health. Ann Am Acad Polit Soc Sci. 2006;604:129–51.

10. Berggren RE, Curiel TJ. After the storm—health care infrastructure in post-Katrina New Orleans. N Engl J Med. 2006 Apr;354(15):1549–52.

11. Madrid PA, Grant R, Reilly MJ, et al. Challenges in meeting immediate emotional needs: short-term impact of a major disaster on children's mental health: building resiliency in the aftermath of Hurricane Katrina. Pediatrics. 2006 May;117(5 Pt 3): S448–53.

12. Leder HA, Rivera P. Six days in Charity Hospital: two doctors' ordeal in Hurricane Katrina. Compr Ther. 2006 Spring;32(1):2–9.

13. Weather L Jr. The Weather family's Hurricane Katrina saga: Leonard Weather Jr., MD of New Orleans. Interview by George Dawson. J Natl Med Assoc. 2006 May; 98(5):779–82.

14. McVey P, Bertolasi S. Katrina and Mississippi nurses—first person accounts. Miss RN. 2005 Winter;67(4):6–7.

15. Hunt D. Hurricane Katrina: stories from the field. Fla Nurse. 2005 Dec;53(4):26–7.

16. Farris KB. Hurricane Katrina: one doctor's journal. J La State Med Soc. 2005 Sep–Oct;157(5):232–7.

17. Delacroix SE Jr. In the wake of Katrina: a surgeon's first-hand report of the New Orleans tragedy. MedGenMed. 2005 Sep 19;7(3):56.

18. Frank IC. Emergency response to the Gulf Coast devastation by Hurricanes Katrina and Rita: experiences and impressions. J Emerg Nurs. 2005 Dec;31(6):526–47.

19. Berggren RE, Curiel TJ. After the storm—health care infrastructure in post-Katrina New Orleans. N Engl J Med. 2006 Apr 13;354(15):1549–52.

20. Kunreuther H. Preparing for the next natural disaster: learning from Katrina. LDI Issue Brief. 2006 Mar–Apr;11(5):1–4.

21. Bourque LB, Siegel JM, Kano M, et al. Weathering the storm: the impact of hurricanes on physical and mental health. Ann Am Acad Pol Soc Sci. 2006;604(1):129–51.

22. Atkins D, Moy EM. Left behind: the legacy of hurricane Katrina. BMJ. 2005 Oct 23;331(7522):916–8.

23. Cova TJ, Church. RL. Modeling community evacuation vulnerability using GIS. Int J Geogr Inf Sci. 1997;11(8):763–84.

24. Litman T. Lessons from Katrina and Rita: what major disasters can teach transportation planners. Journal of Transportation Engineering. 2006 Jan;132(1):11–18.

25. Travis J. Hurricane Katrina. Scientists' fears come true as hurricane floods New Orleans. Science. 2005 Sep 9;309(5741):1656–9.

26. Norris FH, Friedman MJ, Watson PJ, et al. 60,000 disaster victims speak: Part I. An empirical review of the empirical literature, 1981–2001. Psychiatry. 2002 Fall; 65(3):207–39.

27. Brown OW. Using international practice techniques in Texas: Hurricane Katrina experiences: receiving patients in Longview, Texas, 350 miles from ground zero. Pediatrics. 2006 May;117(5 Pt 3):S439–41.

28. Carus WS. Bioterrorism and biocrimes: the illicit use of biological agents since 1900. (Working paper.) Washington, DC: National Defense University, 2001.

29. Cefalu WT, Smith SR, Blonde L, et al. The Hurricane Katrina aftermath and its impact on diabetes care: observations from "ground zero": lessons in disaster preparedness of people with diabetes. Diabetes Care. 2006 Jan;29(1):158–60.

30. Arnold JL. Disaster myths and hurricane Katrina 2005: can public officials and the media learn to provide responsible crisis communication during disasters? Prehospital Disaster Med. 2006 Jan–Feb;21(1):1–3.

31. La Greca A, Silverman WK, Vernberg EM, Prinstein MJ. Symptoms of post-traumatic stress in children after Hurricane Andrew: a prospective study. J Consult Clin Psychol. 1996 Aug;64(4):712–23.

32. Miles N. Crime spike hits Katrina evacuees. Washington, DC: BBC News, 2006 Aug 15.

33. Palm RI, Hodgson ME. Earthquake insurance: mandated disclosure and homeowner response in California. Ann Assoc Am Geogr. 1992 Jun;82(2):207–22.

34. Palm RI. Natural hazards: an integrative framework for research and planning. Baltimore: John Hopkins University Press, 1990.

35. Steady FC. Women and children first: environment, poverty and sustainable development. Rochester: Schenkman Books, 1993.

36. Cutter SL. The forgotten casualties: women, children and environmental change. Glob Environ Change. 1995;5(3):181–94.

37. Massey D. Space, place and gender. University of Minnesota Press, 1994 Aug.

38. Fordham MH. Making women visible in disasters: problematising the private domain. Disasters. 1998 Jun;22(2):126–43.

39. Curtis A, Leitner M, eds. Geographical information systems and public health: eliminating perinatal disparity. Hershey: IRM Press, 2005.

40. Centers for Disease Control and Prevention (CDC). Surveillance in hurricane evacuation centers—Louisiana, September–October 2005. MMWR. Morb Mortal Wkly Rep. 2006 Jan 20;55(2):32–5.

41. Cohen S, Herbert TB. Health psychology: psychological factors and physical disease from the perspective of human psychoneuroimmunology. Annu Rev Psychol. 1996;47:113–42.

42. Kelly S, Hertzman C, Daniels M. Searching for the biological pathways between stress and health. Annu Rev Public Health. 1997;18:437–62.

43. Collins JW Jr, David RJ, Symons R, et al. African-American mothers' perception of their residential environment, stressful life events, and very low birthweight. Epidemiology. 1998 May;9(3):286–9.

44. Shiono PH, Klebanoff MA, Rhoads GG. Smoking and drinking during pregnancy. Their effects on preterm birth. JAMA. 1986 Jan 3;255(1):82–4.

45. Jaakola JJ, Jaakkola N, Zahlsen K. Fetal growth and length of gestation in relation to prenatal exposure to environmental tobacco smoke assessed by hair nicotine concentration. Environ Health Perspect. 2001 Jun;109(6):557–61.

46. Brooke OG, Anderson HR, Bland JM, et al. Effects on birth weight of smoking, alcohol, caffeine, socioeconomic factors, and psychosocial stress. BMJ. 1989 Mar 25;298(6676):795–801.

47. Chasnoff IJ. Cocaine and pregnancy: clinical and methodological issues. Clin Perinatol. 1991 Mar;18(1):113–23.

48. England GC, Verstegen JP, Hewitt DA. Pregnancy following in vitro fertilisation of canine oocytes. Vet Rec. 2001 Jan 6;148(1):20–2.

49. Fergusson DM, Horwood LJ, Northstone K. Maternal use of cannabis and pregnancy outcome. BJOG. 2002 Jan;109(1):21–7.

50. Shiono PH, Klebanoff MA, Nugent RP, et al. The impact of cocaine and marijuana use on low birth weight and preterm birth: a multicenter study. Am J Obstet Gynecol. 1995 Jan;172(1 Pt 1):19–27.

51. Centers for Disease Control and Prevention (CDC). Health concerns associated with mold in water-damaged homes after Hurricanes Katrina and Rita—New Orleans area, Louisiana, October 2005. MMWR. Morb Mortal Wkly Rep. 2006 Jan 20; 55(2):41–4.

52. Falk H, Baldwin G. Environmental health and Hurricane Katrina. Environ Health Perspect. 2006;114(1):A12–3.

53. Norris FH, Friedman MJ, Watson PJ. 60,000 disaster victims speak: Part II. Summary and implications of the disaster mental health research. Psychiatry. 2002 Fall; 65(3):240–60.

54. Phillips BD. Cultural diversity in disasters: sheltering, housing, and long-term recovery. Int J Mass Emerg Disasters. 1993;11(1):99–110.

55. Satcher D, Fryer GE Jr, McCann J, et al. What if we were equal? A comparison of the black-white mortality gap in 1960 and 2000. Health Aff (Millwood). 2005 Mar–Apr;24(2):459–64.

Chapter 11
A Mobile Medical Care Approach Targeting Underserved Populations in Post–Hurricane Katrina Mississippi

David M. Krol, MD, MPH
Michael Redlener
Alan Shapiro, MD
Ania Wajnberg, MD

Background

On August 29, 2005, Hurricane Katrina struck the Gulf Coast of Mississippi, causing widespread and catastrophic damage to the lives, homes, and businesses of the region. There was extensive physical damage to the medical infrastructure that severely limited access to hospitals and their emergency departments, private clinics, public community health centers, dental and mental health clinics, pharmacies, and many other health-related facilities. This destruction, coupled with the displacement and loss of medical personnel, created a vacuum of care, almost eliminating acute, primary, and tertiary care in the immediate period after the hurricane hit land.

In spite of the overall chaos, medical emergency response teams were able to set up critical care and triage locations at key sites throughout Southern Mississippi, and local and volunteer emergency medical services managed to transport the critically ill and injured. However, in this environment, patients with chronic medical problems lost access to the resources that existed prior to the storm and were left on their own. Medicines were lost, equipment was damaged, and phone service and transportation were eliminated by the hurricane's destruction. Previously manageable health conditions became dangerous, as diabetes, hypertension, asthma, and other chronic diseases went untreated. In a number of limited health assessments, these medical problems topped the list of health concerns for people affected or displaced by Katrina.[1,2]

A primary care disaster response team, Operation Assist (OA), was launched as a joint effort by the Children's Health Fund (CHF) and the Mailman School of Public Health at Columbia University to respond to the immediate health care needs of the region

DAVID KROL *was the Director of Medical Affairs and Clinical Evaluation for The Children's Health Fund and is now Associate Professor and Chair of the Department of Pediatrics at the University of Toledo (UT) College of Medicine.* **MICHAEL REDLENER** *is a medical student at Albert Einstein College of Medicine (AECOM) in the Bronx;* **ALAN SHAPIRO** *is an Assistant Professor of Pediatrics at AECOM, Montefiore Medical Center, where* **ANIA WAJNBERG** *is affiliated with the Primary Care/ Social Medicine Residency Program.*

and to restore lost health care resources.* Two mobile units staffed by clinical teams from the CHF network were deployed to the Gulfport-Biloxi areas of Mississippi and arrived in the region on September 5, 2005.[4] Designed for self-sufficiency, the mobile units are recreational vehicles outfitted with two fully functional examination rooms, a nursing station, a registration area, storage areas for medications and supplies, and refrigeration for medications and vaccines.† The CHF clinical teams have an expertise in providing primary care to underserved communities, such as homeless shelters and public housing communities, in both urban and rural settings.[3]

Operation Assist teams focused their medical outreach efforts on populations known to be medically underserved prior to Katrina's landfall. The versatility of the mobile medical units allowed the teams to reach these people who were otherwise cut off from health services. They afforded great flexibility in providing clinical care to shifting geographic areas of need post-Katrina and to a wide variety of locations, such as indigent neighborhoods, public housing complexes, shelters, motels, houses of worship, community centers, demolition/construction sites, and relief centers. Mobile units allow for immediate and ongoing provision of care to a large number of people as was needed in post-Katrina Mississippi.[5]

This chapter will examine the role of mobile medical units in disaster scenarios, contextualize and quantify patient visit data, examine the most common diagnoses encountered, chronic illness in particular, in this patient population, and draw lessons for future disaster relief situations. The knowledge gained from such an analysis can help responders prepare not only for the acute health care needs resulting from a disaster, but also for those medical needs of the chronically ill that are exacerbated by the loss of the health care infrastructure.

Methods

Data collection. Data were collected from two Children's Health Fund (CHF) mobile medical units at 23 sites for all patient visits in the Gulfport/Biloxi area between September 5–20, 2005. Each patient visit was recorded in a chart that included information on the reason for visit (chief complaint), a brief description of the problem, physical exam, assessment/diagnosis, and plan. The reason for visit was collected to identify any vaccine or pharmaceutical needs that might not have been identified had only the diagnoses been collected. Two reviewers examined each chart and collected data that were consistently available: age, sex, race, reason for visit (chief complaint), diagnoses,

---

* The CHF is a nonprofit organization dedicated to the health and well being of underserved children and families in the United States. The CHF network provides direct clinical care, regardless of ability to pay, at 21 sites throughout the nation. The CHF has developed a model of health care delivery in which a mobile medical program becomes the medical home within the community served. Each mobile program is affiliated with an academic medical center or community health center, which functions as a resource for referral and specialty care. Columbia University's Mailman School of Public Health is an academic public health institution dedicated to the understanding and development of policy and practice to better the health of people worldwide.

† The CHF deployed similar mobile medical unit-based teams to the Baton Rouge/New Orleans and Houston areas during this same time period.

vaccines administered, medications and/or prescriptions given, referrals made. All data were compiled into a Microsoft Excel spreadsheet form.

Data consolidation. In order for the data to be more easily analyzed, understood, described, and compared with previously published data on health care needs and services provided to similar populations after Katrina, the authors consolidated the data points into reproducible categories. The final categories agreed upon by the research team were similar to those used in a previous Centers for Disease Control and Prevention (CDC) publication,[6] but also included categories that were more detailed than those used by the CDC. A similar process was used with the variable of race, wherein the authors consolidated a variety of self-identified race designations into categories used by the U.S. Census.

Data analysis. Counts and frequencies for each of the categories were determined using the pivot table and statistical and function capabilities of the Excel program. In addition to the counts and frequencies of the consolidated categories, counts and frequencies of specific reasons for visit and diagnoses for the whole set of patient visits as well as for each of three age groupings (0–21 years, 22–65, older than 65) were examined.

Results

Demographics. Between September 5–20, 2005, a total of 1,205 patient encounters occurred (Table 1). Fifty-four and four tenths percent (n=611) of encounters that had a sex documented (n=1,123) were female. Of those encounters that had a documented age (n=1,057), 29.0% (n=296) were between the ages of 0–21 years, 64.2% (n=677) between 22–65 years, and 6.8% (n=72) were over age 65 years. Encounters that had a documented race (n=839) included 61.9% (n=519) African Americans, 19.7% (n=165) Asians, 11.8% (n=99) Caucasians, 5.7% (n=48) Hispanic/Latinos, and 1% (n=8) other. The majority (98%) of individuals in the Asian category identified as Vietnamese. The Hispanic/Latino category included individuals who identified themselves as Mexican, Honduran, Guatemalan, Chilean, and Brazilian. The other category was made up of individuals who identified as biracial, brown, and Native American.

Reasons for visit. There were a total of 1,187 patient encounters with a documented reason for visit that generated 1,428 reasons for visit, as many individuals had multiple reasons (data not shown). The most frequently documented reasons that individuals visited the mobile units was for vaccines (53.7% of all persons with a reason for visit, n=638) and pharmacy needs (12.6%, 149). Within each of the three age groups, vaccination was the number one reason for visit. Pharmacy needs were more frequently a reason for visit in the two older age groups. The vast majority (98%) of vaccines requested and distributed to individuals were tetanus (Td). Hepatitis A vaccines were also requested and distributed, but to a smaller number of individuals (n=22, 2.8%). The category of pharmacy visits includes all individuals who requested refills on medications, the majority of which were for chronic illnesses that existed prior to the storm.

Diagnoses. The most frequent diagnoses in those individuals who had at least one diagnosis documented were respiratory, circulatory, minor injury, skin conditions, and endocrine (Table 2). In the circulatory category, the most common specific diagnosis

Table 1.

DEMOGRAPHIC CHARACTERISTICS
OF PATIENTS ENCOUNTERED

Patient characteristics	Patient encounter with documented characteristic	
	n	(%)
Total	1205	100.0
Sex (n=1123)		
Female	611	54.4
Age (n=1055)		
0–21 years	296	29.0
22–65 years	677	64.2
>65 years	72	6.8
Race (n=839)		
African-American	519	61.8
Asian	165	19.6
Caucasian	99	11.8
Hispanic/Latino	48	5.7
Native American	1	.1
Other	7	.8

was hypertension. Upper respiratory tract infection and asthma were the two most common specific diagnoses of the respiratory category. Minor injury diagnoses included abrasions, lacerations, and puncture wounds. Skin condition diagnoses included mostly dermatitis, fungal, and bacterial skin infections. The endocrine diagnoses were primarily diabetes mellitus.

The top three diagnosis categories for the 0–21 years age group included respiratory conditions, skin conditions, and minor injury (Table 3). For the 22–65 age group the top three diagnosis categories were circulatory conditions, respiratory conditions, and minor injury. Members of the older than 65 age group were most commonly diagnosed with circulatory, endocrine, and respiratory problems.

The proportion of patients with chronic diseases (e.g., diabetes mellitus, high blood pressure and other cardiovascular disease, and asthma or chronic obstructive pulmonary disorder)[7] increased with age (Table 4). Of the 0–21 year old age group, 18.1% had a chronic disease diagnosis (mainly asthma). In the 22–65 year old age group, 39.2% had at least one chronic disease (primarily hypertension and diabetes). Two-thirds (67.3%) of individuals older than 65 years had at least one chronic disease diagnosis (primarily hypertension and diabetes).

Table 2.

TEN MOST COMMON DIAGNOSIS CATEGORIES

Diagnosis categories	n	% All diagnosis categories	% All persons with a diagnosis
Respiratory	175	17.1	27.8
Circulatory	174	17.1	27.8
Minor injury	120	11.8	19.2
Skin conditions	117	11.6	18.8
Endocrine	68	6.7	10.9
Other	62	6.1	9.9
Gastrointestinal	56	5.5	8.9
Mental health	41	4.0	6.5
Environmentally induced illness	35	3.4	5.6
Neurologic	29	2.8	4.6

Table 3.

PERSONS WITH AT LEAST ONE OF MOST COMMON DIAGNOSIS CATEGORIES BY AGE GROUP

0–21 Years	n	%	22–65 Years	n	%	>65 Years	n	%
Respiratory	78	41.5	Circulatory	131	34.5	Circulatory	38	77.6
Skin conditions	59	31.4	Respiratory	84	22.1	Endocrine	13	26.5
Minor injury	38	20.2	Minor injury	73	19.2	Respiratory	9	18.4

Discussion

Population served. The OA clinical teams sought the assistance of a local community health center partner, community leaders, government officials, the Red Cross, and the Salvation Army in finding communities largely isolated from ongoing relief efforts. These communities were often found in public housing complexes or at houses of worship that doubled as relief centers. The populations found at these sites were predominantly African American and Vietnamese.

As a result, the demographics of the patient population served in this effort diverged significantly from the demographics of Harrison County, Mississippi, where this effort took place. For 2005, the population of Harrison County was 71.1% Caucasian, 22.5% African American, 2.9% Asian, and 2.5% Hispanic or Latino.[8] The population that

Table 4.

CHRONIC ILLNESS DIAGNOSES BY AGE GROUP

	0–21 Years		22–65 Years		>65 Years	
	n	%[a]	n	%[a]	n	%[a]
Asthma	31	16.5	28	7.4	0	.0
COPD	0	.0	1	.3	2	4.1
Diabetes	2	1.0	46	12.1	13	26.5
Hypertension	1	.5	99	26.1	29	59.2
Other cardiovascular diseases	0	.0	13	3.4	6	12.2

[a]Percentage of individuals with at least one diagnosis.

sought services in this study were predominantly African American with nearly 6-fold higher percentage of Asians and 2-fold higher Hispanic/Latino population than that found in the pre-hurricane general population.

It is possible that the most economically disadvantaged populations were less able to escape the destruction of Hurricane Katrina, a circumstance seen in New Orleans. If those populations were also primarily made up of minority group members it would explain why a larger percentage of minorities sought care from the mobile units.

Reasons for visit. The predominant reason individuals visited the OA mobile medical teams was vaccination (44%), primarily for tetanus (Td). This seems to be a high percentage, though it is difficult to find a comparison in the literature. In one study of post-Katrina illness and injury, 11.6% of visits were for tetanus immunization only, but the publication does not comment on what percentage of individuals with other reasons for visit were immunized.[6] The high percentage of tetanus vaccination in this study is likely due to multiple causes. A combination of health official recommendations and lost vaccination records led to many patients seeking tetanus protection. It is unclear how many patients were over-immunized by this drive. Many so-called *worried well* patients came to the mobile medical units healthy, but seeking out vaccinations and post-disaster health information for themselves and their families. One last factor that may explain the large number of requests for tetanus vaccination is the fact that the Operation Assist teams provided care to a significant number of the demolition/construction crews. Many of these patients were undocumented laborers with no history of previous vaccination.

Another important finding is that 12.6% of people came with a specific request for medication(s) or medication refill. This is not surprising considering the number of individuals with chronic diseases. With the flooding of residences, hurried evacuations, and widespread population displacements, medications were frequently destroyed or lost. Access to pharmacies immediately after the storm was very limited due to damage, destruction, and/or inaccessibility due to loss of public and private transportation. Access to information on where and how to get medication replacement and refill was limited after the storm as well. A retrospective review of clinical and pharmaceutical records from a Red Cross shelter in Jackson, Mississippi showed that 43% of visits to the clinic were for prescriptions only, primarily for chronic disease, with cardiovascular drugs topping the list at 30.8% of prescriptions given. Interestingly, the population served was predominantly African American, 79% from Louisiana and, of those that listed health insurance status, 53% uninsured.[9]

Diagnoses. Key phenomena emerge from the information gathered in this effort: the frequent presentation, exacerbation, and vulnerability of chronic medical problems after a disaster, and, thus, the importance of primary care in a post-disaster setting. A large percentage (35.0%) of the overall patient population seen had at least one chronic disease diagnosis (such as hypertension, asthma, or diabetes). Even more striking was that the older the patient, the more likely they were to have one or more chronic illnesses, and the care they sought was directly related to that chronic illness. Our findings were consistent with surveillance data in evacuation centers[10] though with a slightly lower proportion of chronic illness than that found in a survey of Orleans and Jefferson Parish, Louisiana households.[11] These findings underscore the point that, though experts in disaster, emergency, and trauma medicine may be valuable in a post-disaster setting, primary care clinicians knowledgeable in the treatment of common acute and chronic disease are as important for the short and long-term recovery of populations, especially underserved populations, after a disaster.

Limitations. The areas of service and thus the populations focused on by the mobile medical teams were mission-driven. Therefore, a selection bias towards minority, low-income, and previously underserved populations was expected. While this limits the generalizability of the findings to all socioeconomic and racial/ethnic groups, it still gives important information that can guide health care providers who will serve populations left behind in areas with massive infrastructure disruption.

The initial data were collected by clinicians making up the medical teams from multiple locations around the country utilizing non-standardized data collection tools and various permutations of medical records. Thus, there was wide variability in quantity, quality, and consistency of data reporting. For both of these reasons, missing data or inconsistencies in data were found when collecting information to enter into the database.

The study team attempted to address these problems by standardizing categories for race, reason for visits, and diagnoses via a consensus process. This grouping and categorizing may have obscured more specific information. It is also possible that cases may have been misclassified, particularly for conditions that could be classified under multiple diagnostic categories; however, all original data prior to categorization were still available to the study team for analysis.

Implications

The utility of mobile medical care. As a mobile medical program, Operation Assist filled a specific niche in the chaotic post-Katrina environment. In Mississippi, the hurricane put public and private transportation out of commission, making it difficult for residents to seek assistance beyond their neighborhoods. The Operation Assist mobile medical units had a distinct advantage in providing access during the post-Katrina period. The mobile medical units

- allowed for community outreach to identify people in need of health care who might have suffered adverse health consequences and bring care to their doorstep;
- had the ability to search for patient populations who had become isolated from the wider community after the disaster;
- were self-contained and brought a wide range of medical services and medical supplies, including medications and vaccinations, to populations cut off from care;
- served for a long period of time as a substitute until permanent clinics were up and running.

As an example, the Gulfport, Mississippi mobile medical unit has now become a permanent site in the CHF network, serving the underserved in Harrison County.

It is important, also, to mention that there were some disadvantages to the mobile medical approach. External factors such as disruption of roadways (due to flooding and downed trees, for example) and availability of gas affected provision of care. Likewise, internal mechanical problems and availability of mechanics knowledgeable in the repair of such vehicles also limited their use at times. Finally, due to space constraints, limited supplies could be carried at one time so storage facilities and supply lines had to be identified and maintained.

Disaster-based primary care medicine. In conjunction with the limited data available from surveillance and operational studies of the post-Katrina medical environment, our data emphasize the need to address patients with chronic medical problems and primary care medicine in disaster situations.[9,12–14] *Disaster-Based Primary Care Medicine* is one way in which to organize thinking and planning for a robust medical response to natural or man-made disasters, in particular those that cause widespread destruction (I.E. Redlener, personal communication). The term implies an array of services designed to meet (a) the on-going primary care needs (preventive services and health education, as well as the diagnosis and management of acute and chronic conditions) and (b) the special needs created by the particular health risks and consequences of the disaster and by the deterioration in the availability of health services in general. Whether patients are located in isolated neighborhoods, in shelters, or at home, medical providers must recognize that chronic health problems are widespread and that, in general, the patients with the least resources will be the people who require the most care. There is a role for community medicine and primary care doctors with experience in low-resource settings to play in disaster planning and response.

Systemic reform. In the United States, it is necessary to address chronic disease in disaster preparedness, since chronic disease has become the highest cause of morbidity for the general population. Researchers at the Chronic Diseases and Vulnerable Populations in Disasters Working Group have suggested that the recognition and development of strategies for addressing chronic disease must be incorporated into disaster planning.[14,15] These strategies include identifying pre-disaster disease burden, creating a list of essential medications for providers, ensuring individual and family preparedness, and understanding systemic support for chronic disease.

Our experience and the findings reported here reflect the need expressed by this group. With increasing patient age, providers saw a population increasingly affected by chronic disease. Although mobile medical units were successful in providing stopgap measures, systemic preparedness will better serve the population as a whole.

Conclusions

While it is impossible to predict accurately the exact nature of medical needs after major natural or man-made disasters, we do know that there exists a baseline level of significant health disparities and barriers to care. In the setting of a disaster, many of these disparities and barriers to care become more recognizable if not exacerbated. The communities that suffer most, given this baseline, are those with the fewest resources to withstand the major disruption disasters can bring to a fragile health care system connection. Greater effort must be made to help such communities prepare for disasters and avoid the disastrous consequences seen after Katrina.

In the absence of a concerted nationwide effort to decrease health disparities and remove barriers to care for the underserved, we will most certainly face again the disproportionate needs of the underserved in times of disaster. Mobile medical care is a delivery model developed to reach those with the greatest barriers to receiving traditional medical services. Mobile medical units staffed by clinicians experienced in dealing with the clinical and social needs of the underserved and comfortable working in a resource-poor environment can make a positive contribution to post-disaster care. We hope that lessons learned by Operation Assist in the Mississippi Gulf will strengthen this model.

Acknowledgments

The authors would like to acknowledge all those who volunteered to participate in the provision of health care services during Operation Assist. The sacrifices made by those who gave their time and effort are greatly appreciated by your colleagues and those you served.

Notes

1. Centers for Disease Control and Prevention (CDC). Update on CDC's response to Hurricane Katrina. Atlanta, GA: CDC, 2005 Sep 19. Available at http://www.cdc.gov/od/katrina/09–19–05.htm.

2. Henry J. Kaiser Family Foundation. The Washington Post/Kaiser Family Foundation/Harvard University Survey of Hurricane Katrina evacuees. Washington, DC: The Henry J. Kaiser Family Foundation, 2005 Sep 16. Available at http://www.kff.org/newsmedia/upload/7401.pdf.

3. Redlener I, Redlener K. System-based mobile primary pediatric care for homeless children: the anatomy of a working program. Bull N Y Acad Med. 1994 Summer; 71(1)49–57.

4.   Shapiro A, Seim L, Christensen RC, et al. Chronicles from out-of-state professionals: providing primary care to underserved children after a disaster: a national organization response. Pediatrics. 2006;117(5 Pt 3):S412–5.

5.   Kasis I, Lak L, Adler J, et al. Medical relief operation in rural northern Ethiopia: addressing an ongoing disaster. Isr Med Assoc J. 2001 Oct;3(10):772–7.

6.   Centers for Disease Control and Prevention (CDC). Surveillance for illness and injury after hurricane Katrina—three counties, Mississippi, September 5–October 11, 2005. MMWR. Morb Mortal Wkly Rep. 2006 Mar 10;55(9):231–4.

7.   Centers for Disease Control and Prevention (CDC). Surveillance in hurricane evacuation centers—Louisiana, September–October 2005. MMWR. Morb Mortal Wkly Rep. 2006 Jan 20;55(2):32–5.

8.   U.S. Census Bureau. Fact sheet: Harrison County, Mississippi—2000, 2005 American Community Survey data profile highlights. Washington, DC: U.S. Census Bureau, 2006. Available at http://factfinder.census.gov/servlet/ACSSAFF-Facts?_event=&geo_id=05000US28047&_geoContext=01000US%7C04000US28%7C05000US28047&_street=&_county=harrison&_cityTown=harrison&_state=04000US28&_zip=& _lang=en&_sse=on&ActiveGeoDiv=&_useEV=&pctxt=fph&pgsl=050&_submenu Id=factsheet_1&ds_name=null&_ci_nbr=null&qr_name=null&reg=null%3Anull&_keyword=&_industry=.

9.   Currier M, King DS, Wofford MR, et al. A Katrina experience: lessons learned. Am J Med. 2006 Nov;119(11):986–92.

10. Centers for Disease Control and Prevention (CDC). Morbidity surveillance after hurricane Katrina—Arkansas, Louisiana, Mississippi and Texas, September 2005. MMWR. Morb Mortal Wkly Rep. 2006 Jul 7;55(26):727–31.

11. Centers for Disease Control and Prevention (CDC). Assessment of health-related needs after Hurricanes Katrina and Rita—Orleans and Jefferson Parishes, New Orleans area, Louisiana, October 17–22, 2005. MMWR. Morb Mortal Wkly Rep. 2006 Jan 20; 55(2):38–41.

12. Sirbaugh PE, Gurwitch KD, Macias CG, et al. Caring for evacuated children housed in the Astrodome: creation and implementation of mobile pediatric emergency response team: regionalized caring for displaced children after a disaster. Pediatrics. 2006 May;117(5 Pt 3):S428–38.

13. Connelly M. IMERT deployment to Baton Rouge, Louisiana in response to Hurricane Katrina, September 2005. Disaster Manag Response. 2006 Jan–Mar;4(1):4–11.

14. Mokdad AH, Mensah GA, Posner SF, et al. When chronic conditions become acute: prevention and control of chronic diseases and adverse health outcomes during natural disasters. Prev Chronic Dis. 2005 Nov;2 Spec no:A04. Available at http://www.cdc.gov/pcd/issues/2005/nov/05_0201.htm.

15. Ford ES, Mokdad AH, Link MW, et al. Chronic disease in health emergencies in the eye of the hurricane. Prev Chronic Dis. 2006 Apr;3(2):A46. Available at http://www.cdc.gov/pcd/issues/2006/apr/05_0235.htm.

Chapter 12
Wading in the Waters: Spirituality and Older Black Katrina Survivors

Erma J. Lawson, PhD, RN
Cecelia Thomas, PhD, LMSW-AP

Coping with distress following a hurricane has been a major research interest in public health and sociology.[1-3] Researchers have often viewed such coping in terms of psychological resources, cognitive strategies, and behavioral techniques.[4] For example, hardiness is a positive psychological coping trait; interpretations of an event are considered a cognitive technique;[5] behavioral strategies include yoga and biofeedback, among many others.[6] Notably, previous studies have often paid little attention to how older Black hurricane survivors cope.[4-8]

Katrina, at its height a category 5 hurricane, caused catastrophic damage.[9-11] Breached levees flooded 80% of New Orleans and resulted in $75 billion in damages.[9-11] Katrina was responsible for at least 1,417 deaths; between 3,000 and 5,000 people remain missing and 1.5 million were displaced.[12] Although it is unclear how many will return, as of October 2005, approximately 50,000 households comprising mostly poor, Black American residents had no plans to return to New Orleans.[12] If that number is accurate, Katrina-induced migration will be the largest internal migration in a generation.[11-13]

As sections of the New Orleans levee system collapsed, the natural disaster of Katrina deteriorated into a social debacle. Thousands of people, mostly Black and poor, many of them elderly, were trapped in the New Orleans Superdome and the city's convention center, or on rooftops, without electricity or food.[10-12] Many bodies that emerged from the floodwaters were of people aged 50 years or older,[10-13] evidence of their low priority in the nation's response to Katrina.[11] Moreover, the consequences of this natural disaster are grave: 1.5 million people had to meet the challenge of where they would live or work, and pondered if they would ever return to their homes after such massive, widespread suffering.[10-13] They faced the shock of losing loved ones while dealing with confusion over federal policies regarding disaster relief.

This chapter explores the coping of older Katrina survivors and seeks to stimulate innovative theoretically driven strategies to redefine Katrina-related coping mechanisms prominent for an older Black population. It briefly reviews the literature on coping. It presents a qualitative study of how Katrina survivors coped to reestablish their lives.

ERMA LAWSON *is an Associate Professor of Medical Sociology at the University of North Texas (U-NT).*
CECELIA THOMAS *is an Assistant Professor in the Department of Rehabilitation, Social Work, and Addictions at U-NT.*

Religious and spiritual coping. Beliefs in a Higher Power have influenced every aspect of the Black experience.[14-16] Religion provided hope and group identity throughout 250 years of slavery[14-16] and previous research has extensively documented that religious institutions are important sources of support for Blacks.[14-17] Specifically, an analysis of several national data sets by Chatters and colleagues found that 8 out of 10 Blacks reported that religious beliefs are very important to them, and 43.6% said they "almost always" sought spiritual comfort through religion.[18]

This is particularly true for older adults.[19-21] For example, Keonig and colleagues in 1988 found that 45% of older Blacks coped with stressful life events through religious activity.[20] Around the same time, Krause and Tran also found that older Blacks relied on involvement in religious activities to buffer the effects of negative life events.[22] Participation in church programs provided positive self-worth, thereby reducing psychological distress.

Furthermore, numerous studies have shown that Black use prayer as a resource.[17-28] According to Chatters and Taylor, 78% of a nationally-based representative sample of Blacks reported praying almost daily.[29] A significant number of Blacks believe in healing power of prayer compared with Whites and other racial/ethnic groups;[24-25] approximately 50% of Blacks report requesting that others pray for them daily.[29] In 1995, McAddo found that 72% of Black women engaged in prayer for emotional support.[30] This is consistent with Hill et al., who found that Black mothers living in urban areas used prayer to cope with such problems as pervasive criminality.[31] Similarly, Bryant-Davis found that Black survivors of childhood violence incorporated prayer and spiritual beliefs as a preferred method of coping with the associated trauma.[32] A study of coping during the 9-11 terrorist attacks found that Black respondents, compared with other racial/ethnic groups are most likely to have reported praying to cope with the trauma of those events.[33] Prayers, Cook and Wiley suggest, are understood by Blacks (as well as others) as a direct link to God about problems in daily life.[34]

Extensive research has also reported that Blacks rely on spiritual practices and religious beliefs to cope with chronic and acute illness.[30,35-38] For example, Blacks use prayer to cope with breast cancer,[38-39] and to practice health prevention behavior;[40-41] and to live with HIV[42] and recovery from alcohol addiction.[43] Becker and Newsome found that religion influenced older Blacks to perform instrumental activities of daily living, irrespective of gender, age, education, and self-rated health status.[44]

Older Blacks' tendency to seek spiritual comfort through prayer during personal crises operates irrespective of socioeconomic status.[45-48] These findings underscore the prevalence of spirituality and prayer as a preferred means of coping with problems in this population.[28,30-35,40-41,48-49]

Although researchers have documented the influence of religious practices and spiritual beliefs of Blacks, few studies have explored how religion and spirituality enable older Blacks to rebound following a natural disaster.

Methods

The research team recruited study participants from a residential adult senior citizen Texas facility that housed some Katrina survivors. Other residents at this facility were mostly upper-middle class, White senior citizens. The facility offered apartments that provided Katrina survivors with one- or two-bedroom (one-bathroom) units as needed and as available.

Subjects. The investigators purposefully selected study participants who had been dislocated by Hurricane Katrina. The inclusion criteria were no mental or physical disability, no previous suicide attempts, and no current use of illicit drugs.

Data procedures. Before the data collection began, the research team obtained institutional review board (IRB) approval from the University of North Texas and held an informational meeting with the facility's director. The director presented the idea of the research study to the Katrina survivors who fit the inclusion criteria. Approximately 20 Katrina residents resided at the facility; 12 respondents met the inclusion criterion and 8 respondents volunteered to participate. However, as the study progressed, other residents approached the team to tell their stories. All of the respondents completed informed consent forms and were told that this was an exploratory study to understand Katrina survivors' coping and to make service delivery recommendations.

Data collection. Limited demographic information was obtained from participants via a data sheet and the research team collected qualitative data using focus groups. However, following the first interview, it was apparent that this was not the best method to use with the study population due to the inordinate time required for each member to relate his or her experiences. Consequently, the team decided to conduct interviews with one or two individuals at a time. All the interviews were tape-recorded and transcribed verbatim by the research team or by a doctoral student. The research team crosschecked transcriptions.

Most of the respondents participated in three interviews and the researchers made an effort to select times and a location convenient for the respondents. All of the interviews took place in the study participants' living rooms and often lasted much longer than expected, from 1–3 hours. The investigators collected data over a 10-month period.

Interview guide. The research team collected data using interviews to understand the experiences of older Katrina survivors. The first question established rapport, and follow-up questions focused on coping and the failure of the federal, state, and local governments to coordinate service delivery. The first interview included some the following items as prompts:

- A number of people have coped with traumatic events. Tell us how you have coped with previous traumatic situations.
- Walk us through your experiences of Hurricane Katrina.
- Tell us how you coped with each phase of Katrina.

The first interviews generated as much as 52 pages of transcription; the transcriptions averaged approximately 32 pages each. The third interviews averaged approximately 40 pages, as the themes were re-defined and re-conceptualized.

Data analysis. The investigators read the transcripts, and each member of the team used open coding to generate an emergent set of categories. Grounded theory was used to develop the codes for categories that the data might fit.[50–51] The team members analyzed the data line-by-line, yielding a total of about 60 codes on spirituality themes. The principal investigator collapsed the coding schemes using Ethnograph V5.0 for

Windows PC (Qualis Research Associates, P.O. Box 50437, Colorado Springs, CO 80949), a computerized qualitative analysis program, to determine the consistency of those schemes, to search and note segments within the data, and to mark codes. A coding paradigm was developed for conditions and strategies of the major themes; regular comparison across interviews was made of themes. Box 1 depicts sample coding of interview responses, collapsed by theme. An audit trail, peer reviews, and member checks were incorporated in the study to ensure the trustworthiness of the data.

Participant observation. In addition to interviewing the study participants, the researchers actively observed the respondents in their social worlds. During the study, a few of the respondents requested specific favors, such as rides to church or to the local shopping mall to help relieve their social isolation. Throughout the study processes, the researchers recorded their observations of significant events affecting the participants as memos. According to Denzin, the emphasis of qualitative research is on in-depth understanding of the social context.[52] Participant observation created a holistic understanding of coping among older Black Katrina survivors.

Reflexivity in the study. The participant observation memos were distinct from the field notes recorded following data collection. Although a researcher conducts a preliminary data analysis during data collection, reflexive analyses sensitize the researcher to particular themes and thus inform data analysis and interpretation. Murphy et al. emphasize the role of *reflexivity* in how researchers' own socialization and personal biography influence data analysis.[53]

Acknowledging reflexivity ensures that researchers' assumptions are to some degree explicit. In the present study, the researchers achieved this aim by exploring their own racial/ethnic identities (Black) and early socialization. As researchers we perceived ourselves as members of the Black community and as having much in common with the Katrina survivors. As women of color, we, too, sensed heightened vulnerability in the view of the government's response to Katrina. Although we realized that differences exist between the Katrina survivors and us, many of the study participants grew up in the South and reported strong religious traditions similar to our own experiences. According to Murphy et al., researchers may be blinded to the data if they fail to recognize differences and similarities between the researcher and respondents.[53] Thus, the researchers concentrated on not losing sight of their own identities and how they might be playing a role during the interpretation phase of the study.

Results

Sample demographics. The sample comprised 10 adults, 2 men and 8 women. SPSS was used to analyze descriptive information of respondents. The sample consisted of Katrina survivors 55 years and older, with the oldest aged 67. The majority were widowed; one participant experienced the Katrina-related death of a spouse. Most of the respondents relocated to Texas from the poorest parish of New Orleans. All of the respondents grew-up in two parent households. One respondent was raised by a stepmother. Eight respondents completed high school; one completed 10 years of education; and one

Box 1.

RESEARCH THEMES OF COPING STRATEGIES: SEPTEMBER, 2005–JUNE, 2006

Theme description and coding	Sample coping responses by respondents
Constant divine communication	"I knew me and my family was going to be alright because of the power of prayer."
	"Prayer helps me to know what God wants me to do."
	"I talk to God daily and say the Lord's Prayer and ask the Lord to watch over me, because I feel I am favored by God."
Miracles of faith	"I've come this far by faith and trust in God."
	"God does not put any more on us than we can bear."
	"Believe me, there is a God and He is in control."
	"Faith and God got me through. I knew I was going to be alright."
Inspirational reading	"Every morning is my quiet time with God."
	"Daily I read the scripture and spend at least a good half hour every day reading."
	"I read meditations every day, a little meditation in order to survive and to go on."
Coping by helping and assisting others	"There was a lady sitting there, and I asker her, where is your family? She said her family dropped her off. She was outside the Superdome so we took her in and took care of her until the last day. She was in her 70s."
	"God had me there for a reason. I had to get an ambulance for a guy who made the newspapers by looking for his wife, but he died on the 19th."
	"A meal is the tie that binds, so I cooked and distributed food to those who needed it."
	"One of the girls I was with, mother could not walk, she was crippled, so someone had to carry her on their back and walk through the water."

completed four years of college. The typical respondent was approximately 58.3 years of age, female, widowed, with 12 years of education.

Identified themes. *Prayer throughout the day.* Prayer throughout the day is defined as talking to God minute to minute as a personal and intimate habit. A distinctive one-on-one relationship to a Higher Power was incorporated into the respondents' daily lives. For example, they reported praying throughout the day and seeking Divine guidance. Often, these prayers were composed spontaneously, or offered in silence, and involved thanking God for the positive experiences that occurred during Katrina. For instance, the respondents reported thanking a Higher Power for the rescue from rooftops, appropriate sleeping space in shelters, and moving to permanent housing. According to the respondents, a Higher Power was involved in every activity; they believed that God always spoke to them, and they always listened. As Anne, a 55-year-old woman, who experienced a great deal of trauma at the Superdome stated, "I talk to God constantly 'cause He will love and protect you every step of the way."

The respondents' continual communication with God involved a personal relationship with Him, and not necessarily church membership. For instance, Celeste, a 55-year-old middle-class Katrina survivor whose husband died about 5 years before the hurricane struck, described her personal relationship with God as follows: "I don't go to church. I stopped going to church years earlier. I pray and talk to God every day, and constantly. There is not a minute which goes by that I do not talk to God." Elaborating on this theme of persistent communication, Carl a 65-year-old male and retired school teacher explained: "I talk to God daily and say the Lord's Prayer and ask the Lord to watch over me, because I feel that I am favored by God." According to Carl, "favored by God" translates into viewing God as gracious, caring, and ever-present. In the midst of what they viewed as unjust FEMA treatment and their painful awareness of an unmerciful society, the respondents reported that they believed God was just, loving, and merciful, and would exert the final judgment and deliver them from FEMA.

Rita, a 57-year-old woman who had a history of drug addiction, recalled the incident of misplacing her grandchildren. She reported:

> I freaked out and prayed, 'God please work it out for me.' Work it out, cause I could not go and get my grandbabies. People said if I went back, I would drown. When we got to the Superdome, we sat and then I started to pray.

Rita paused and tearfully noted, "I said Jesus, it is in your name. What is this here? Is the world coming to an end?' And I asked God for forgiveness for all that I have done 'cause I did not know what I was 'bout to face." She emphatically added, "It looked as though I was facing the last days of my life."

These findings are consistent with research that documents that private religious practices such as prayer often mediate the impact of stress for a large number of Black women.[24–25,27,35–36,38]

Divine miracles. The findings showed that the respondents' experiences of miracles represented a form of coping defined by participants as God's power flowing to people who pray. The respondents perceived miracles as unpredictable daily occurrences that solve apparently insoluble problems. For instance, Beth, aged 60, who slept outside of the Superdome on hard concrete for hours, believed that God performed miracles throughout the experience. She remarked: "Even though we didn't have control of where we were going, I thought God was controlling where I needed to end up. You can't figure out what God's purpose is, but you know the purpose was for you to be here."

Numerous narratives illustrated the survivors' profound belief in miracles. For instance, Diane, a 55-year-old female survivor recalled her belief in miracles. She stated: "God was there. He blessed me. My home is safe. A tree could have fell on it or anything. And then when I got to the shelter, I was the first one to leave. You see the good Lord removed me from there before I was hurt."

Essie, a 61-year-old widow, also reported her view of a miracle that allowed a short wait for the bus to Texas as well as seats for her family. She explained: "It only took 20 minutes to get on the bus to leave New Orleans. Other families waited hours. Before we got on the bus, they were separating whole families. Then when it was my turn, they put families together on one bus." According to Essie, a miracle occurred that decreased the wait time as well as provided space on the bus to travel to Texas, which reaffirmed her belief in miracles. Other respondents also reported miracles surrounding finding family members; locating the right church to attend; determining an appropriate physician; and even discovering suitable beauty/nail salons or barber shops.

Inspirational reading and coping. Although the hurricane and subsequent breached levees undermined the respondents' sense of control, they often regained it through the use of religious reading—the Bible, inspirational books, and daily devotional meditation books—to cope with Katrina. Carl reported that while he was in the Superdome, he read the Bible daily to gain strength. Another survivor, 59-year-old Jim, explained the effects of reading the scriptures as he awaited rescue from his rooftop. He reported:

> Every day, I read Psalm 91—'He who dwells in the shelter of the Most High will abide in the shadow of the Almighty. I will say to the Lord, My refuge and my fortress, My God, in whom I trust.' I did not read the Bible daily, so now reading the Bible bolsters my faith.

The respondents reported receiving comfort from readings from the Old Testament, which speaks of God dwelling among and caring for His people. Jim also said, "I can look back where God was working in my life like Psalms 91:11–16: 'For He shall give His angels charge over you to keep you in all your ways." Approximately 80% of the respondents reported that reading the Bible allowed them to increase their understanding of God.

The respondents also read inspirational books and materials to develop a "closer, more fruitful walk with God." For example, *Guideposts,* a devotional magazine, provided inspiration and encouragement, and the respondents reported they experienced the Spirit connecting them to God through the words of that magazine. Rita explained:

> I read meditations every day, a little meditation in order to survive and to go on. For instance, [reading from the magazine] this one reads, 'I want to be worthy of

Thy blessings of happiness and good fortune. So, please let me walk each day in Thy presence.' These verses help me to stay cool 'cause I have to concentrate on me.

Assisting others and coping. To further assist them in coping with Katrina, the respondents devoted much time to helping others. The act of assisting people less fortunate than themselves is rooted in the respondents' religious beliefs. One respondent recited his philosophy: "Giving to others and helping those in need is how God blesses you." Frequently, the respondents exchanged clothing, food, and various services in a spirit of cooperation and assistance.

The respondents typically reordered their priorities, giving low priority to mundane concerns and high priority to helping others, and reported gaining positive meaning from the experience. Beverly, age 55, for example, described how many individuals helped others reach the Superdome. She remarked, "One of the girls I was with, her mother could not walk; she was crippled. So someone had to carry her and pick her up on their back and walk through the water."

Beverly also recalled that, on seeing a woman sitting alone outside the Superdome, she felt compelled to help. She explained,

We made a homeless shelter, like with cardboards, and stayed there until we left. There was a lady sitting there, and I asked her, 'Where is your family?' And she said, 'I don't know. My family dropped me off.' She was outside the Superdome, so we took her in. She was in her seventies, and we took care of her until the last day. I asked people to take her to the hospital because she had problems. So, they took her, and I was happy.

In some cases, the respondents related helping to divine purpose and, ultimately, to coping. Rita stated; "There was a guy here who was sick, . . . like I said, God has me here for a reason. I had to get an ambulance for him, but later he died." Rita arranged transportation to church for the deceased man's widow and provided assistance to completing FEMA money voucher forms. Respondents valued helping individuals in worse shape than themselves. Another male respondent recalled distributing food to and cooking for other survivors, actions symbolizing the spiritual component of collective Katrina survivorship. Indeed, according to one respondent, a meal is the tie that binds and through the preparation and serving of New Orleans gumbo and fried okra, as well as other services, Katrina survivors helped and comforted each other. Others described helping those who had poor reading and writing skills to complete extensive FEMA documentation for housing vouchers as well as passing on information about the latest FEMA deadlines. As Carl, Jim, Rita, and other respondents stated, "When I help another person, it helps me to take my mind off my problems."

Participant observation results. The participant observations confirmed the results found in the interviews. First, the respondents were observed talking to God throughout the day and relying on Divine guidance when deciding where to live, or which church to attend. Second, the observations revealed that a number of respondents not only read daily mediations, but purchased various television ministers' books and called 800 numbers for prayer. Third, often the respondents voiced deep disappointment over the loss of family Bibles due to the storm and the fact that most shelters failed to provide Bibles upon their arrival. Fourth, a large majority of the respondents expected miracles after FEMA failures.

Follow-up. Thirteen months after Hurricane Katrina made landfall in the United States, most of the respondents reported that they were still dealing with some of the same issues as in the first interviews, such as the FEMA deadlines for housing support. One respondent remarked, "A lot of people are still having housing problems and a lot of them cannot live alone. New Orleans is still stalling in rebuilding." They described themselves as having their lives on hold and seemed to be grieving for the loss of their city: "There is nothing to go back to, no jobs or homes." Yet that respondent's belief in a Higher Power remains: "I am trusting in the Lord. He will guide. I pray, and reading helps keep me spiritually uplifted."

Discussion

This exploratory analysis examined the coping of older Black Katrina survivors. In this sample, there was extensive reliance on a Higher Power to cope with the hurricane and its aftermath. Unceasing communication with a Higher Power represented an integral dimension of the respondents' faith and resulted in spiritual strength. Indeed, ongoing communication with a Higher Power has typically played a central role in Blacks' efforts to endure and respond to life's challenges.[14-16,25,45-46] The respondents in the present study viewed their relationship with God as personal, essential, and unique, providing comfort, inspiration, and guidance. Importantly, the respondents' spiritual practices and behaviors were not dependent on church attendance, or participation in organized church activities.

The continual talk with a Higher Power can be viewed as an expansion of prayer, and the respondents reported it as the most frequently used coping strategy. Clearly, unceasing communication with a Higher Power assisted the respondents in gaining control over threatening events. As a result, they often exhibited courage and determination to cope with the dislocation of Katrina. This is consistent with previous literature that documented that while other sources of well-being decline with age, relationship with a supreme being may become more important over time.[19-20,22]

A majority of the respondents reported that miracles had occurred in their lives during the hurricane and its aftermath. Understanding the respondents' belief in miracles when they prayed requires viewing their experiences from a particular perspective. Historically, Blacks have believed in and practiced the paradox of faith—the certainty of the uncertainty[14-16,51]—and reported having had spiritual experiences involving unexplainable coincidences.[25] Although the respondents in the present study experienced a great deal of pain and loss, these survivors expressed an unfaltering belief that the reality of miracles springs from living as people who are united with God.

The study also found that scriptures and inspirational materials served as sources of coping. Although, historically, Blacks have engaged in Bible-reading, the study finding that many of the respondents read inspirational books written by non-Black authors suggests some convergence of traditionally Black religious materials with those of their White American counterparts. The message is that the world is in a crisis, but that belief in old-time religion results in divine protection. This message was expressed by a large proportion of the participants.

The data reported here reveal that the tradition among Blacks of helping others, including older people, clearly helped these Katrina survivors cope. This is reminiscent of such historical practices as mutual benefit societies of early churches,[15] care-giving and support of neighbors, and the exchanges of goods, services, and shared bathrooms in depression-era Chicago tenements[14,54] Helping others less fortunate than themselves provided relief and the capacity to adjust and cope with the tragedy. These findings tie in with a more general body of literature indicating that, when faced with a threat, individuals will usually help others to bolster their self-esteem as well as to find emotional healing.[2,4,14,23-25] It is important to recognize that the act of assisting others combines a faith-based motive with psychological processes, resulting in the respondents' assisting others to cope with problems. Although people generally assist each other when a natural disaster strikes, in this sample, Blacks' religious faith guided their actions to help others.

Overall, the respondents' lifestyles and ethos can be viewed as important elements of social capital in view of the fact that Blacks' spiritual practices and religious beliefs often reflect positive coping. According to the World Health Organization, social capital is embodied in social norms and beliefs to facilitate support.[55] In this way, social capital enhances health. Consequently, in this sample, the positive effects of non-organizational spiritual practices may counterbalance some of the negative distress associated with Katrina.

Additional research is needed to clarify how different types of religious involvement may mediate the effects of a natural disaster. For instance, researchers must investigate how speaking in tongues, divine revelations, divine healing, visions, fasting, prophecies, and tithing as well as the usage of prayer cloths, praise dance, and listening to gospel music relate to the mental health of Blacks and others. Future research must address how physiological measures, spirituality, and coping are interrelated. Expressions of spirituality through service to others or passing on information to other older natural disaster survivors also deserves future research consideration. Understanding Blacks' spirituality provides an opportunity for assessing coping and for planning culturally appropriate disaster responses.

Limitations. The limitations of this study are the following: First, the respondents retrospectively recalled the Katrina experience. Second, the sample size is small and findings cannot be generalized without great caution to any larger group. Third, only one research site was utilized. It is unclear whether Katrina survivors in other housing arrangements (e.g., single family housing, traditional apartments) might recall different experiences. Fourth, the sample was homogeneous, mostly women of lower socioeconomic status. However, the sample is consistent with the demographics of Katrina survivors. The strength of this study is the use of in-depth interviews to discover perceived coping mechanisms immediately on the survivors' arrival in Texas.

Acknowledgments

We would like to thank the courageous survivors of Katrina who shared their stories with honesty, pain, and compassion. We would also like to thank the director of the residential facility who allowed us to conduct this study. The names used are pseudonyms.

Notes

1. Campanella TJ. Urban resilience and the recovery of New Orleans. Journal of the American Planning Association. 2006 Spring;72(2):141–7.
2. Bolin RC. Long-term family recovery from disaster. Boulder, CO: University of Colorado, 1982.
3. Pearlin LI, Schooler C. The structure of coping. J Health Soc Behav. 1978 Mar; 19(1):2–21.
4. Lazarus RS, Folkman S. Stress, appraisal and coping. New York: Springer, 1984.
5. Kobasa SC. Stressful life events, personality, and health: an inquiry into hardiness. J Pers Soc Psychol. 1979 Jan;37(1):1–11.
6. Weiss LG, Lonngquist, LE. The sociology of health, healing, and illness. Upper Saddle River, NJ: Prentice Hall, 2000.
7. Pescosolido BA. Beyond rational choice: the social dynamics of how people seek help. Am J Soc. 1992 Jan;97(4):1096–38.
8. Lazarus RS. Coping theory and research: past, present, and future. Psychosom Med. 1993 May–Jun;55(3):234–47.
9. Select Bipartisan Committee to Investigate the Preparation for and Response to Hurricane Katrina. Testimony of Major General Harold A. Cross, the Adjutant General of Mississippi. In: Select Bipartisan Committee to Investigate the Preparation for and Response to Hurricane Katrina. Hearing—Hurricane Katrina: preparedness and response by the Department of Defense, the Coast Guard, and the National Guard of Louisiana, Mississippi, and Alabama. Washington, DC: 109th Congress, Select Bipartisan Committee, 2005 Oct 27.
10. U.S. Senate Subcommittee on Bioterriosm and Public Health Preparedness (SBPHP). Hearing on Hurricane Katrina: public health and emergency preparedness. Washington, DC: 109th Congress, SBPHP, 2006 Feb 9.
11. Horner K. Evacuee survey gauges storm's mental toll. Dallas Morning News. 2006 March 10:A1, A5.
12. Select Bipartisan Committee to Investigate the Preparation for and Response to Hurricane Katrina. A failure of initiative: final report of the Select Bipartisan Committee to Investigate the Preparation for and Response to Hurricane Katrina. Washington, DC: U.S. Government Printing Office, 2006 Feb 15.
13. Louisiana Division of the Arts. In the wake of hurricanes: a coalition effort to collect our stories and rebuild our culture. Baton Rouge: Louisiana Division of the Arts, 2005. Available at http://www.louisianafolklife.org/katrina.html.
14. Meier A, Rudwick EM. From plantation to ghetto: an interpretive history of American negroes. New York: Hill and Wang, 1970.
15. Foner PS. History of Black Americans: from the emergence of the cotton kingdom to the eve of the compromise of 1850. Westport, CT: Greenwood Press, 1983.
16. DuBois WEB. Black reconstruction in America, 1860–1880. New York: Athenum, 1977.

17. Newlin K, Knafl K, Melkus GD. African-American spirituality: a concept analysis. ANS Adv Nurs Sci. 2002 Dec;25(2):57–70.

18. Chatters LM. Religion and health: pubic health research and practice. Annu Rev Public Health. 2000 May;21:335–67.

19. Koenig HG. Research on religion and aging: an annotated bibliography. Westport, CT: Greenwood, 1995.

20. Koenig HG, McCullough ME, Larson DB. Handbook of religion and health. New York: Oxford University Press, 2001.

21. Koenig HG, George LK, Seigler IC. The use of religion and other emotion-regulating coping strategies among older adults. Gerontologist. 1988 Jun;28(3):303–10.

22. Krause N, Van Tran T. Stress and religious involvement among older blacks. J Gerontol. 1989 Jan;44(1):S-13.

23. Brown DR, Keith V, Robinson Brown D, eds. In and out of our right minds: the mental health of African American women. New York: Columbia University Press 2003.

24. Klonoff, EA, Landrine H. Belief in the healing power of prayer: prevalence and health correlates for African Americans. West J Black Stud. 1996;20(4):207–10.

25. Watson W, ed. Black folk healing: the therapeutic significance of faith and trust. New Brunswick: Transaction Publishers, 1984.

26. Nelson-Becker, H. Religion and coping in older adults: a social work perspective. J Gerontol Soc Work. 2005;45(1–2):51–67.

27. Brown DR, Ndubuisi SC, Gary LE. Religiosity and psychological distress among Blacks. J Relig and Health. 1990 Mar;29(1):55–68.

28. Johnson KS, Elbert-Avila KI, Tulsky JA. The influence of spiritual beliefs and practices on the treatment preferences of African Americans: a review of the literature. J Am Geriatr Soc. 2005 Apr;53(4):711–19.

29. Chatters LM, Taylor RJ. Life problems and coping strategies of older Black adults. Soc Work. 1989;34:313–19.

30. McAdoo H. Stress levels, family help patterns, and religiosity in middle- and working-class African American single mothers. J Black Psychol. 1995;21(4):424–49.

31. Hill HM, Hawkins SR, Raposa M, et al. Relationship between multiple exposures to violence and coping strategies among African American mothers. Violence Vict. 1995 Spring;10(1):55–71.

32. Bryant-Davis T. Coping strategies of African American adult survivors of childhood violence. Prof Psychol Res Pr. 2005;36(4):409–14.

33. Constantine MG, Alleyne VL, Caldwell LD, et al. Coping responses of Asian, Black, and Latino/Latina New York City residents following the September 11, 2001 terrorist attacks against the United States. Cult Divers Ethnic Minor Psychol. 2005 Nov;11(4):293–308.

34. Cook DA, Wiley, CY. Psychotherapy with members of African American churches and spiritual traditions. In: Richards SP, Bergin AE, eds. Handbook of psychotherapy and religious diversity. Washington, DC: American Psychological Association, 2000.

35. Taylor RJ, Chatters LM, Jayakody R, et al. Black and White differences in religious participation: a multisample comparison. J Sci Study Relig. 1996 Dec;35(4):403–10.

36. Banks-Wallace J, Parks L. It's all sacred: African American women's perspectives on spirituality. Issues Ment Health Nurs. 2004 Jan–Feb;25(1):25–45.

37. Lawson EJ. A narrative analysis: a black woman's perceptions of breast cancer risks and early breast cancer detection. Cancer Nurs. 1998 Aug;21(6):421–9.

38. Bourjolly J. Differences in religiousness among black and white women with breast cancer. Soc Work Health Care. 1998;28(1):21–39.

39. Culver JL, Arena PL, Antoni MH, et al. Coping and distress among women under treatment for early stage breast cancer: comparing African Americans, Hispanics, and non-Hispanic Whites. Psychooncology. 2002 Nov–Dec;11(6):495–504.

40. Chester DN, Himburg SP, Weatherspoon LJ. Spirituality of African-American women: correlations to health-promoting behaviors. J Natl Black Nurses Assoc. 2006 Jul;17(1):1–8.

41. Waite PJ, Hawks SR, Gast JA. The correlation between spiritual well-being and health behaviors. Am J Health Promot. 1999 Jan–Feb;13(4):159–62.

42. Simoni JM, Martone MG, Kerwin JF. Spirituality and psychological adaptation among women with HIV/AIDS: implications for counseling. J Couns Psychol. 2002;49(2): 139–47.

43. Brome DR, Owens MD, Allen K, Vevaina T. An examination of spirituality among African American women in recovery from substance abuse. J Black Psychol. 2000; 26(4): 470–86.

44. Becker G, Newsom E. Resilience in the face of serious illness among chronically ill African Americans in later life. J Gerontol B Psycho Sci Soc Sci. 2005 Jul;60(4): S214–23.

45. Billingsley A. Climbing Jacob's ladder: enduring legacy of African American families. New York: Simon & Schuster, 1992.

46. Lincoln CE, Mamiya LH. The Black church in the African American experience. Durham, NC: Duke University Press, 1990.

47. Tully MA. Lifting our voices: African American cultural responses to trauma and loss. In: Nader K, Dubrow N, Stamm H, eds. Honoring differences: cultural issues in the treatment of trauma and loss. Philadelphia: Brunner/Mazel, 1999.

48. Joseph M. The effect of strong religious beliefs on coping with stress. Stress and Health. 1998 Oct;14(4):219–24.

49. Cohen H, Thomas C, Williamson C, et al. Meaning of religion and spirituality for older adults: Jewish, African American and Caucasian perspectives. J Gerontol Soc Work. (In press.)

50. Glaser BG, Strauss AL. The discovery of grounded theory. Chicago: Aldine Transaction, 1967.

51. Glaser BG, Strauss AL. Time for dying. Chicago: Aldine Transaction, 1967.

52. Denzin NK. Interpretive ethnography. Thousand Oaks, CA: Sage, 1997.

53. Murphy E, Dingwall R, Greatbatch D, et al. Qualitative research methods in health technology assessment: a review of the literature. Health Technol Assess. 1998 Aug; 2(16):iii–ix, 1–274.

54. Giddings PJ. When and where I enter. The impact of Black women on race and sex in America. New York: Bantam Books, 1984.

55. Baum F. Social capital, economic capital and power: further issues for a public health agenda. J Epidemiol Community Health. 2000 Jun;54(6):409–10.

PART II: Assessment

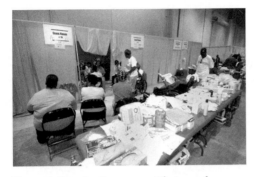

Figure 6. Examination rooms. Photograph courtesy of the Baylor College of Medicine Office of Public Affairs.

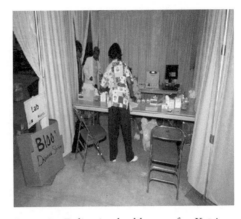

Figure 7a. Delivering health care after Katrina. Photograph courtesy of the Baylor College of Medicine Office of Public Affairs.

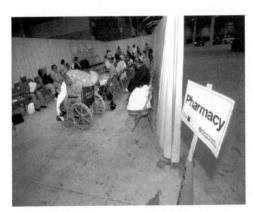

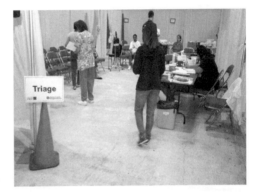

Figures 7b–d. Delivering health care after Katrina. Photographs courtesy of the Baylor College of Medicine Office of Public Affairs.

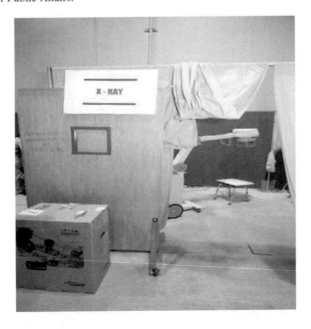

Chapter 13
The Hurricane Choir: Remote Mental Health Monitoring of Participants in a Community-based Intervention in the Post-Katrina Period

Robin Harvey, PhD
Michael Smith, BSc
Nicholas Abraham, PhD
Sean Hood, MD, PhD, FRCAP
Dennis Tannenbaum, MD, FRCAP

Introduction

Natural disasters such as the hurricanes that struck the coast of southern Louisiana, Mississippi, and Texas in 2005 are synonymous with the destruction of the physical environment and the depletion of material assets of individuals and whole communities. They are unique in that the widespread destruction they cause often results in collective trauma in which whole communities find themselves engulfed in severe shock.[1] In the case of the 2005 hurricane season, the rapid succession of a number of large and destructive hurricanes is likely to have intensified the psychological impact of the disasters, as infrastructure that survived previous storms was destroyed, rebuilding efforts were restricted, and stressors on survivors were exacerbated and drawn out over a long period.

Typically, post-disaster stress symptoms include (among others) recurrent nightmares, intrusive memories, hypervigilant arousal, impaired concentration, depression, emotional detachment from others, and disengagement from parts of life that were previously rewarding.[1,2] With exposure to such severe psychological distress, post-traumatic stress disorder (PTSD) can develop, having a severe impact on healthy functioning and making emergence from the effects of a disaster much more difficult.[3] For example, David and colleagues[4] demonstrated that 51% of survivors who were exposed to Hurricane Andrew developed a new-onset psychiatric disorder. Of these, PTSD was the most common (at 36%), followed by major depression (30%) and generalized anxiety

ROBIN HARVEY *is a registered psychologist and Research and Development Manager at Sentiens Pty Ltd. and an External Research Associate at the University of Western Australia (UWA) in Perth.* **MICHAEL SMITH,** *the corresponding author, is a Research Officer at Sentiens and a doctoral candidate in the School of Psychology at UWA.* **NICHOLAS ABRAHAM** *is a counsellor and Chief Executive Officer of the Abraham Group LLC in Washington, DC.* **SEAN HOOD** *is a consultant psychiatrist at Sentiens and a Senior Lecturer at UWA.* **DENNIS TANNENBAUM** *is a consultant psychiatrist at Sentiens.*

disorder (11%). Moreover these researchers found significant co-morbidity, with 68% of PTSD sufferers also satisfying the clinical criteria for major depression.

In the case of the hurricane disaster of 2005, it is possible that the prevalence rates of psychological trauma are likely to be associated with the presence or absence of community risk factors. Prior to Hurricane Katrina, data from the U.S. Census (2000) highlighted the fact that New Orleans had an 18% poverty rate and was one of the poorest metropolitan centers in the country.[5] Nationally, New Orleans was ranked in the bottom 20% for the educational qualifications of its residents. Class and race divisions were prevalent, with two thirds of the Black population living in the inner city of New Orleans in contrast to a predominantly White suburban population. In short, the region of New Orleans was growing slowly, struggling with issues such as segregation, concentrations of chronic poverty in Black communities, and underemployment.[6] Given these disadvantages, it is probable that the region was particularly ill-equipped to tackle the devastating impact of Hurricane Katrina.

The Hurricane Choir. Being a member of a functional community can have broad benefits to mental health.[7-11] As suggested by Norris and colleagues, it is necessary to develop ongoing assistance and interventions that provide mental health care to disaster victims in a way that is "culturally appropriate and feasible."[12,p.291] Given the musical heritage of South Louisiana, a culturally appropriate community initiative in the post-hurricane period was a choir, organized by Australian choral leader Martin Meader in Baton Rouge, Louisiana. The choir (called the *Hurricane Choir*) comprised hurricane disaster evacuees and survivors who rehearsed and performed to live audiences. The choir commenced six months after the hurricane disasters and had a 12-week intensive rehearsal period that culminated in three public performances in the American Spring of 2006. Rehearsals were held three times a week in local churches, community centers, and evacuee villages.

The organizers of the Hurricane Choir were keen for the mental health outcomes of choir participants to be monitored during rehearsals. Subsequently, researchers from Sentiens, an Australian health care company, and the University of Western Australia were invited by the choir organizers to collaborate in the project and develop a strategy to track the mental health outcomes of choir participants.

Ours was a naturalistic research project and we did not attempt to influence the planning and processes involved with the formation of the choir. A web-based monitoring system was used to record the experiences of participants before and after the hurricane disaster and to measure self-reported levels of psychological distress. The platform technology of the online system was developed by Sentiens and has been used successfully in mental health clinical applications in Perth, Western Australia, since 2002.[13-14]

Enrollment and procedure. Choir members had a window of one month to enroll into the research. The project was promoted to existing choir members at rehearsal nights in which they were directed to a web-based enrollment page hosted by the researchers. Informed consent was sought at choir rehearsals and electronically via a web page. Incorporated into the enrollment phase was some basic data collection on demographics, medical histories (including incidence of past psychiatric disorders), and social networks. Access to the Internet was provided at the choir rehearsal facility on donated computers. Alternatively, participants were encouraged to complete the questionnaires at home if they had access to the Internet.

It was a requirement that all participants have an e-mail address; however, it was recognized that not all participants would have e-mail addresses and would not be skilled at using computers. A guide to setting up e-mail accounts was provided and volunteers were available to assist those who required help with the technology. In addition, participants could request extra assistance in completing the project. This assistance included help with the technology and help comprehending and understanding the content delivered to them.

While the web-based system has the facility to deliver evidence-based therapy (e.g., cognitive behavioral therapy), this feature was not used for this project as researchers wanted to measure only the impact of the Hurricane Choir on mental health. Prior approval by the University of Western Australia Human Research Ethics Committee was obtained and a local counselor was on hand to provide extra assistance to any distressed participants (although no participants required this assistance during the study). Access to brochures promoting mental health literacy was also supplied.

Data were collected at scheduled sessions, each of which covered a period of 5 days in which measures were administered. Automatically generated e-mail reminders notified and encouraged participants to adhere to the research schedule. If a participant logged on during a session week, they were directed to the measures that were scheduled. In addition to administration of questionnaires, an e-diary was available to participants to enter any thoughts and feelings they may have had.

Data collection. Measures were taken prior to the initial rehearsals for the choir with repeated measures occurring midway through the rehearsal period and immediately before the final performances. Eighty five percent of the original 150 choir participants consented to participate in the research project (n=127). Eighty per cent of those who gave their consent (n=102) subsequently completed online enrollment and one or more scheduled sessions. Standardized mental health and attitudinal measures included:

- Depression, Anxiety, and Stress Scales (DASS)[15]
- Davidson Trauma Scale[16]
- Life Orientation Test Revised (LOT-R)[17]
- Hurricane Coping Self-Efficacy Scale (HCSE)[18]
- A modified version of the Inventory of Socially Supportive Behaviours (ISSB)[19]

Additional data were collected to identify risk and resilience factors for individual participants. These included:

- age, sex, marital status, dependents, level of education;
- level of resource loss (including financial loss and loss of housing and employment);
- availability of family support and social networks;
- impact of the hurricane on the individual in the first week after the disaster;
- experiences of loss (including bereavement);

- perceived level of social and community support, including religious commitment; and
- presence/absence of pre-existing mental health and other medical conditions.

Preliminary outcomes. A complete analysis of the full set of data is planned when the follow-up data are collected. Some preliminary outcomes are presented here. First, at the beginning of the choir, disruption to family functioning, loss of optimism, and drug and mental health problems were the most common problems (Table 1). To expand upon this, it should be noted that losses were severe: a substantial number of choir members had lost a friend or family member in the disaster. Second, qualitative feedback from participants and volunteers indicated that those who were initially anxious about using computers for the research grew to enjoy it when they realized that they would be supported through the early learning process. Finally, local government and non-government agencies in the disaster zone recognized the value of the project in tracking mental health remotely, provided sponsorship and support, and expressed particular interest in using the system to monitor the mental health of their aid workers and to provide accessible, online psycho-education in the area of stress management.

Unfortunately, the project was not without some limitations. It is possible that early disorganization by choir organizers in the establishment phase of the choir discouraged individuals who were highly stressed from joining the choir. For example, coping with change is very challenging to individuals with PTSD and there were frequent changes to rehearsal dates and venues in the early stages of choir recruitment. Coupled with this, transportation difficulties reduced choir participation rates for evacuees despite their enthusiasm for the project. However, despite the above problems, the paradigm employed in this study provided the opportunity for disadvantaged and traumatised members of a community to utilize online monitoring, enabling tracking of mental health outcomes in the context of disaster recovery.

Table 1.

PRESENCE OF STRESSORS CAUSED BY 2005 HURRICANE SEASON, BEGINNING OF REHEARSALS, N=102

Risk variable	Percentage of choir participants
Loss of family or friend in the hurricane disaster	11
High or moderate level of family disruption	18
Disruption to family functioning	88
Pre-existing medical conditions that had not received appropriate care	35
Loss of optimism	75
Drug problems and mental health problems	41
Loss of control	37
Loss of psychological resources	26
Loss of monetary resources	20

A Final Comment

This summary introduces a novel naturalistic research project using Internet-based monitoring to track the mental health outcomes of participants in a community choir following Hurricane Katrina. To a large extent this project succeeded; researchers from Australia were able to engage and recruit the majority of participants from the choir and monitor their mental health during their rehearsals in Louisiana.

It should be recognized that the choir provided a strategy to assist survivors of the hurricanes who might not otherwise have been able to get direct psychological support from mental health professionals. Although there were federal funds directed to crisis counselling, these were underutilized by survivors of the hurricane.[20] It is difficult to know why this was the case but examination of the tracking data provided by the Brookings Institution suggests that, despite high levels of trauma, there were lower percentages of health professionals available to provide support to survivors in New Orleans and Louisiana than are available in the U.S. more generally. In addition many people may have found it hard to acknowledge their vulnerability and seek mental health support. The choir provided a non-stigmatised and supportive environment in which individuals could find support and develop social networks. It is hoped such projects assist disaster survivors to feel increased social support and a greater sense of community cohesion, and lead to improved coping skills that may increase resilience to PTSD. Further analysis of longitudinal data from the project will aim to find evidence for this.

Notes

1. Benight CC, Bandura A. Social cognitive theory of posttraumatic recovery: the role of perceived self-efficacy. Behav. Res Ther. 2004 Oct;42(10):1129–48.
2. Williams R. The psychosocial consequences for children and young people who are exposed to terrorism, war, conflict and natural disasters. Curr Opin Psychiatry. 2006 Jul;19(4):337–49.
3. McMillen JC, North CS, Smith EM. What parts of PTSD are normal: intrusion, avoidance, or arousal? Data from Northridge, California, earthquake. J Traumatic Stress. 2000 Jan;13(1):57–75.
4. David D, Mellman TA, Mendoza LM, et al. Psychiatric morbidity following Hurricane Andrew. J Traumatic Stress. 1996 Jul;9(3):607–12.
5. U.S. Census Bureau. United States and States—percent of people below poverty level in the past 12 months (for whom poverty status is determined): 2002. Washington, DC: U.S. Census Bureau, American FactFinder, 2003.
6. The Brookings Institute. New Orleans after the storm: lessons from the past, a plan for the future. Washington, DC: Brookings Institution, 2005.
7. Goenjian AK, Steinberg AM, Najarian LM, et al. Prospective study of posttraumatic stress, anxiety, and depressive reactions after earthquake and political violence. Am J Psychiatry. 2000 Jun;157(6):911–6.
8. Middleton KL, Willner J, Simmons KM. Natural disasters and posttraumatic stress disorder symptom complex: evidence from the Oklahoma tornado outbreak. International Journal of Stress Management. 2002;9(3):229–36.

9.   U.S. Department of Health and Human Services. Developing cultural competence in disaster mental health programs: guiding principles and recommendations. (DHHS Pub. No. SMA 3828.) Rockville, MD: Center for Mental Health Services, Substance Abuse and Mental Health Services Administration, 2003.

10. Ziersch AM, Baum FE, MacDougall C, et al. Neighbourhood life and social capital: the implications for health. Soc Sci Med. 2005 Jan;60(1):71–86.

11. Aneshensel CS, Sucoff CA. The neighborhood context of adolescent mental health. J Health and Soc Behav. 1996 Dec;37(4):293–310.

12. Norris FH, Kaniasty K. Received and perceived social support in times of stress: a test of the social support deterioration deterrence model. J Pers Soc Psychol. 1996 Sep;71(3):498–511.

13. Robertson L, Smith M, Tannenbaum D. Case management and adherence to an online disease management system. J Telemed Telecare. 2005;11 Supp 2:S73–5.

14. Robertson L, Smith M, Castle D, et al. Using the Internet to enhance the treatment of depression. Australas Psychiatry. 2006 Dec;14(4):413–7.

15. Lovibond PF, Lovibond SH. The structure of negative emotional states: comparison of the Depression Anxiety Stress Scales (DASS) with the Beck Depression and Anxiety Inventories. Behav Res Ther. 1995 Mar;33(3):335–43.

16. Davidson JR, Book SW, Colket JT, et al. Assessment of a new self-rating scale for posttraumatic stress disorder. Psychol Med. 1999 Jan;27(1):153–60.

17. Scheier MF, Carver CS, Bridges MW. Distinguishing optimism from neuroticism (and trait anxiety, self-mastery, and self-esteem): a reevaluation of the Life Orientation Test. J Pers Soc Psychol. 1994 Dec;67(6):1063–78.

18. Benight CC, Ironson G, Durham RL. Psychometric properties of a hurricane coping self-efficacy measure. J Trauma Stress. 1999 Apr;12(2):379–86.

19. Barrera M Jr, Sandler IN, Ramsay TB. Preliminary development of a scale of social support: studies on college students. Am J Community Psychol. 1981 Aug;9(4): 435–47.

20. Katz B, Fellowes M, Mabanta M. Katrina index: tracking variables of post-Katrina reconstruction. Washington, DC: The Brookings Institute, 2006 Feb 1.

Chapter 14
Rapid Needs Assessment among Hurricane Katrina Evacuees in Metro-Denver

Tista S. Ghosh, MD, MPH
Jennifer L. Patnaik, MSPH
Richard L. Vogt, MD

O n August 29, 2005, Hurricane Katrina, a category 4 hurricane, struck the Gulf Coast of the United States, causing massive destruction and population displacement throughout the region.[1,2] As a result, hundreds of thousands of Gulf Coast residents were evacuated to at least 18 different states.[1-3] On September 3, 2005, Colorado was officially asked to provide assistance to Gulf Coast evacuees. By September 4, 2005, the first planeloads of evacuees arrived in metropolitan Denver, and were housed in dormitories at the former Lowry Air Force Base. Over the next four weeks, 3,600 evacuees registered at Lowry, with an average of 400 people in residence per day. To identify medical and non-medical service needs in this population, Tri-County Health Department (TCHD), Colorado's largest local health department, conducted a rapid needs assessment among a sample of evacuee households at Lowry, who arrived during the week of September 4, 2005. The results were used to meet the identified needs of the evacuee population as a whole and also to identify differential needs among evacuee sub-populations.

Methods

From September 4 to 9, 2005, during the first week of the evacuees' arrival, a rapid needs assessment was conducted among a sample of newly arriving evacuees. The aim was to prepare for the needs of these evacuees and of future evacuees expected to arrive in the following weeks. All evacuees who registered at Lowry during the first week were sent by bus to a Red Cross Family Assistance center to register with the Federal Emergency Management Association (FEMA). Out of eight buses sent from Lowry to the Assistance Center that week, two buses were randomly selected. Every household represented in these two buses was surveyed. Trained TCHD personnel conducted structured, standardized interviews of the heads of each household. The interview questionnaire was designed by TCHD to assess evacuee demographics, self-reported acute and chronic medical conditions, service needs, and plans to remain in

TISTA GHOSH is the Medical Advisor at the Tri-County Health Department in Greenwood Village, Colorado, where JENNIFER PATNAIK is the Epidemiology Program Manager and RICHARD VOGT is the Executive Director.

Colorado. This methodology, as part of a preliminary report on evacuee surveillance, has been described elsewhere.[4]

The data from this survey were analyzed in SAS 9.1. to assess the distribution of evacuee needs. Analyses comparing the needs of non-Hispanic Black and non-Hispanic White evacuees were also conducted, using unadjusted chi-square analyses. Other races were excluded from this comparison due to small numbers.

Results

A total of 106 households were surveyed. No heads of households refused to participate, resulting in a 100% response rate. Among heads of households surveyed, the majority (54.6%) were non-Hispanic Blacks (Table 1). There were a mean number of 3.8 family members per household. The majority of evacuee households (83.2%) arrived from Louisiana, and 61.4% were from New Orleans. Common chronic medical conditions among households included hypertension (28.4%), depression/psychiatric illnesses (23.2%), asthma/chronic lung disease (21.1%), cardiovascular disease (17.9%), and diabetes (13.7%) (Table 2).

The most common acute medical symptoms among households seemed consistent with altitude sickness, including excessive thirst (33.7%), dizziness/lightheadedness (21.8%), and difficulty breathing (18.8%) (Table 2). These symptoms remained prevalent even when households including people with asthma or chronic lung conditions were removed from the analysis. Among households without any members with asthma or chronic lung diseases, 31% had members with excessive thirst, 20% dizziness/light-headedness, and 16% difficulty breathing.

Among all households surveyed, 60.2% had one or more family members requiring prescription medications. Of those households requiring prescriptions, 38.8% were lacking them at the time of the survey, and 42.7% had members who had gone without their prescriptions at some point as a result of Hurricane Katrina. The most common long-term service needs included medical services, health insurance, housing assistance, and clothing, particularly winter clothes (Table 3). While most services were already being offered, many evacuees seemed unaware of their availability. Among those surveyed, 49.1% of households planned to stay in Colorado permanently, suggesting the need to provide these services over an extended period of time.

Several racial differences were noted in this assessment. Non-Hispanic Blacks were significantly more likely to be from Louisiana than non-Hispanic Whites (92.3% of Blacks versus 70.6% of Whites, p=0.01). Blacks were significantly more likely than Whites to require employment services (43.4% of Blacks versus 17.1% of Whites, p=0.01). They were also significantly more likely to require housing assistance (58.5% of Blacks versus 34.3% of Whites, p=.03) and dental services (62.3% of Blacks versus of 37.1% Whites, p=.02) (Table 3). No significant racial differences were seen in acute medical conditions or in prescription needs. Furthermore, Blacks were not more likely than Whites to want to remain in Colorado.

Table 1.

DEMOGRAPHICS OF HEADS OF HOUSEHOLDS, N=106

	N	%
Sex		
Male	58	54.7
Female	48	45.3
Race/ethnicity[a]		
Non-Hispanic Black	53	54.6
Non-Hispanic White	35	36.1
Hispanic White	6	6.2
Asian/Pacific Islander	2	2.1
Native American	1	1.0
Home state[b]		
Louisiana	84	83.2
Mississippi	17	16.8

[a] Nine (9) people did not provide information on race/ethnicity.
[b] Five (5) people did not provide information on their home state.

Discussion

Disasters can lead to illness, injury, devastation of homes, disruptions of essential services, and the displacement of populations. In post-disaster settings, it is important to gather real-time data on the characteristics and needs of the affected population, in order to respond appropriately.[5,6] Rapid needs assessments can provide essential information on medical and non-medical needs in post-disaster situations.[7-9] This is true, not only in the disaster setting itself, but also in locations outside the disaster area to which displaced people go.[10,11]

Traditionally, public health assessments among displaced populations have focused on infectious disease-related issues, since evacuees are often subject to unclean living conditions that can facilitate infectious diseases transmission.[6,12] However, needs assessments should also focus on chronic diseases within displaced populations. Chronic diseases can be exacerbated in post-disaster settings, due to stress, injury, and disrupted access to health care.[6,12] The TCHD rapid needs assessment provided insight into the types of chronic medical conditions affecting evacuees, along with related needs. For instance, it identified a large need for prescription medications, which was accommodated mainly through a clinic established on-site at the Lowry base. It was important to meet this prescription need quickly, in order to control chronic illnesses and avoid complications.

The TCHD rapid needs assessment also proved useful in identifying a unique region-specific need for altitude sickness education. Altitude sickness is seen during rapid ascents to higher elevations, and is associated with symptoms of dizziness, shortness

Table 2.

SELF-REPORTED ACUTE AND CHRONIC MEDICAL CONDITIONS AMONG HURRICANE KATRINA EVACUEE HOUSEHOLDS, N=106

	% of households	Mean no. per household
Acute medical conditions		
Excessive thirst	33.7	2.9
Dizziness/lightheadedness	21.8	1.3
Difficulty breathing	18.8	1.6
Cough	16.8	1.5
Diarrhea or vomiting	11.9	1.4
Skin rashes	11.9	1.0
Cuts and bruises	9.9	1.0
Fever or chills	6.9	1.5
Chest pain	6.0	1.0
Broken bones	3.0	1.0
Eye infection	3.0	1.0
Animal bites	2.0	1.0
Other[a]	10.0	1.3
Chronic medical conditions		
High blood pressure	28.4	2.4
Depression/anxiety	23.2	2.9
Asthma/chronic lung disease	21.1	1.1
Heart disease	17.9	1.1
Diabetes	13.7	1.3
Cancer	6.3	1.0
Pregnancy	5.3	1.0
Stroke	3.2	1.3
Seizures	3.2	1.0
Liver disease	2.1	1.0
Kidney disease	1.1	1.0
Other[b]	9.6	1.3

[a]Other acute conditions included nose bleeds, allergies, acute congestive heart failure, insect bites, back and joint pain, and strep throat.
[b]Other chronic conditions included arthritis, gout, hypothyroidism, and glaucoma.

of breath, nausea, and headache.[13] Symptoms of dehydration, such as excessive thirst, can also be worsened with increasing elevation.[13,14] The rapid arrival of the evacuees from sea level to the altitude of the Denver area (5,280 feet) may thus have accounted for the high prevalence of lightheadedness, excessive thirst, and difficulty breathing among evacuee households, including in households without any chronic lung con-

Table 3.

SERVICE NEEDS AMONG HURRICANE KATRINA EVACUEES: NON-HISPANIC BLACK VS. NON-HISPANIC WHITE HOUSEHOLDS

Type of service	Total households % (n=106)	Black households % (n=53)	White households % (n=35)	P-value[a]
Medical services	51.0	50.9	54.3	.76
Health insurance	47.2	49.1	42.9	.57
Housing assistance	46.2	58.5	34.3	**.03**
More clothing	45.3	54.7	37.1	.11
Dental services	45.3	62.3	37.1	**.02**
Vision services	43.3	47.2	34.3	.23
Employment	34.0	43.4	17.1	**.01**
Transportation	32.1	41.5	22.9	.07
Schools	20.8	22.6	14.3	.33
Immunizations	19.8	20.1	17.1	.67
WIC services	15.1	11.3	25.7	.08
Birth control	14.2	13.2	17.1	.61
Child care	13.2	17.0	8.6	.26
More food/water	13.2	17.1	23.1	.55
Legal services	12.3	17.0	5.7	.12
Grief counseling	12.3	11.3	8.6	.68
Religious	10.3	11.3	11.4	.99
Pet services	6.6	3.8	4.6	.16

[a] P-values are based on unadjusted chi-square analyses of responses from Black heads of households versus White heads of households. Bolded values are considered statistically significant ($p<.05$).

ditions. These findings prompted TCHD to raise evacuee awareness of the effects of Denver's altitude. Health department nurses began to provide altitude sickness education to all evacuees during their initial registration at Lowry. Health department nurses also began to educate evacuees on the availability of a variety of services during their initial registration, since the needs assessment indicated a lack of evacuee awareness of services being offered.

The TCHD rapid needs assessment also provided useful information regarding the racial/ethnic distribution of the evacuee population. In this instance, the predominant racial group identified among evacuees (55% non-Hispanic Black) was vastly different from that of the native population (3.8% non-Hispanic Black) in Colorado.[15] This marked difference helped TCHD and partner agencies recognize the need for culturally competent individuals to interact with the evacuees. Thus, to meet the needs of this predominantly Black population in a culturally appropriate manner, Black church groups and other Black community leaders were asked to participate in evacuee-service efforts.

The TCHD rapid needs assessment was also helpful in identifying differential needs based on race. Non-Hispanic Black households were more likely than non-Hispanic White households to require employment, housing, and dental services, although they were just as likely to plan to stay in Colorado long-term. These differences may reflect racial disparities in the state of Louisiana, from where the majority of Black households arrived, or they may be related to socioeconomic class differences or other factors. The TCHD needs assessment was designed under urgent circumstances to identify acute medical and service needs and was therefore limited in its ability to identify the reasons behind these racial disparities. The survey did not ask about income, education level, previous use of government services, or other variables that may have played a role. A more in-depth assessment of these racial disparities might have helped TCHD and its partner agencies better meet the needs of the non-Hispanic Black evacuees. In future post-disaster situations, it is important that public health agencies like TCHD consider the importance of disparities in race, class, and gender when designing and conducting needs assessments in displaced populations, particularly when dealing with groups that are less familiar to or less prevalent in the native population.

Another limitation of the TCHD needs assessment was its sampling method. Designed during emergent, rapidly changing circumstances, the sampling method may have limited the survey's representativeness of the entire evacuee population at Lowry. Furthermore, the needs assessment was conducted during a one-week period among the first group of evacuees arriving at Lowry. The needs of evacuees arriving in the following three weeks may have differed from those of this initial group. Moreover, the initial group's needs may have changed over time. In future post-disaster settings, public health agencies like TCHD should consider repeating needs assessments to identify changing characteristics and needs in the affected populations.

Rapid needs assessments can serve as a valuable tool in identifying unique regional, cultural, and other unanticipated needs in displaced populations. These types of assessments should be conducted routinely in emergency settings, both at the site of the disaster and in evacuation areas, since needs may vary based on location.[11] Repeat assessments may also be useful in identifying new or shifting needs. Furthermore, the detection of racial, class, or gender disparities among displaced persons should be an important consideration when designing and conducting rapid needs assessments, in order better to identify and meet the distinctive needs of sub-populations.

Acknowledgments

Stacy Weinberg, Leslie Smith, and Julie Uhernik at Tri-County Health Dept. and Wendy Bamberg at the Colorado Department of Public Health and Environment provided valuable assistance in survey design and data collection.

Notes

1. Centers for Disease Control and Prevention (CDC). Public health response to Hurricanes Katrina and Rita—United States, 2005. MMWR Morb Mortal Wkly Rep. 2006 Mar 10;55(09):229–31.

2. Brodie M, Weltzien E, Altman D, et al. Experiences of hurricane Katrina evacuees in Houston shelters: implications for future planning. Am J Public Health. 2006 Aug; 96(8):1402–8.

3. Centers for Disease Control and Prevention (CDC). Infectious disease and dermatologic conditions in evacuees and rescue workers after Hurricane Katrina—multiple states, August–September, 2005. MMWR Morb Mortal Wkly Rep. 2005 Sep 30; 54(38):961–4.

4. Centers for Disease Control and Prevention (CDC). Illness surveillance and rapid needs assessment among Hurricane Katrina evacuees—Colorado, September 1–23, 2005. MMWR Morb Mortal Wkly Rep. 2006 Mar 10;55(9):244–7.

5. Bradt DA, Drummond CM. Rapid epidemiological assessment of health status in displaced populations—an evolution toward standardized minimum, essential data sets. Prehospital Disaster Med. 2002 Oct–Dec;17(4):178–85.

6. Mokdad AH, Mensah GA, Posner SF, et al. When chronic conditions become acute: prevention and control of chronic diseases and adverse health outcomes during natural disasters. Prev Chronic Dis. 2005 Nov;2 Spec no:A04.

7. Ogden CL, Gibbs-Scharf LI, Kohn MA, et al. Emergency health surveillance after severe flooding in Louisiana, 1995. Prehospital Disaster Med. 2001 Jul–Sep;16(3):138–44.

8. Centers for Disease Control and Prevention (CDC). Community needs assessment and morbidity surveillance following an ice storm—Maine, January 1998. MMWR Morb Mortal Wkly Rep. 1998 May 8;47(17):351–4.

9. Centers for Disease Control and Prevention (CDC). Rapid community health and needs assessments after Hurricanes Isabel and Charley—North Carolina, 2003–2004. MMWR Morb Mortal Wkly Rep. 2004 Sep 17;53(36):840–2.

10. Bennett C, Mein J, Beers M, et al. Operation Safe Haven: an evaluation of health surveillance and monitoring in an acute setting. Commun Dis Intell. 2000 Feb 17; 24(2):21–6.

11. Toole MJ. The rapid assessment of health problems in refugee and displaced populations. M & GS (Medicine and Global Survival). 1994;1:2007.

12. Greenough PG, Kirsch TD. Hurricane Katrina. Public health response—assessing needs. N Engl J Med. 2005 Oct 13;353(15):1544–6.

13. Dennie ML, Bayley EW. Into thinner air. Am J Nurs. 2002 Sep;Suppl:8–12.

14. Cumbo TA, Basnyat B, Graham J, et al. Acute mountain sickness, dehydration, and bicarbonate clearance: preliminary field data from the Nepal Himalaya. Aviat Space Environ Med. 2002 Sep;73(9):898–901.

15. U.S. Census Bureau. 2000 Census. Table DP-1. Profile of General Demographic Characteristics: 2000. Geographic Area: Colorado. Washington, DC: U.S. Census Bureau, 2000.

Chapter 15
Displacement of the Underserved: Medical Needs of Hurricane Katrina Evacuees in West Virginia

Marilyn L. Ridenour, BSN, MBA, MPH
Kristin J. Cummings, MD, MPH
Julie R. Sinclair, DVM
Danae Bixler, MD

On August 29, 2005, Hurricane Katrina made landfall as a Category 4 storm near Buras, Louisiana, 60 miles south of New Orleans.[1] Because Hurricane Katrina was very large, it pushed record storm surges onshore, affecting the entire Mississippi Gulf Coast and parts of Alabama. Unprecedented flooding, particularly in New Orleans and surrounding parishes ensued. As of October 6, 2005, a total of 1,185 Gulf Coast fatalities due to Hurricane Katrina had been confirmed and property damage was estimated to be $200 billion, topping 1992's Hurricane Andrew as the most expensive in the U.S. history.[2]

Hurricane Katrina displaced approximately one million people from the Gulf Coast region.[3] Evacuation centers were established in the affected states as well as neighboring Texas, which sheltered an estimated 250,000 evacuees in the days following the storm.[4] The response ultimately took on a national scope, with over 1,000 evacuation centers in 27 states involved.[5] This chapter reports on the experiences at one of those evacuation centers in the state of West Virginia.

West Virginia is a landlocked, mountainous state approximately 1,000 miles from the Gulf Coast. Evacuees arrived in the state capitol of Charleston by air, and then traveled approximately 165 miles by bus to the evacuation center. The evacuation center was established at an Army National Guard Training Site Command with ongoing activities and provided temporary housing for the evacuees. More than 300 evacuees arrived at

Disclaimer: The findings and conclusions in this report are those of the authors and do not necessarily represent the views of the National Institute for Occupational Safety and Health or the Centers for Disease Control and Prevention.

MARILYN RIDENOUR is an Epidemic Intelligence Service Officer (EISO) with the Centers for Disease Control and Prevention (CDC), National Institute for Occupational Safety and Health (NIOSH), Division of Safety Research (DSR). **KRISTIN CUMMINGS** is also an EISO with NIOSH, in the Division of Respiratory Disease Studies, in Morgantown. **JULIE SINCLAIR** is a Career Epidemiology Field Officer with the CDC and is also with the U.S. Public Health Service in the Philadelphia Department of Public Health. **DANAE BIXLER** is the Director of Infectious Disease Epidemiology with the West Virginia Bureau of Public Health in Charleston, West Virginia.

the evacuation center between September 4–7, 2005. Relief workers at the evacuation center included Red Cross volunteers; local, state, and national public health personnel; and representatives of other community groups. The center was operational until October 1, 2005, at which point all evacuees had, with Red Cross assistance, found alternative housing.

At the center, evacuees were housed in communal barracks by family status, sex, and special needs. The barracks had communal showers, bunk beds, and large lockers. Two Red Cross volunteers per floor monitored the barracks. There were two hand-washing stations (four spigots per station) outside of the mess hall, where meals were served cafeteria-style. Bus service to local shopping centers was provided periodically. West Virginia University (WVU) health care providers established a temporary on-site medical clinic to provide basic diagnostic and therapeutic services, prescription medications, and referrals. The clinic was operational from the time of the evacuees' arrival.

To provide appropriate medical, dental, mental health and social services to the evacuees, the West Virginia Department of Health and Human Resources (WVDHHR) and the U.S. Centers for Disease Control and Prevention (CDC) conducted a medical needs assessment from September 9–12, 2005. The objective was to identify current needs and to coordinate the provision of care and services in collaboration with state and local partners.

Methods

The WVDHHR requested assistance from the CDC to assess the medical, dental, mental health, and social service needs of evacuees at this center. Two Epidemic Intelligence Service Officers (EISOs) from the National Institute for Occupational Safety and Health (NIOSH) were assigned to collaborate with an EISO stationed at the WVDHHR. Using a CDC surveillance instrument and a WVU medical screening tool, personnel from WVDHHR and the CDC designed a needs assessment and health status questionnaire (see Appendix). The questionnaire covered: 1) acute conditions, including physical symptoms, mental health symptoms, and recent injuries; 2) chronic medical conditions, including prescription medication use and pre-existing disabilities; and 3) current needs. The current needs section of the questionnaire addressed assistive devices, medical and dental care, and mental health services including assistance with substance abuse problems. On September 9th, the questionnaire was piloted on approximately 5% of the evacuee population. Minor adjustments were made to the questionnaire (such as reordering some of the questions) and the full assessment was conducted on September 10th–12th. The survey team consisted of WVDHHR and CDC personnel and WVU medical students. Survey team members obtained a convenience sample by approaching evacuees outside the mess hall, in the barracks, at a tuberculosis testing station, and at a meeting with the evacuated families and the West Virginia Department of Education. Interviews were conducted individually with the evacuee, or with the evacuee's parent or guardian, if appropriate. Efforts were made to maintain evacuees' confidentiality in communal settings.

The survey team also obtained Red Cross household registration records. These records provided household demographic information: pre-disaster address, dwelling type, dwelling insurance, and total household income range. Information related to the hurricane, such as extent of dwelling damage and anticipated housing needs, was also included. The household information was linked to the questionnaire by the names and ages of household members.

Data were entered into a Microsoft access database by WVDHHR and CDC personnel and analyses were conducted using Epi Info, Version 3.01 (CDC, 2003).

Results

Red Cross registration records. The Red Cross registered a total of 220 households representing all 323 individuals. Sixty-four percent of the evacuees were male (Table 1). Three percent were under 5 years of age and 8% were over 65 years of age. The mean age of the individuals was 40 years (median 44 years), with a range from 1 year to 83 years. Fifty-five percent had lived in a single family home before the storm and 40% had lived in an apartment, while 2% reported having been homeless or living in a homeless shelter. Twenty-three percent owned their dwellings, while 75% rented. Eighty-four percent suffered major damage or complete destruction of their property. Eighty-seven percent did not have insurance for the dwelling itself and 90% did not have insurance for its contents. Forty percent reported a yearly household income less than $7,500 and 44% reported a household income between $7,500 and $25,000.

WVDHHR and CDC needs assessment. A total of 164 people, or 51% of all evacuees at the center, participated in the assessment (Table 2). Sex and age distributions of respondents were similar to those of all center evacuees. Eighty-one percent were African American and 16% were Caucasian. Twenty-five percent reported an acute illness and 46% reported having at least one chronic medical condition. Almost half (47%) were taking prescription medication. Forty percent reported a mental health symptom. Twenty-eight percent reported being anxious or depressed, while almost a quarter (23%) reported experiencing insomnia. Ten percent reported using street drugs

Table 1.

CHARACTERISTICS OF ALL EVACUEES IN WEST VIRGINIA, SEPTEMBER 2005

Characteristic	n	%[a]	95% CI[b]
Sex (n=323)			
Male	207	64	(59–69)
Female	116	36	(31–41)
Age, in years (n=323)			
<5	11	3	(2–6)
5–17	50	16	(12–20)
56–65	42	73	(68–78)
>65	25	8	(5–11)

Table 1. *(continued)*

Characteristic	n	%[a]	95% CI[b]
Type of housing (n=209)			
Apartment	83	40	(33–47)
Homeless	2	1	(0–3)
Homeless shelter	3	1	(0–4)
Hotel	1	1	(0–3)
Mobile home	6	3	(1–6)
Single	114	55	(48–61)
Ownership (n=203)			
N/A	4	2	(1–5)
Own	47	23	(18–30)
Rent furnished	61	30	(24–37)
Rent unfurnished	91	45	(38–52)
Housing damage (n=203)			
Destroyed	122	60	(53–67)
Major	49	24	(18–31)
Minor	10	5	(2–9)
Unknown	22	11	(7–16)
Estimated housing needs (n=201)			
None	1	1	(0–3)
Permanent	149	74	(68–80)
Temporary	47	23	(18–30)
Unknown	4	2	(1–5)
Structural insurance (n=180)			
No	156	87	(81–91)
Yes	24	13	(8–19)
Contents insurance (n=176)			
No	159	90	(85–94)
Yes	17	10	(6–15)
Income range (n=181)			
$0–7,499	73	40	(33–48)
$7,500–9,999	19	11	(6–16)
$10,000–14,999	34	19	(13–25)
$15,000–24,999	25	14	(9–20)
$25,000–34,999	16	9	(5–14)
$35,000 and over	14	8	(4–13)

[a]Percentages may not add to 100 because of rounding.
[b]Confidence interval.

or alcohol. Five percent had thoughts of harming themselves or others. Thirteen percent had a recent injury. Nine percent reported having a physical disability.

Dental care was the most commonly reported current medical need, at 57%, followed by eyeglasses (34%), dentures (28%), and medical services (25%) (Table 3). Thirteen percent reported needing counseling or psychotherapy.

Table 2.

DEMOGRAPHICS AND RESULTS OF MEDICAL NEEDS ASSESSMENT—WEST VIRGINIA, SEPTEMBER 2005 (N=164)

Characteristic (N=164)	n	%	95% CI[a]
Gender (N=164)			
Male	109	67	(59–74)
Female	55	34	(26–41)
Age, in years (N=164)			
<5	2	1	(0–4)
5–17	26	16	(11–22)
18–65	119	73	(65–79)
>65	17	10	(6–16)
Race (N=160)			
African American	129	81	(74–86)
Asian/Pacific Islander	4	3	(1–6)
Multi-racial	1	1	(0–3)
White	26	16	(11–23)
Medical needs assessment			
Acute illness	41	25	(19–32)
Chronic medical conditions	76	46	(39–54)
Taking prescription medications	77	47	(39–55)
Mental health conditions	65	40	(32–48)
Anxiety/depression	46	28	(21–36)
Insomnia	38	23	(17–30)
Use street drugs/alcohol	17	10	(6–16)
Thoughts of harming self	3	2	(0–5)
Thoughts of harming others	5	3	(1–7)
Recent injury	22	13	(9–20)
Physical disabilities	15	9	(5–15)

[a]Confidence interval.

Discussion

The challenges facing the public health community in the wake of Hurricane Katrina were immense. The Gulf Coast infrastructure was damaged and in many cases destroyed, leaving thousands of people without access to basic necessities (food, clean water, sanitation, and shelter). Under such conditions, evacuees are at risk for infectious diseases, including respiratory and gastrointestinal illnesses.[3,6-7] Injuries (including lacerations, punctures, and animal bites) are also a concern in natural disasters, and wounds can become infected, at times with exotic organisms.[8-9] While epidemics following natural disasters are rare,[10] the prompt provision of medical services, restoration of hygiene, and alleviation of crowding are first steps to avert the spread of communicable diseases. The evacuation center in West Virginia provided a medical clinic capable of diagnosing and treating infectious conditions; full sanitary services, including showering facilities and hand wash stations outside the cafeteria; three hot meals per day; and adequate, clean (though not private) housing units. While, initially, treatment and prevention of infectious diseases were health priorities at the center, the assessment highlighted a prevalence of chronic conditions and acute mental health symptoms of even greater concern. Almost half of the respondents had a chronic medical condition and required prescription medications, and a substantial number had a physical disability. Unexpectedly high proportions of the respondents reported needing durable medical equipment, such as dentures and eyeglasses, as well as dental care (both emergent and non-emergent). A large number endorsed mental health symptoms and requested

Table 3.

RESULTS OF NEEDS ASSESSMENT—WEST VIRGINIA, SEPTEMBER 2005 (N=164)

Most common current needs	n	%	95% CI[a]
Dental care	93	57	(49–64)
Eyeglasses	56	34	(27–42)
Dentures	46	28	(21–36)
Medical services	41	25	(19–32)
Smoking cessation	23	14	(9–20)
Counseling/psychotherapy	22	13	(9–20)
Hearing aid	9	6	(3–10)
Assistance with alcohol/drug issues	6	4	(1–8)
Cane	6	4	(1–8)
Family planning	4	2	(1–6)
Wheelchair	3	2	(0–5)
Walker	2	1	(0–4)
Interpretive needs	1	1	(0–3)

[a]Confidence interval.

counseling services. Thus the assessment permitted an evaluation of the current needs of the evacuees two weeks after the hurricane. We concluded that:

- The medical clinic should continue to provide care for chronic medical conditions, including prescription medication, and make referrals to local hospitals as appropriate.
- Dental services should continue for emergent conditions, and should be expanded to include non-emergent care.
- Arrangements should be made for evacuees to be evaluated and fitted for dentures and eyeglasses.
- Relief workers should continue to provide mental health services, including counseling, and make referrals for psychiatric care, as appropriate.

Relief workers responded by procuring the services needed. The medical clinic continued to operate on a full-time basis until September 18th, serving 20 to 25 evacuees per day, and then on a part-time schedule, serving 10 to 15 evacuees per day. The WVU Dental School was available for urgent dental care needs and a private oral surgeon provided dental services to 4 individuals. In addition, a nationwide denture provider offered one-day service for dentures. The local Lions Club came to the center and screened individuals for eyeglasses. A local eyeglass provider and eye doctor provided services to people who needed eyeglasses. These services were provided free of charge. Counseling was provided by trained Red Cross volunteers, and a referral system with nearby hospitals was established for acute psychiatric care.

The evacuees describing mental health symptoms highlight a common experience of survivors of natural disasters.[11-12] Grief reactions to loss of life and property and anxiety about the future can lead to symptoms of depression (tearfulness, apathy, and change in sleep patterns) in the days and weeks following a disaster. The aftermath of a natural disaster can also bring traumatic experiences with mental health sequelae. Reports of violence following the flooding in New Orleans, for instance, circulated in the press and were anecdotally reported by the evacuees. One mother described her 6 year old son's mental state upon arriving at the evacuation center this way: "He won't let me out of his sight. He is worried by soldiers." While the majority of such symptoms can be expected to remit with time, some represent exacerbations of pre-existing mental health conditions and others are likely to progress to chronic post-traumatic disorders.[11] The inclusion of mental health services in the public health response to disasters has many advocates,[13-14] though some have expressed concerns about the potential risks of iatrogenic harm.[15] Follow-up of Katrina survivors who did and did not receive mental health services will be necessary to assess the long-term effectiveness of such interventions.

The needs for dental care and dentures were particularly prevalent among the evacuees. While some of these needs related directly to the disaster, such as dentures lost or left behind, others reflected poor dental health that predated the hurricane. An analysis of the National Health and Nutrition Examination Survey (NHANES III) limited to African Americans found that dental health was worse for those individuals who were poor, unemployed, and uninsured than for their counterparts; furthermore, those living in the South of the U.S. reported poorer dental health than those living elsewhere.[16] Other studies have confirmed such racial and socioeconomic disparities.[17-18] Poor dental health can negatively affect nutrition, is linked to some chronic diseases, and affects self-esteem and appearance.[19] The evacuees at the center in West Virginia were from some of the areas of New Orleans hardest hit by Hurricane Katrina. Many would not be able to return to their homes and jobs for months, if not longer, and would have to seek housing, employment, and a social support system in a new location. Like any chronic disease with external manifestations, poor dental health could complicate their reintegration. Thus dental health care needs were an unexpected but important target for intervention at this center and should be considered in future disasters.

There were several limitations to our assessment. It relied on self-reporting both for household and health information, which may have introduced a recall bias for some questions. People with current health concerns may have been more likely to participate in the health assessment than those without such concerns, leading to overrepresentation. The assessment was obtained from a convenience sample so the results cannot be generalized to other evacuees. If any individuals had medical conditions of a sensitive nature (such as HIV), they may have avoided the assessment due to concerns about confidentiality. While efforts were made to include the less mobile by visiting their living quarters within the barracks, this group also may have been underrepresented. Only half of the evacuees participated in the needs assessment, which may reflect "questionnaire-fatigue" on the part of evacuees following the detailed registration process, as well as reluctance to discuss the harrowing disaster they had so recently experienced.

Public health personnel have successfully conducted needs assessments to evaluate the health status and immediate needs of communities following hurricanes,[20-23] a tropical storm,[24] and an ice storm.[25] Conducting an assessment soon after the evacuees arrived at the center in West Virginia was critical for evaluating the health status and needs of the evacuees. The data obtained from the needs assessment were used by decision-makers to direct response activities, and provide appropriate services to this population during their stay at this evacuation center in West Virginia.

Acknowledgments

This report is based, in part, on contributions by the West Virginia Red Cross. We would like to acknowledge, in particular, the work of L. Haddy, PhD; H. Zappia, MS; M. Del-Rosario, MD; T. Shwe, MBBS; S. Hill; S. Stowers; J. Morgan; J. Takarsh; W. VonDollen; C. Leach, WVDHHR; D. M. Deci, MD; B. VanDyke; C. Teba; N. Roidad; K. Moore; O. Carrick; S. Shreve, WVU School of Medicine; and Denise Knoebel, Preston County Health Department.

Appendix

Family Name _____

Last Name, First Name (Head of Household) _____

MEDICAL NEEDS ASSESSMENT:

Last Name _____   First Name _____

Date of Birth ____/____/____

Gender: ___Male ___Female

Race: ___ Asian/Pacific Islander
___ African-American
___ White
___ MultiRacial
___ Unknown

City of Permanent Residence _____   State of Permanent Residence _____

PART I—Acute Conditions

Do you feel ill or sick today?	Yes/No
If no, skip to PART II.	
Gastrointestinal illness (gut problems)	Yes/No
Watery diarrhea/runs	Yes/No
Bloody diarrhea/runs	Yes/No
Vomiting/throw-up	Yes/No
Other, specify _____	
Respiratory illness (breathing problems)	
Upper respiratory tract infection (cold, runny nose)	Yes/No
Influenza-like illness (fever and cough or sore throat)	Yes/No
Lower respiratory tract illness (pneumonia)	Yes/No
Tuberculosis (TB), suspected	Yes/No
Pertussis (whooping cough), suspected	Yes/No
Other, specify _____	
Dehydration	Yes/No
Heat related injury (heat exhaustion, heatstroke)	Yes/No
Neurologic illness	Yes/No
Meningitis/encephalitis, suspected (stiff neck, headache)	Yes/No
Disorientation/confusion	Yes/No
Other, specify _____	
Dermatologic (skin problems) condition	Yes/No
Varicella (chickenpox), suspected	Yes/No
Rubella (German measles)/measles, suspected	Yes/No
Scabies (bugs, "the itch")	Yes/No
Rash, acute onset + fever	Yes/No
Other, specify _____	

Other infectious disease condition	Yes/No
Fever >100.4° F (38°C) ALONE without localizing signs	Yes/No
Jaundice (viral hepatitis, suspected)	Yes/No
Lice	Yes/No
Wound infection, specify site	Yes/No
Conjunctivitis (red eyes, gunk in eyes)	Yes/No
Other, specify _____	

PART II—Chronic and Other Conditions

Are you pregnant?	Yes/No
# weeks _____ or #months _____	
Chronic (ongoing, long term) medical conditions	Yes/No
Do you have any heart disease/high blood pressure?	Yes/No
Hypertension (high blood pressure)	Yes/No
Other, specify _____	
Do you have any lung disease?	Yes/No
COPD/emphysema	Yes/No
Asthma	Yes/No
Other, specify _____	
Do you have any kidney disease?	Yes/No
Dialysis dependent	Yes/No
Other, specify _____	
Do you have diabetes?	Yes/No
Insulin	Yes/No
Oral medication	Yes/No
Other, specify _____	
Do you have problems with your immune system?	Yes/No
Cancer	Yes/No
HIV/AIDS	Yes/No
Hepatitis B or C	Yes/No
Chronic or high dose steroid use	Yes/No
Other, specify _____	
Do you have any neurological problems?	Yes/No
Stroke/paralysis	Yes/No
MS (multiple sclerosis)	Yes/No
Other, specify _____	
Do you have any problems with your blood?	Yes/No
Sickle-cell anemia	Yes/No
Hemophilia	Yes/No
Requires blood products	Yes/No
Other, specify _____	
Known allergies (medications, food, seasonal), specify _____	
Are you taking any prescription medications?	Yes/No

Do you have any disabilities?	Yes/No
Physical disabilities	Yes/No
Mobility impairment (wheelchair, walker, etc.)	Yes/No
Other, specify _____	
Sensory disability	Yes/No
Visually impaired (blindness, limited vision)	Yes/No
Hearing impaired	Yes/No
Other, specify _____	
Cognitive disability (learning problems)	Yes/No
Mental retardation	Yes/No
Autism	Yes/No
Attention Deficit Hyperactivity Disorder (ADHD)	Yes/No
Other, specify _____	
Resided in a group home, nursing home or assisted care facility	Yes/No
Other, specify _____	

Mental health condition (nerves)	Yes/No
Anxiety/depression	Yes/No
Trouble sleeping?	Yes/No
Use street drugs/alcohol dependence/withdrawal	Yes/No
Thoughts of harming yourself?	Yes/No
Thoughts of harming others?	Yes/No
Other, specify _____	

A recent injury?	Yes/No
Self-inflicted injury—intentional (violence)	Yes/No
Assault-related injury—intentional (violence)	Yes/No
Unintentional injury (accidents)	Yes/No
Other, specify _____	

What insurance and other assistance were you on at the time of the hurricane?	
Medicaid	Yes/No
Medicare	Yes/No
Private insurance	Yes/No
Worker's Comp	Yes/No
Veteran assistance	Yes/No
Other, specify _____	

	Currently Using	Need
Do you need any of the following or are you currently using?		
Cane	Yes/No	Yes/No
Walker	Yes/No	Yes/No
Seeing eye dog	Yes/No	Yes/No
Hearing aid	Yes/No	Yes/No
Wheelchair	Yes/No	Yes/No
Eyeglasses	Yes/No	Yes/No
Dentures	Yes/No	Yes/No
Dental care	Yes/No	Yes/No
Interpretive needs (signing or translation services)	Yes/No	Yes/No
Family planning services	Yes/No	Yes/No
Medical services	Yes/No	Yes/No

Counseling/psychotherapy	Yes/No	Yes/No
Assistance with alcohol or drug issues	Yes/No	Yes/No
Smoking cessation	Yes/No	Yes/No
Other, specify _____		

Date of Questionnaire: 09/   /2005   Interviewer initials: _____

Notes

1. Medlin J, Ball R, Beeler G; National Weather Service. Extremely powerful Hurricane Katrina leaves a historic mark on the Northern Gulf Coast. Mobile, AL: National Weather Service Forecast Office: Mobile-Pensacola, 2006 Jul 7. Available at www.srh .noaa.gov/mob/0805Katrina/.

2. Anonymous. Estimates in Swiss Re sigma study confirm 2005 as costliest ever. Insurance Journal. 2005 Dec: International News. Available at http://www.insurancejournal .com/news/international/2005/12/21/63327.htm.

3. Centers for Disease Control and Prevention (CDC). Infectious disease and dermatologic conditions in evacuees and rescue workers after Hurricane Katrina—multiple states, August–September, 2005. MMWR Morb Mort Wkly Rep. 2005 Sep 30; 54(38):961–4.

4. Office of the Governor: Rick Perry. Summary of key State of Texas actions in response to Hurricane Katrina. Austin, TX: Office of the Governor, 2005 Sep 3. Available at http://www .governor.state.tx.us/divisions/press/pressreleases/PressRelease.2005-09-03.3607.

5. American Red Cross. Facts at a glance: American Red Cross response to Hurricane Katrina and Rita. Washington, DC: American Red Cross, 2006 Jan 19. Available at http://www.redcross.org/news/ds/hurricanes/katrina_facts.html.

6. Conolly MA, Gayer M, Ryan MJ, et al. Communicable diseases in complex emergencies: impact and challenges. Lancet. 2004 Nov 27–Dec 3;364(9449):1974–83.

7. Lim JH, Yoon D, Jung G, et al. Medical needs of tsunami disaster refugee camps. Fam Med. 2005 Jun;37(6):422–8.

8. Centers for Disease Control and Prevention (CDC). Surveillance for injuries and illness and rapid health needs assessment following Hurricanes Marilyn and Opal, September–October 1995. MMWR Morb Mortal Wkly Rep. 1996 Feb 2;45(04):81–5.

9. Centers for Disease Control and Prevention (CDC). Vibrio illnesses after Hurricane Katrina—multiple states, August–September 2005. MMWR Morb Mortal Wkly Rep. 2005 Sep 23;54(37):928–31.

10. Alexander D. The health effects of earthquakes in the mid-1990s. Disasters. 1996 Sep; 20(3):231–47.

11. Gray MJ, Maguen S, Litz BT. Acute psychological impact of disaster and large-scale trauma: limitations of traditional interventions and future practice recommendations. Prehospital Disaster Med. 2004 Jan–Mar;19(1):64–72.

12. Woersching JC, Snyder AE. Earthquakes in El Salvador: a descriptive study of health concerns in a rural community and the clinical implications: Part III—Mental health and psychosocial effects. Disaster Manag Response. 2004 Apr–Jun;2(2):40–5.

13. Holloway HC, Norwood AE, Fullerton CS, et al. The threat of biological weapons. Prophylaxis and mitigation of psychological and social consequences. JAMA. 1997 Aug 6;278(5):425–7.

14. Susser ES, Herman DB, Aaron B. Combating the terror of terrorism. Sci Am. 2002 Aug;287(2):70–7.

15. Everly GS Jr. Early psychological intervention: a word of caution. Int J Emerg Ment Health. 2003 Fall;5(4):179–84.

16. Green BL, Person S, Crowther M, et al. Demographic and geographic variations of oral health among African Americans based on NHANES III. Community Dent Health. 2003 Jun;20(2):117–22.

17. Gilbert GH, Duncan RP, Shelton BJ. Social determinants of tooth loss. Health Serv Res. 2003 Dec;38(6 Pt 2):1843–62.

18. Gilbert GH. Racial and socioeconomic disparities in health from population-based research to practice-based research: the example of oral health. J Dent Educ. 2005 Sep;69(9):1003–14.

19. U.S. Department of Health and Human Services (HHS). Oral health in America: a report of the Surgeon General. Rockville, MD: U.S. Department of Health and Human Services, National Institute of Dental and Craniofacial Research, National Institutes of Health, 2000.

20. Centers for Disease Control and Prevention (CDC). Rapid health needs assessment following Hurricane Andrew—Florida and Louisiana, 1992. MMWR Morb Mortal Wkly Rep. 1992 Sep 18;41(37):685–8.

21. Centers for Disease Control and Prevention (CDC). Needs assessment following Hurricane Georges—Dominican Republic, 1998. MMWR Morb Mort Wkly Rep. 1999 Feb 12;48(5):93–5.

22. Centers for Disease Control and Prevention (CDC). Rapid assessment of the needs and health status of older adults after Hurricane Charley—Charlotte, Desoto, and Hardee Counties, Florida, August 27–31, 2004. MMWR Morb Mort Wkly Rep. 2004 Sep 17;53(36):837–40.

23. Centers for Disease Control and Prevention (CDC). Rapid community health and needs assessment after Hurricanes Isabel and Charley—North Carolina, 2003–2004. MMWR Morb Mort Wkly Report. 2004 Sep 17;53(36):840–2.

24. Centers for Disease Control and Prevention (CDC). Tropical Storm Allison rapid needs assessment—Houston, Texas, June, 2001. MMWR Morb Mortal Wkly Rep. 2002 May 3;51(17):365–9.

25. Centers for Disease Control and Prevention (CDC). Community needs assessment and morbidity surveillance following an ice storm—Maine, January 1998. MMWR Morb Mortal Wkly Rep. 1998 May 8;47(17):351–4.

Chapter 16
Hurricane Katrina's Impact on Pediatric and Adult Patients with Sickle Cell Disease

Nicole A. Karras, MD
Charles S. Hemenway, MD, PhD

Sickle cell disease (SCD) is the most common inherited genetic disorder in African Americans. It comprises multiple genotypes expressing variable, often serious, clinical sequelae. Complications may occur as early as infancy, and SCD ultimately leads to profound morbidity and shortened life expectancy.[1-3,7-14] However, significant improvements in the care of individuals with SCD have evolved over the past two decades.[3] One of the mainstays of treatment for SCD is regular health maintenance throughout the patient's lifetime.[1,2] In most states, once the presence of SCD is detected, typically through newborn screening, infants are referred to a comprehensive SCD clinic or a specialist. The health maintenance schedule is intense, with more frequent visits to the specialist during early childhood than to the general pediatrician (see Table 1).[1,2,4] Regular visits to a medical hematologist (or other practitioner with expertise in treating adult patients with SCD) continue once the patient is 18 years old. The National Institutes of Health recommend the health maintenance schedule listed in Box 1.[2] The importance of establishing and maintaining a medical home for SCD patients has been clearly described by Lane et al.[1] The medical home should include a comprehensive sickle cell clinic that coordinates all aspects of multidisciplinary care in collaboration with the patients' primary physician. Notably, there is evidence that proper health maintenance decreases morbidity and mortality among patients with SCD.[1,2,5,10]

Prior to August 2005, the delivery of health care to adults and children with SCD in the greater New Orleans metropolitan area differed in important ways. The great majority of children with SCD were treated at one of three private, medical school-affiliated hospitals and their clinics. For reasons largely related to insurance reimbursement rates, adults with SCD in the New Orleans area who lacked private medical insurance (including those with Louisiana Medicaid) were referred to the SCD clinic at the Medical Center of Louisiana in New Orleans (MCLNO, also known as Charity Hospital). As children reached early adulthood (18–21 years of age), their care was almost always transferred to the SCD clinic at MCLNO. Thus, the MCLNO was the primary provider of health care to adult patients with SCD in greater New Orleans prior to Hurricane Katrina.

NICOLE A. KARRAS is a Resident in Training in the Department of Pediatrics at Tulane University. CHARLES S. HEMENWAY is an Associate Professor of Pediatrics, also at Tulane.

Table 1.

PEDIATRIC SCD[a] HEALTH MAINTENANCE SCHEDULE

Age	Routine visits, immunizations	Lab tests/medications
Birth–6 mo	Every 2 months, Pneumococcal Vaccine at 2, 4, 6 months	CBC every visit, Pen VK
6 mo–2 yrs	Every 3 months, Pneumococcal vaccine booster at 15 months, and flu vaccine	CBC every 3–6 months, Ferritin serum FE and TIBC once at 1–2 yrs BUN, Cr and LFTs once at 1–2 yrs Continue Pen VK, Folic Acid
2–5 yrs	Every 6 months, 23 valent pneumococcal vaccine at 2 yrs and booster at 5, flu, Meningococcus vaccines	Increase Pen VK, CBC and UA yearly, periodic BUN, CR and LFTs Folic Acid
>5 yrs	Every 6–12 months, hearing, vision screening, continue influenza, pneumococcal and Meningococcus vaccines	Folic Acid, Pen VK, continue labs

[a]SCD = sickle cell disease
Source: Wethers DL. Sickle cell disease in childhood: Part 1. Laboratory diagnosis, pathophysiology and health maintenance. Am Fam Physician. 2002 Sep 1;62(5):1013–20, 1027–8.

The Sickle Cell Center of Southern Louisiana (SCCSL) is a state-sponsored organization that provides services to patients with SCD in southeastern Louisiana, including the New Orleans metropolitan area as well as parts of southern Mississippi. In addition to providing community education, patient teaching, and social work services, the SCCSL maintains a database of patient demographics and contact information. The SCCSL follows and is available to patients with SCD regardless of the institution that provides their care. An important objective of the SCCSL is to ensure that patients with SCD have a medical home.

In August 2005, Hurricane Katrina destroyed much of the city of New Orleans. That destruction fell on buildings, as well as services such as mail delivery. Moreover, it led to a large emigration of both physicians and other health care professionals away from the city and the closure of many area hospitals. Two of the three primary hospitals caring for children with SCD were temporarily closed but reopened no later than two months after the storm (the third hospital remained open). At the time of this study, however, the MCLNO was closed to inpatients, and all outpatient services were severely curtailed. With this background, it was imperative that we begin to assess the SCD patient population in greater New Orleans to determine the effects of a damaged medical infrastructure on their access to a level of care appropriate for their illness.

Box 1.

ADULT SCD[a] HEALTH MAINTENANCE SCHEDULE

Initial health maintenance visit
- Opportunity to establish rapport with the patient and family
- Determine medical needs
- Compile complete database including psychological strengths, historical information, pertinent medical issues

Ongoing health care visits
- Initially a few visits every 1 to 2 weeks should develop rapport, develop problem list and care plan
- Routine medical evaluations are scheduled every 2 to 6 months depending on phenotype and active problems
- Blood counts, reticulocyte counts, urinalysis are repeated at each visit
- Pulse oximetry is also helpful at each visit
- Patient education
- Pen VK is typically discontinued after the age of 18 years

[a]SCD = sickle cell disease
Source: Adams R, Ataga KI, Ballard H, et al. National Institute of Health. The management of sickle cell disease. 4th Ed. (NIH Pub. No. 02-2117.) Washington, DC: National Institutes of Health, National Heart, Lung, and Blood Institute, Division of Blood Diseases and Resources, 2002 Jun.

Specifically, we wished to learn directly from patients whether they perceived that their medical care was compromised eight months after Hurricane Katrina.

Methods

An anonymous survey was conducted with the approval of Tulane University's Institutional Review Board. Due to the anonymous and voluntary nature of the survey, informed consent was not required. The purpose and significance of the survey was explained to participants prior to beginning the survey. The survey took place during May 2006, eight months after Hurricane Katrina. The survey was primarily conducted over the telephone using the SCCSL's patient registry. Mailings were avoided due to the suspension of regular mail delivery in the city at the time of the study. Printed copies of the survey were also made available at Tulane University Hospital's emergency room as well as area pediatric hematology clinics (equivalent adult clinics did not exist) with instructions that if the participant completed the survey over the telephone, he/she was not to submit a duplicate. The survey was written in easily comprehensible language in order to be understood by as many patients as possible. It covered both pediatric and adult populations, with a parent/guardian completing the pediatric surveys. Questions were phrased with the intention of having participants identify weaknesses and shortcomings in the post-Katrina health care environment. To do this, patients were sometimes asked to compare their health status and access with that to which they were accustomed prior to Katrina. For example, the survey included these items: "Are you waiting longer at emergency room visits?" and "Is your overall health better or worse since the hurricane?" There was room for the participant to freely elaborate on his/her response to the question, "Are you happy with your medical care?" The purpose for gathering responses to this question was to determine possible improvements to provide more satisfactory health care as well as to determine which parts of the system were working well.

The pediatric population included SCD patients who were 18 years old and younger. The remainder constituted the adult population. Patients with all types of SCD (Hb SS, Hb SC, Hb S-Beta+ Thalassemia) were included. Individuals with the sickle cell trait only were not included. Occasionally, participants could not answer every question in the survey because some were not applicable to them.

Results

Of 459 adult patients registered with the SCCSL, 235 telephone calls reached numbers that had been disconnected. Of 379 pediatric patients in the registry, 215 telephone calls reached disconnected numbers. Some other telephone numbers did not receive incoming calls and, in a small number of cases, telephone contact information was not available from the registry. During the one-month survey period, we were able to recruit a total of 24 pediatric and 22 adult participants. The participants' responses to the questions are represented graphically in Figures 1–9. The title of each figure corresponds to a question from the survey. A chi-square analysis was used to detect significant differences between the groups of adult and pediatric patients. Finally, representative quotations from responses to the open-ended opinion question from patients/guardians are listed in Box 2. In brief, compared with pediatric patients, a statistically significantly larger portion of the adult population reported having a difficult time seeing a hematologist, dissatisfaction with their current medical care and a subsequent feeling that their overall health was worse than before Hurricane Katrina. In contrast, the majority of the pediatric population (or their parents/guardians) reported satisfaction with the health care available to them and found it comparable to the health care they received prior to the hurricane. Notably, the reported number of emergency room visits between the two age groups was similar; the number of visits did not appear to correlate with the patient's overall self-health assessment.

Discussion

This survey of patients in the New Orleans metropolitan area with SCD focuses on patient-perceived differences in the quality of health care eight months after Hurricane Katrina. We note significant differences between the responses of adult and pediatric patients, with adults reporting greater dissatisfaction with the current state of their medical care. Thus, it seems as though the adult population with SCD suffered dispro-

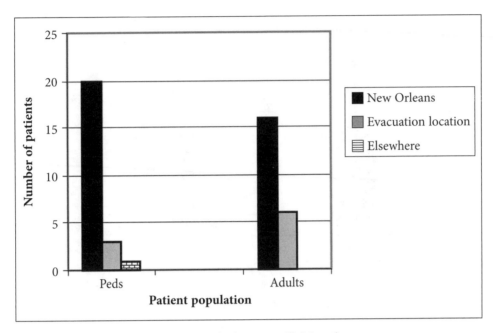

Figure 1. "Where are you living since the hurricane?" (N=46)

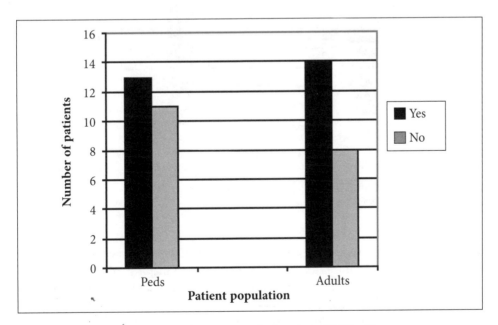

Figure 2. "Have you seen a new doctor since the hurricane?" (N=46, Chi-square = 0.424567310532223, $p \leq 1$)

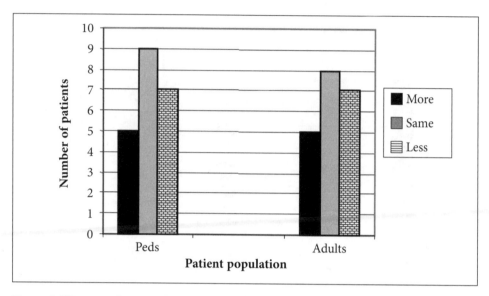

Figure 3. "Have you been to the emergency room more or less than a typical year?" (N=41)

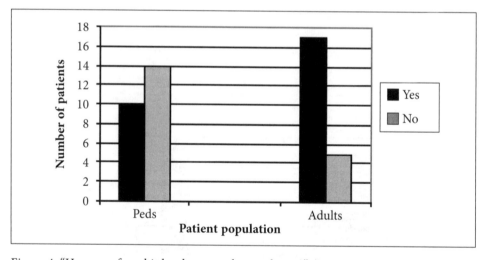

Figure 4. "Have you found it hard to see a hematologist?" (N=46, Chi-square = 6.00236280938035, $p \leq .025$)

portionately in comparison with the pediatric population. We attribute these differences to the severely limited choices for medical care faced by a majority of adults with SCD in the New Orleans area after Hurricane Katrina. The reduction in medical services did not extend to the pediatric population.

In May of 1736, Charity Hospital, later renamed the Medical Center of Louisiana of New Orleans, opened its doors. Until Hurricane Katrina, it was the second oldest continuously operating public hospital in the United States.[6] The 2,680 bed institu-

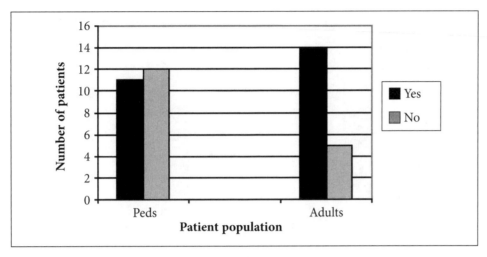

Figure 5. "Are you waiting longer at office visits or emergency room visits?" (N=42, Chi-square = 2.88759186969982, $p \leq .10$)

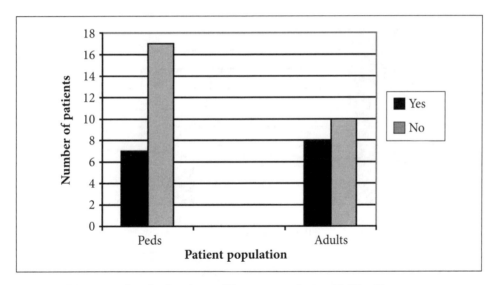

Figure 6. "Have you found it harder to fill your prescriptions?" (N=42, Chi-square = 1.04567901234568, $p \leq 1$)

tion was the primary teaching hospital for 2 medical schools in the city and provided both primary and tertiary care to a large uninsured population. Remarkably, with the exception of newborns and a pediatric emergency room, MCLNO served relatively few children. Louisiana regulations make Medicaid available to most children whose families lack medical insurance, and pediatric subspecialists at the city's private hospitals accept patients with Louisiana Medicaid. However, adult patients, including those with SCD, face more restrictive eligibility requirements for Louisiana Medicaid. Furthermore, according to surveys conducted by the SCCSL, a large percentage of subspecialists in

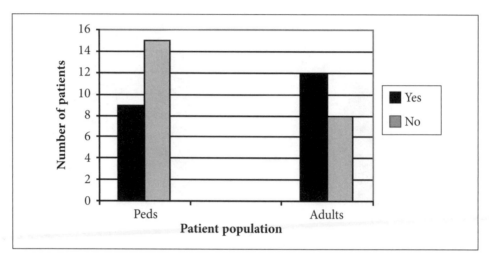

Figure 7. "Are you traveling further to see a hematologist" (N=44, Chi-square = 2.21366459627329, $p \leq .2$)

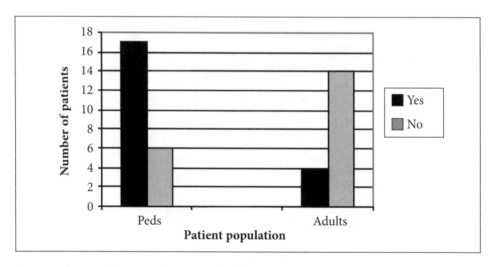

Figure 8. "Are you happy with your medical care?" (N=41, Chi-square = 10.7984587071544, $p \leq .01$)

internal medicine in the New Orleans area do not accept adult patients with SCD and Louisiana Medicaid (unpublished survey results). In practical terms, MCLNO was the only institution providing unencumbered access to regular care for adults with SCD.

During the past two or more decades, a *de facto* system of health care has evolved for patients with SCD in metropolitan New Orleans. Children have enjoyed relatively easy access to primary and subspecialty care at any one of at least three private hospitals. MCLNO/Charity Hospital became the primary source of care for the uninsured in the region as well as for Louisiana Medicaid-insured adult patients who were unable to establish themselves with a provider elsewhere. The dominant role of a single institution

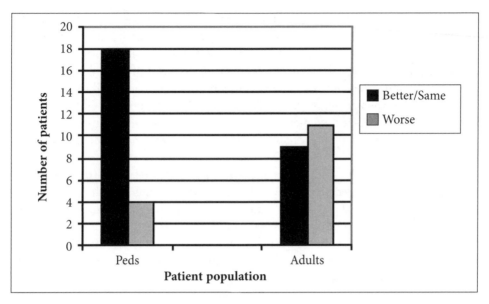

Figure 9. "Do you feel your overall health is better/same or worse since the hurricane?" (N=43, Chi-square = 6.18545454545455, $p \leq .025$)

Box 2.

DIRECT QUOTES FROM PARTICIPANTS/GUARDIANS

Pediatric population
- "I'm too far from the Sickle Cell Center, so I wait in the ER for them [ER Doctors] not to help her"—From Leesville, LA.
- "I'm not satisfied with the general pediatrician's management [of Sickle Cell Disease] or the absence of a hematologist"—From Gulfport, MS.

Adult population
- "I am having a hard time getting proper pain medicines and seeing proper doctors"—New Orleans, LA (NOLA).
- "Doctors don't know about how to control pain or how to access my port properly. They don't follow Tulane protocol and don't give proper prescriptions"—rural Georgia.
- "Disappointed by care in Alexandria, LA. They gave me pain medicines that didn't work because they didn't have my medical records"—Alexandria, LA.

---

in caring for adults with SCD appears to have placed these individuals with a chronic illness at risk. Our survey results suggest that the prolonged closure of MCLNO in the aftermath of Hurricane Katrina has exposed one or more shortcomings of a highly centralized hospital system that is charged with caring for the poor.

The reality after Hurricane Katrina is that many patients are not receiving the care to which they were previously accustomed, an opinion expressed by patients in the interviews we conducted. Furthermore, these adult patients, who are familiar with subspecialty management of their SCD, report unhappiness with their current treatment and relay that their overall health is suffering. As a result, patients report seeing primary care and emergency medicine doctors not specifically trained in the intricacies of SCD management. It is unsettling that participants reported being accused of narcotic-medicine-seeking at emergency rooms by medical staff in outlying hospitals (who were less familiar than specialists with the extensive and debilitating pain of a SCD crisis).

It is plausible that the general anxiety, stress, and anger resulting from the storm were expressed in the specific open-ended responses of patients regarding their health care. However, we would expect that adults with SCD as well as parents/guardians of children with SCD would be equally affected by this phenomenon. It is noteworthy that there were no differences between the two groups with respect to the difficulty reported in filling prescriptions. This is an important component of health care that is largely independent of hospitals and clinics. We propose that the differences between adult and pediatric patients reported in this survey stem largely from the reliance of adults with SCD on a centralized state-sponsored hospital in metropolitan New Orleans. The pediatric population is satisfied with their care because they have had uninterrupted access to care, while the adult population's dissatisfaction may stem from the storm-imposed limitations to subspecialty care. The other regrettable outcome is that the lines of communication between the Sickle Cell Center and most of its patients have been severed. With so many patients losing their homes and belongings, and with the immediate post-hurricane malfunction of the New Orleans area cell phone towers, most of the population changed their telephone numbers and are now unreachable. Given this situation, the necessary task of informing patients of the possibility of reestablishing care in New Orleans is daunting.

Notably, "better" and "worse" health or medical care were not defined other than by participants' opinions. There were no specific medical criteria to lend to those descriptions other than the participants self-evaluation or evaluation of their children.

The present study was hindered by a small sample size due to an inability to contact the majority of patients in the SCCSL database. This was a result of the relocation of much of the population of New Orleans, with people living in shelters and hotels, and with relatives. No speculations are made here about the care that evacuees received in their new locations, only about the care that was provided in the New Orleans area to those that returned to the city. Although many of the comparisons made are statistically significant for the sample obtained, it is plausible that if a larger sample size were included, the results and conclusions would be substantially different.

Conclusion

Now that the worst natural disaster to strike American soil is in the recovery phase, there are potentially important lessons to be learned from the findings in this survey. First, the public health office should recognize the urgent need for subspecialty clinics and respond by sponsoring them at existing medical facilities. Next, the disaster points to the potential utility of a web-based electronic medical record system. For patients with SCD, this would facilitate treatment at remote facilities, clarify medical histories, and possibly prevent medication-seeking accusations. Third, it highlights the possibility that in some settings, adult patients may be more vulnerable than children with identical medical conditions.

Acknowledgments

The authors would like personally to express tremendous gratitude to the staff of the Sickle Cell Center of Southern Louisiana for their efforts, enthusiasm, and assistance.

Notes

1. Section on Hematology/Oncology Committee on Genetics; American Academy of Pediatrics. Health supervision for children with sickle cell disease. Pediatrics. 2002 Mar;109(3):526–35.
2. Adams R, Ataga KI, Ballard H, et al. National Institute of Health. The management of sickle cell disease. 4th Ed. (NIH Pub. No. 02-2117.) Washington, DC: National Institutes of Health, National Heart, Lung, and Blood Institute, Division of Blood Diseases and Resources, 2002 Jun.
3. Castro O. Management of sickle cell disease: recent advances and controversies. Br J Hematol. 1999 Oct;107(1):2–11.
4. Wethers DL. Sickle cell disease in childhood: Part 1. Laboratory diagnosis, pathophysiology and health maintenance. Am Fam Physician. 2002 Sep 1;62(5):1013–20, 1027–8.
5. Embury SH, Vichinsky EP. Overview of the management of sickle cell disease. Version 14.1. Waltham, MA: UpToDate, 2005 Sept 19.
6. Medical Center of Louisiana New Orleans (MCLNO). History: charity's beginnings. New Orleans, LA: MCLNO, 2006. Available at http://www.mclno.org/MCLNO//Menu/Hospital/History/history.aspx?node=131.
7. Downes SM, Hambleton IR, Chuang EL, et al. Incidence and natural history of proliferative sickle cell retinopathy: observations from a cohort study. Ophthalmology. 2005 Nov;112(11):1869–75.
8. Sebire G, Tabarki B, Saunders DE, et al. Central venous sinus thrombosis in children: risk factors, presentation, diagnosis and outcome. Brain. 2005 Mar;128(Pt 3): 477–89.
9. Buchanan GR, DeBaun MR, Quinn CT, et al. Sickle cell disease. Hematology Am Soc Hematol Educ Program. 2004:35–47.
10. Wojciechowski EA, Hurtig A, Dorn L. A natural history study of adolescents and young adults with sickle cell disease as they transfer to adult care: a need for case management services. J Pediatr Nurs. 2002 Feb;17(1):18–27.
11. Yardumian A, Crawley C. Sickle cell disease. Clin Med. 2001 Nov–Dec;1(6):441–6.
12. Bruno D, Wigfall DR, Zimmerman SA, et al. Genitourinary complications of sickle cell disease. J Urol. 2001 Sep;166(3):803–11.
13. Knight J, Murphy TM, Browning I. The lung in sickle cell disease. Pediatr Pulmonol. 1999 Sep;28(3):205–16.
14. Hoppe C, Styles L, Vichinsky E. The natural history of sickle cell disease. Curr Opin Pediatr. 1998 Feb;10(1):49–52.

Chapter 17
Media Use and Information Needs of the Disabled during a Natural Disaster

Patric R. Spence, PhD
Ken Lachlan, PhD
Jennifer M. Burke, PhD
Matthew W. Seeger, PhD

Natural disasters and similar cataclysmic events are becoming both more harmful and more common, which magnifies the need to examine the most effective ways citizens can obtain crisis and risk information.[1-4] Research in this area on people with disabilities* is primarily in the area of evacuation, with frequent comparisons drawn between the disabled and the elderly.[5-6] This study attempts to go beyond these limited investigations by comparing the effectiveness of risk messages, crisis preparation, media choice, and information-seeking behaviors of disabled and non-disabled populations directly affected by Hurricane Katrina. Recommendations are offered concerning how disaster personnel can use this information to minimize harm and facilitate effective responses for disabled populations.

Preparing for a crisis. The public will often base its assessment of the risks associated with potential disasters on sensory perception.[7] The sense of risk is typically visceral and the risks themselves well understood; thus, if members of the public have received appropriate information in a timely manner they will likely take action to protect themselves.

In the area of disabilities and evacuations, research suggests that impairments and health problems can affect disaster response.[6,8] People who are disabled may be unable to respond quickly or to take proper protective action during crisis events and therefore may be more likely to experience harm.[5,8] More people now live with disabilities of some kind than ever before, a direct result of improved medical care and rising

---

*There has been considerable debate surrounding the appropriate terminology to be used in reference to those with physical conditions that limit their activities. While the term handicapped has been largely abandoned, some are comfortable with the term disabled, while others prefer the term differently-abled. This article will use the term disabled, given its use in communication science.

PATRIC SPENCE *is an Assistant Professor in the Department of Communication Arts and Sciences at Calvin College in Grand Rapids, Michigan.* KEN LACHLAN *is an Assistant Professor at Boston College,* JENNIFER BURKE *is an Assistant Professor at Prairie View A&M University, and* MATTHEW SEEGER *is a Professor at Wayne State University.*

survival rates from birth defects, life-threatening and chronic diseases, and accidents.[9] U.S. Census information from 2000 reports that 15.6% (n=63,913) of the occupants of metropolitan New Orleans reported having disabilities. The present study sought to compare the seriousness of the hazards posed by Katrina as perceived by disabled and non-disabled New Orleans residents. The following research question was posed:

RQ1: To what extent was there a difference between the disabled and the non-disabled in taking preparations to survive the storm?

Information-seeking and the role of uncertainty. After the onset of a crisis, individuals seek information.[10-11] The dominant source of information is usually the mass media.[11-14] The news media is generally thought to be a valuable and timely source of information;[15] crises necessitate that the messages provided be ordered, specific, and distributed through accessible channels. To explore how disabled and non-disabled people might differ in this connection, the following research questions are proposed:

RQ2: Were there differences between the disabled and the non-disabled in information seeking behaviors?

RQ3: Were there differences between the disabled and the non-disabled in the use of traditional media?

Information sources. Television and interpersonal networks are the most commonly used sources for acquiring information about important news events.[16-18] Television may be the preferred medium if a crisis erupts in the evening, while a crisis triggered during normal working hours may lead people to rely on interpersonal channels and radio.[11,14,18] It may also be the case that crises that explode during night or non-waking hours would lead people to rely on interpersonal networks, especially if they are not actively consuming media at this time.

Interpersonal networks (particularly outside of the immediate family) are critical for individuals with disabilities, providing a type of validation in that they are perceived as different from non-voluntary family relationships.[19] Given the past research concerning the importance of various information sources, the following research question is offered:

RQ4: What channel will be reported as the primary medium used to learn about evacuation notices among people with disabilities?

New media and information. In examining the use of new media in the context of a crisis, it was noted that when a crisis erupts during the business day, mobile telephones may replace interpersonal interactions, as people call friends and family to obtain information.[18] Because Katrina was tracked for days, the drawn-out timeframe may have made new media a viable option for information gathering. Given the lack of knowledge surrounding new media by the disabled during crises with prolonged trigger events, the following research question is offered:

RQ5. How important were new media and cellular telephones in comparison with interpersonal interactions and traditional media for those with disabilities before and after Hurricane Katrina?

Methods

Participants and measures. Surveys were administered to Katrina evacuees in relief centers in Cape Cod, Massachusetts; Lansing, Michigan; and at federal emergency aid distribution centers in Texas during the weeks following the evacuation of New Orleans (see Tables 1 and 2 for sample demographics).

Disability was measured by a three-part Likert-type question asking the state of physical health. Almost half (40.7%, n=232) of the respondents reported some type of physical disability. Of the 232 that reported some type of physical disability, 162 described it as *minor* and 70 respondents described it as *major*. This variable was collapsed into a binary variable simply describing the presence or absence of a physical disability.

Crisis preparation. Two items were designed to measure the participants' efforts to prepare for a disaster of this kind. For both items, participants were simply asked to check a box indicating *yes* or *no*. The first item was designed to address emergency preparation in the home, and the second item addressed evacuation efforts.

Information-seeking. Ten items addressed individual information-seeking characteristics. Respondents were asked to "indicate what information you most wanted immediately following the storm," with response categories of *strongly agree, agree, neutral, disagree,* and *strongly disagree.* Reliability analyses indicated α=.93 for the ten item index.

Information sources. Another series of items examined the medium through which respondents first learned about the evacuations. Respondents were asked to "indicate how you first learned of evacuation notices," and were given 10 categories from which to choose.

Results

Descriptive analyses were used to address research question one. Of the 283 non-disabled respondents answering the question, 133 (46.9%) reported having some kind of emergency kit or supplies set aside in case of an emergency. Furthermore, 113 (40.4%) reported having some kind of evacuation plan in place. Looking at the physically disabled subpopulation there is little difference with respect to the first measure, with 101 (43.5%) reporting some sort of emergency kit or supplies. However, disabled respondents were somewhat less likely than the non-disabled to report having an evacuation plan, with only 78 (34.1%) indicating an in-place plan.

Table 1.

SAMPLE DEMOGRAPHICS

	Disabled		Non-disabled	
	Frequency	Valid %	Frequency	Valid %
Age, in years				
<25	34	15.4	44	19.4
26–30	44	19.9	43	19.0
31–35	24	10.9	47	16.8
36–40	18	8.1	31	11.1
41–45	25	11.3	27	9.7
46–50	31	14.0	27	9.7
51–55	21	9.5	20	7.1
56–60	11	5.0	11	4.0
61–65	2	.9	6	2.1
66+	11	5.0	3	1.1
Missing	11		6	
Sex				
Male	67	29.4	97	34.0
Female	161	69.4	185	65.6
Missing	4		3	
Race				
African-American	207	90.8	229	82.4
Caucasian	9	3.9	24	8.6
Other	12	5.3	25	9.0
Missing	4		7	
Total	232		285	

Demographic Characteristics, Storm Preparation, and Information-Seeking

Crisis preparation. The predictive power of disability (controlling for demographics) in crisis preparation was evaluated using logistic regression. Demographic characteristics and whether or not the respondent was disabled were entered as a single block predicting the presence or absence of an emergency supply kit. Significant results for the model were detected, chi-square (5, N=554)=33.54, p<.001, Nagelkerke R^2=.11. Regression coefficients indicated that older respondents, those in higher income brackets, African Americans, and the disabled were less likely to have such a kit available. Similar analyses were repeated for the presence or absence of an evacuation plan in case of a hurricane or other emergency. Entering the same variables into the predictor block produced a

Table 2.

INCOME ACROSS DISABLED AND NON-DISABLED

Income	Disabled		Non-disabled	
	Frequency	Valid %	Frequency	Valid %
<$10,000	79	42.0	84	33.9
$10–15,000	29	15.4	28	11.3
$15–20,000	13	6.9	15	6.0
$20–25,000	18	9.6	29	11.7
$25–30,000	7	3.7	15	6.0
$30–35,000	12	6.4	12	4.8
$35–40,000	8	4.3	19	7.7
$40–45,000	6	3.2	13	5.2
$45–50,000	2	1.1	3	1.2
$50–60,000	8	4.3	10	4.0
$60–75,000	4	2.1	10	4.0
$75–100,000	1	.5	4	1.6
$100,000 +	1	.5	6	2.4
Missing	44		37	
Total	232		285	

Table 3.

CRISIS PREPARATIONS ACROSS
DISABLED AND NON-DISABLED RESPONDENTS

Preparation	Disabled		Non-disabled	
	Frequency	Valid %	Frequency	Valid %
Possessed emergency kit				
Yes	101	43.5	133	46.9
No	127	55.7	150	53.1
Missing	4		2	
Had evacuation plan				
Yes	78	34.1	113	40.4
No	151	65.9	167	59.6
Missing	3		5	
Total	232		285	

significant overall model, chi-square (5, N=554)=29.05, p<.001, Nagelkerke R^2 =.094. Older respondents, those in higher income brackets, and the disabled were less likely to have developed an evacuation plan (see Table 4).

Information-seeking. To explore the impact of disability on information-seeking, disability was entered into a linear regression model along with demographic characteristics, predicting the value for the information seeking index score. This model was statistically significant, F (5, 403)=3.09, p=.01, R^2 =.04. Women and African Americans reported slightly higher index scores for aggregate information-seeking, while the disabled reported slightly lower scores (see Table 5).

To further explore the patterns of information-seeking across the two populations, *post hoc* tests examined differences in the individual items that made up the information-seeking index (see Table 6). Mean comparisons indicate that the disabled were less likely to place importance on information concerning the scope of the damage, government response, rescue operations, the larger impact of the storm, who else was affected, and friends and family.

Critical sources of information. Research questions three and four addressed the importance of different media in seeking out information about the disaster. The results point to television as the dominant medium. A total of 101 (43.9%) of the 230 respondents reported that television was their primary source of information. A total of 61 disabled respondents (26.5%) reported that face-to-face communication with acquaintances was most critical, while 9 (3.9%) reported relying on interpersonal communication with strangers (see Table 7).

Research question five examined the relative importance of new media in information seeking about the storm. The results indicate that new media were almost entirely insignificant in providing information about the storm. Out of 230 respondents, only

Table 4.

LOGISTIC REGRESSION ANALYSES—PREDICTORS OF PREPARATIONS TAKEN BEFORE STORM, *EXP (B)* FUNCTIONS FOR DEMOGRAPHICS AND DISABILITY

Predictor	Model 1 (emergency kit)	Model 2 (evacuation plan)
Age	.965***	.970***
Sex	.872	1.06
Race	.664**	.814
Income	.938*	.919***
Disability	.669*	.664*
Note: Nagelkerke R^2	.110	.094
X^2	33.54***	29.05***
*p<.06, **p<.01, ***p<.001		

Table 5.

LINEAR REGRESSION ANALYSES—DEMOGRAPHIC PREDICTORS OF INFORMATION SEEKING, STANDARDIZED REGRESSION COEFFICIENTS FOR DEMOGRAPHIC PREDICTORS AND DISABLITY

Predictor	Model 1 (information seeking)
Age	.033
Sex	.115
Race	.127*
Income	.034
Disability	−.100*

$R^2 = .030$
$F (5,403) = 3.09$, p=.01
*p<.05, **p<.01, ***p<.001

Table 6.

DIFFERENCES IN INFORMATION IMPORTANCE— T-TESTS FOR MEAN COMPARISONS

Information category	Disabled	Non-disabled	t	p-value
Scope of the damage	1.46	1.23	2.85	<.005
Government response	1.60	1.41	2.06	<.048
Food/water distribution	1.55	1.51	.41	n.s.
Evacuation	1.63	1.52	1.08	n.s.
Shelters	1.62	1.67	−.45	n.s.
Rescue operations	1.69	1.39	3.74	<.002
Larger impact of storm	1.70	1.48	2.23	<.027
Who was affected	1.47	1.24	2.91	<.004
Friends and family	1.33	1.14	2.81	<.005
Healthcare/medicine	1.54	1.56	−.21	n.s
Other	1.91	1.88	.09	n.s.

Note: Items were reverse scored; lower means indicate greater perceived importance.
n.s. = not significant

2 reported finding out about the hurricane and evacuation from the Internet. Only 25 disabled respondents (10.9%) reported communication over the phone as being the most important.

Table 7.

PRIMARY INFORMATION SOURCES FOR
DISABLED AND NON-DISABLED RESPONDENTS

Medium	Disabled		Non-disabled	
	Frequency	Valid %	Frequency	Valid %
Television	101	43.9	133	47.3
Face-to-face (friend)	61	26.5	55	19.6
Telephone	25	10.9	26	9.3
Radio	21	9.1	44	15.7
Face-to-face (stranger)	9	3.9	5	1.8
Posted info	2	.9	4	1.4
Internet	2	.9	1	.4
Newspapers	0	.0	2	.7
Other	6	2.6	4	1.4
Missing	2		4	
Total	232		285	

Discussion

Preparations. One reason the disabled community may be less likely than others to evacuate is the need for particular services which many disabled people may believe are not provided at safety centers, or a lack of awareness of centers that provide such services. Further, some individuals with disabilities receive aid from others *via* a formal or informal arrangement. Evacuation may be seen as something that would disrupt this relationship. Disabled adults are twice as likely as non-disabled adults to live alone, thus leading to greater need for assistance.[20] Coordinating that assistance during a crisis, may be difficult. Given all of this, some disabled people may see little prospect of evacuation or simply may not know how to make arrangements for it; they may, therefore, see the possession of an emergency supply kit and supplies as their best chance of surviving the crisis.

It has been noted that age is often closely tied to disability, and that individuals with physical disabilities often live at the lower end of the socioeconomic spectrum.[21] However, the mean age in this sample was 36.09 ($SD=12.00$) for non-disabled respondents and 38.06 ($SD=14.04$) for the disabled respondents. Given that there is little difference in age between the disabled and the non-disabled respondents in this sample, emergency management organizations must ascertain for any given group whether the needs of the disabled can be adequately addressed in the same way as the needs of the elderly.

Information-seeking. Results indicated that women and African Americans were significantly more likely to engage in information-seeking than their counterparts, while the disabled population was less likely to do so than the non-disabled. It was also found that the disabled respondents were less likely than the non-disabled to place importance on information concerning the scope of the damage, government response, rescue operations, the larger impact of the storm, who else was affected, and friends and family. Although there is not a body of past literature examining the crisis information-seeking habits of disabled populations, it appears that the disabled may have a different set of informational needs that may not have been adequately addressed. Information will not be persuasive if the messages do not meet the desired needs.[22]

Critical sources of information and use of new media. Overall, respondents indicated that the most important information source was television; there was little difference between the two populations with regard to preferred medium. There was also little difference between the populations in use of new media, as neither group used new media to any appreciable extent. While past research has suggested that electronic media (such as television) are somewhat brittle in times of natural disaster, it may be the case that new media and Internet resources are even more so; for example, simply losing power would render a home computer useless, while battery operated televisions and radios may still work.[23–25]

Implications. Effective communication is a key element in understanding how best to prevent, prepare for, respond to, and learn from risks and crises. Scientists still have much to learn about the most effective means of communicating critical information to vulnerable populations during a crisis. The current study suggests specific message areas in need of such attention, such as crisis preparation, evacuations, and information distribution.

The disabled subpopulation in this study was somewhat more likely to have an emergency kit ready for the hurricane but less likely than the non-disabled sub-population to have an evacuation plan. This suggests that some sizeable part of the disabled population may not see evacuation as feasible. Hurricanes have longer warning periods than many other crises, which may allow for relatively advanced notice. Therefore, the need for messages designed to motivate disabled people to conduct pre-crisis planning may be even more pressing than is suggested by the disastrous outcomes of Katrina. Such planning would improve the safety of thousands of people and save lives.

More effort is needed in examining the evacuation of the disabled. This may include expanded registration efforts to allow emergency officials to know where disabled people live and to coordinate the arrival of help before a storm arrives. Typically, evacuation of low mobility groups is the responsibility of public agencies. However, in practice, administrators may not be familiar with evacuation procedures. Encouraging community members to pledge to care for disabled individuals in the case of an emergency may help prevent harm. Further, if relationships with others are developed over time, when an evacuation is required, the disabled individual may be more comfortable leaving and may be more likely to have the resources to do so.

Finally, new media has not emerged as a strong source of information dissemination in a crisis event. Although new media and its role in crisis and risk communication is an attractive area of study, the media have not yet achieved a point of critical adoption to warrant focus during a crisis event. From a message placement standpoint, it appears as though television may still be the best place for initial alerts for all populations.

Future research. While the current study examined responses to Hurricane Katrina, not all the results are hurricane-specific. Further research must examine issues that affect the disabled in crises in order to provide service providers with more information concerning crisis response and message design for disabled people.

The results of the present study suggest a difference in willingness between disabled and non-disabled individuals' responses to evacuation notices. While the disabled seem likely to make preparations for a natural disaster such as Hurricane Katrina, they may be among those most in need of supplies, evacuation planning, and information due to a limited capacity to adapt to rapidly changing and threatening conditions. A future goal in research concerning the disabled should be discovering how best to target and to assist disabled people in crisis preparations. Similarly, research should address effective means of motivating disabled individuals to seek information in order to minimize harm and promote better crisis awareness.

Conclusion

A clear need exists for effective crisis and risk messages targeted at disabled populations. As crises occur more frequently and become larger in scope, frequency, harm, and duration, the need for these messages increases correspondingly. Attention must be given to populations that may have unique needs or who may have been overlooked in the existing literature. Although there is much left to learn about communication, risk, and crisis in relation to those with disabilities, the results of this study may be seen as a starting point and a call for future research.

Acknowledgments

This material is based on work supported by the National Science Foundation (NSF) under grant number 0428216. Any opinions, findings, conclusions, or recommendations expressed here are those of the authors and do not necessarily reflect the views of NSF.

Notes

1. Quarantelli EL. Disasters: theory and research. Beverly Hills, CA: Sage Publications, 1978.
2. Sellnow TL, Seeger MW, Ulmer RR. Chaos theory, informational needs and the North Dakota floods. J Appl Commun Res. 2002 Nov;30(4):269–92.
3. Coombs WT. Ongoing crisis communication: planning, managing, and responding. London: Sage Publications, 1999.
4. Seeger MW, Sellnow T, Ulmer RR. Communication and organizational crisis. Westport, CT: Praeger Publishers, 2003.
5. Chou YJ, Huang N, Lee CH, et al. Who is at risk of death in an earthquake? Am J Epidemiol. 2004 Oct 1;160(7):688–95.
6. Morrow BH. Identifying and mapping community vulnerability. Disasters. 1999 Mar; 23(1):1–18.
7. Helsloot I, Ruitenberg A. Citizen response to disasters: a survey of literature and some practical implications. Journal of Contingencies and Crisis Management. 2004;12(3):98–111.

8. Boyce JK. Let them eat risk? Wealth, rights and disaster vulnerability. Disasters. 2000 Sep;24(3):254–61.

9. Tierney KL, Petak WJ, Hahn H. Disabled persons and earthquake hazards. (Monograph No. 46.) Boulder, CO: University of Colorado, Institute of Behavioral Science, 1988.

10. Brashers DE, Neidig JL, Haas SM, et al. Communication in the management of uncertainty: the case of persons living with HIV or AIDS. Commun Monogr. 2000; 67(1):63–84.

11. Spence PR, Westerman D, Skalski P, et al. Proxemic effects on information seeking following the 9/11 attacks. Communication Research Reports. 2005;22(1):39–46.

12. Murch AW. Public concern for environmental pollution. Public Opin Q. 971;35: 100–6.

13. Greenberg BS, Hofschire L, Lachlan K. Diffusion, media use and interpersonal communication behaviors. In: Greenberg BS, ed. Communication and terrorism: public and media responses to 9/11. Cresskill, NJ: Hampton Press, 2002;3–16.

14. Spence PR, Westerman D, Skalski PD, et al. Gender and age effects on information-seeking after 9/11. Communication Research Reports. 2006;23(3):217–23.

15. Heath RL, Liao S, Douglas W. Effects of perceived economic harms and benefits on issue involvement, information use and action: a study in risk communication. Journal of Public Relations Research. 1995;7:89–109.

16. Greenberg BS. Diffusion of news of the Kennedy assassination. Public Opin Q. 1964;28(2):225–32.

17. Spitzer SP, Spitzer NS. Diffusion of news of the Kennedy and Oswald deaths. In: Greenberg BS, Bradley S, Parker EB. The Kennedy assassination and the American public: social communication in crisis. Stanford, CA: Stanford University Press, 1965; 99–111.

18. Bracken CC, Jeffres L, Neuendorf KA, et al. How cosmopolites react to messages: America under attack. Communication Research Reports. 2005 Feb;22(1):47–58.

19. Lyons RF, Sullivan MJL, Ritvo PG, et al. Relationships in chronic illness and disability. Thousand Oaks, CA: Sage Publications, 1995.

20. Kaye HS. Disability watch: the status of people with disabilities in the United States. Volcano, CA: Volcano Press, 1997.

21. Kennedy J, LaPlante MP. A profile of adults needing assistance with activities of daily living, 1991–1992. (Disability Statistics Report 11.) Washington, DC: U.S. Department of Education, National Institute on Disability and Rehabilitation Research, 1997.

22. Lachlan KA, Spence PR. Hazard and outrage: developing a psychometric instrument in the aftermath of Katrina. Journal of Applied Communication Research. 2007 Feb; 35(1):109–23.

23. Hooke WH. U.S. participation in international decade for natural disaster reduction. Natural Hazards Review. 2000 Feb;1(1):2–9.

24. Kluver AR. The logic of new media in international affairs. New Media & Society. 2002;4(4):499–517.

25. Perez-Lugo M. Media uses in disaster situations: a new focus on the impact phase. Sociol Inq. 2004;74(2):210–25.

Chapter 18
Adverse Health Outcomes after Hurricane Katrina among Children and Adolescents with Chronic Conditions

Barbara Rath, MD

Jessica Donato, MPH

Alyson Duggan, MPH

Keith Perrin, MD

Daniel R. Bronfin, MD

Raoult Ratard, MD, MPH

Russell VanDyke, MD

Manya Magnus, PhD, MPH

Hurricane Katrina made landfall on the Gulf Coast of the United States on August 29, 2005, causing one of the country's most expensive natural disasters in terms of both financial and human losses.[1,2] In New Orleans, the combination of wind, storm surge, and rainfall resulted in an undermining of the levee system and flooding of over 80% of the city by neighboring Lake Pontchartrain.[1] The impact of the hurricane on New Orleans, both immediate and over the subsequent year has been extensively chronicled.[1-12]

Even in the absence of a natural disaster, children and adolescents—especially those with chronic health conditions—have specific needs and vulnerabilities at each developmental stage. Of the 469,032 residents of New Orleans at the time of Hurricane Katrina, an estimated 27% were under 18 years old.[13] While children and adolescents will react differently to a disaster and its aftermath depending on age, developmental level, and prior experiences, much child functioning will be influenced by how parents and other caregivers respond to the stress of the disaster and their states of health. Often a caregiver's own mental state can greatly influence his or her parenting behaviors.[14] In the face of stress, children can develop post-traumatic stress disorder (PTSD) and other mental health conditions. These may surface as depression, withdrawal, behavioral problems, hyperactivity, or delinquency. There can also be somatic

BARBARA RATH and RUSSELL VANDYKE are both affiliated with the Tulane University Health Sciences Center, Department of Pediatrics in New Orleans. JESSICA DONATO, ALYSON DUGGAN, and MANYA MAGNUS are affiliated with The George Washington University School of Public Health and Health Services, Department of Epidemiology and Biostatistics. KEITH PERRIN is affiliated with Children's Hospital of New Orleans, DANIEL BRONFIN with the Ochsner Clinic Foundation, Department of Pediatrics (in New Orleans), and RAOULT RATARD with the Louisiana Office of Public Health in Metairie, Louisiana.

manifestations of chronic stress.[15,16] Children with pre-existing chronic conditions may experience adverse physical and psychological outcomes more than children without them in the face of stressors.

Disaster survivors with pre-existing chronic conditions may be particularly vulnerable when faced with specific disaster-related situations. For example, patients with immunodeficiency and AIDS may face increased susceptibility to opportunistic infections. People with chronic conditions may as a matter of course depend on health care specialists and on complex treatment regimens, diets, and other interventions. Not having shelter or usual routines can create more disruptions than arise for people without such conditions.[17] Children and adolescents dependent on adult caregivers, especially children with special needs, may be particularly prone to adverse effects of evacuation and disruption of support systems and routines. Children and adolescents with special needs experienced increased morbidity and mortality also during Hurricane Andrew, which altered access to medications, physician contact, and routine care.[18] In the United States, approximately 12.8% of children are classified as having special health-care needs, defined by the U.S. Maternal and Child Health Bureau as: "... those who have or are at increased risk for a chronic physical, developmental, behavioral, or emotional condition and who also require health and related services of a type or amount beyond that required by children generally."[19, p.138] In addition, those requiring ventilation or other electronic life-support services may be even more affected, given power outages.[20]

Few studies have been conducted to provide insight into the complicated needs of children and adolescents with pre-existing chronic conditions following natural disasters. The purpose of this study is to identify physical, utilization, and psychological outcomes among such children and adolescents after Hurricane Katrina. An improved understanding of the needs of children and adolescents following disasters may help foster improved continuity of care and more success meeting these patients' needs.

Methods

Data were collected from October to December 2005 by an anonymous cross-sectional survey administered to a convenience sample of children and adolescents. Consenting patients 0 to 24 years of age seen at health care facilities post-Katrina in the metropolitan New Orleans area were eligible if they had not taken the survey previously and they reported age and gender. A multidisciplinary team of pediatricians, researchers, social workers, psychologists, and behaviorists created the instrument, adapting items from several previously validated instruments (i.e., PTSD Questionnaire of the National Child Traumatic Stress Network and Louisiana State University, Department of Psychiatry; Project Liberty of the New York Crisis Counseling Program; the UCLA Reaction Index[14,35]). Medical questions included an extensive checklist for self-reporting of symptoms pre- and post-Katrina. Question items included self-report status of acute and chronic conditions pre- and post-Katrina, health care utilization (i.e., well-child visits, immunizations), and evacuation experiences. Due to the conditions at the time of survey administration, validation with hospital records was not feasible and all data were via self-report by the caregiver or the respondent. All participants were informed of the purpose of the study and asked to participate when presenting at one of the select administration sites in New Orleans. The study sites included: 1) Children's Hospital of New Orleans, 2) Tulane Hospital for Children, 3) Ochsner for Children Ambulatory Care Center, 4) Covenant House (an organization for adolescents in need of care and shelter), and 5) private practices and city health clinics serving 0 to 24 year olds in the New Orleans Metro Area as well as the Charity Hospital Emergency Room (located at the New Orleans Convention Center). The survey was conducted while waiting for provider visits either by 1) the child/participant, 2) the parent/guardian for the child, 3) the child/participant with parent/guardian together, or 4) the child or guardian /parent with assistance by a volunteer/ health care professional. Participants indicating on the form that they had taken the survey before were excluded.

Univariate and bivariate analyses were performed to describe the study sample and evaluate potential confounders. To evaluate unadjusted associations between independent and dependent variables, chi-square tests were used for categorical variables and unpaired t-tests for continuous variables. Logistic regression was used to model unadjusted and adjusted relationships between predictors and outcomes of disruption of care and development of new symptoms or diagnoses. A goodness-of-fit test ($\alpha=0.15$) was used to assess model fit.

An individual was classified as having a chronic condition if they answered *yes* to having, diabetes, asthma, other chronic lung disease, allergies, HIV/AIDS, other immune disease, heart defect/disease, cystic fibrosis, mental retardation, attention deficit/hyperactivity disorder (ADHD), autism, depression, other mental health or behavior problems, seizure disorder, sickle cell disease, kidney failure/dialysis, or liver failure prior to August 2005. Disruption in routine care was defined as when the participant reported *yes* to either missed doctor's visits by self-report, ran out of medications, missed immunizations, or was not current in immunizations. Development of a new symptom or diagnosis occurred if the participant reported not having a condition prior to August 2005 yet had it in any one of the first four months following the hurricane. For the panel of psychological response variables, participants reporting having a particular experience or outcome *much* or *most* of the time were considered to have a positive response. Facility was entered into the regression models as an indicator variable to assess specific differences between facilities. Stata, v. 9.0se (College Station, Texas) was used for all analyses. In this study, all instruments, consents, and modifications were approved prior to implementation by all governing institutional review boards (IRB) (Children's Hospital, Tulane Hospital, George Washington University, and Ochsner Hospital and Clinic).

Results

Between October and December 2005, 601 surveys were completed. Of these, 531 were eligible [reasons for exclusion: invalid age: 42 (7.0%); no gender: 12 (2.0%); taken before: 16 (2.7%)]. As seen in Table 1, the majority of the children were younger than 13 years old (79.8%) [median 5.33 years, mean age 6.9 years (standard deviation 5.6, range 0.08–24)] and seen at the Children's Hospital of New Orleans (one of the first facilities to re-open after the hurricane) (72.9%). The sample was approximately half male (50.2%) and nearly half African American (42.8%). Nearly half of the children were seeking medical care for a new problem (47.1%), and the remainder for an existing problem (28.3%) or a well-child visit (14.5%). Almost half of the children had one or more chronic conditions prior to Hurricane Katrina (43.2%). Most (81.0%) had evacuated their homes due to the hurricane; 78.4% reported living in an environment affected by mold, flood, roof, glass, or storm damage at the time of survey administration.

There were no differences ($p \leqslant .05$) between children with and without pre-existing conditions with respect to person completing the survey, gender, race, ethnicity, facility, immunization status (up to date *vs.* not, as well as having missed an immunization); whether or not they evacuated; or the presence of roof, glass, or storm damage at the current residence. However, children with and without pre-existing chronic conditions differed from one another in several aspects. Children with chronic conditions sought care more often for new health problems than did children without chronic conditions. They were also more likely to visit the clinic for secondary health problems rather than their underlying chronic condition (43.5%). The chronic conditions *per se* were less often the reason for doctor's visits during the first months after the hurricane/evacuation (16.2%, $p < .001$). Children with pre-existing chronic conditions were also more likely to take medication or inhalers to control asthma than those without chronic health conditions (37.4% vs. 3.9%, $p < .001$), to have their asthma worsen (16.3% vs. 1.9%, $p < 0.001$), to have missed a doctor's visit (49.2% vs. 39.8%, $p < .01$), or to have run out of medications (33.9% vs. 7.9%, $p < .001$) since the hurricane or evacuation. Children with chronic conditions were more likely to live in a home with flood damage (19.7% vs. 11.3%, $p < .05$) or mold (23.6% vs. 15.8%, $p < .05$) after their return to post-Katrina New Orleans. While nearly half (43.9%) of the participants had experienced one or more disruptions in medical care (missed medications or doctor's visits, not being up to date on immunizations or having missed at least one immunization), children with pre-existing conditions were more likely than those without to have experienced at least one disruption in care (58.4% vs. 38.3%, $p < .001$). Although older children were more likely to have a pre-existing condition [mean 8.22 (sd 5.49) vs. 6.14 (5.63), $p < .001$], younger children were more likely to have developed new symptoms or diagnoses than older children and adolescents [mean 6.51 (sd 5.46) vs. 7.97 (6.03), $p < .001$].

Among children with pre-existing chronic conditions, all of the HIV-positive participants (n=7) and 90% of the children with pre-existing diagnoses of depression (n=9) experienced one or more disruption in care ($p < .05$). After adjusting for age, race, gender, and facility, children with prior conditions were significantly more likely to experience a disruption in care than were their counterparts (OR 2.62, 95% CI 1.78–3.87, $p < .001$). Of the 102 children who reported having asthma (either as a chronic or non-chronic condition), 80 (78.4%) reported that they required more asthma medication or inhalers during the first three months after the hurricane than pre-Katrina. Of these, 30 (39.5%) reported that their asthma had worsened since September 2005. Of the 379 children who did not need asthma medication or inhalers prior to the hurricane, 12 (3.2%) began using such medication since September 2005, and nearly 2% of these children reported a worsening of symptoms since that time.

Specific symptoms were evaluated to compare children with and without pre-existing chronic conditions with respect to their development of new symptoms following

Table 1.

CHARACTERISTICS OF PEDIATRIC PATIENTS (N=531)

	n	%[a]
Gender		
Male	268	50.5
Female	263	49.5
Race		
Caucasian/White	227	42.8
African American/Black	215	40.5
Other	89	16.7
Age		
<1 year	69	13.0
1 to <5 years	179	33.7
5 to <13 years	176	33.2
13 to 24 years	107	20.2
Health care facility		
Children's Hospital New Orleans	387	72.9
Ochsner for Children	88	16.6
Tulane Hospital for Children	27	5.1
Other facilities	29	5.5
Clinic/ER visit purpose		
For a new health problem	250	47.1
For a physical/check-up or well-child visit	77	14.5
For a problem that existed before hurricane	150	28.3
Other	54	10.2
Chronic conditions prior to Hurricane Katrina[b]	209	39.4
Diabetes	17	3.2
Asthma or other chronic lung disease	93	17.5
Used asthma medication or inhalers prior to Hurricane Katrina	107	20.2
Self-report: Worsened asthma since Hurricane Katrina	33	6.2
Allergies	65	12.2
HIV/AIDS or other immune disease	10	1.9
Heart disease or heart defect	11	2.1
ADHD	20	3.8
Depression	10	1.9
Other mental health or behavioral disorder	19	3.6
Seizure disorder	15	2.8
Other conditions	50	9.4
Missed physician visit due to hurricane	182	41.1
Ran out of medications since the hurricane	84	19.7
Missed immunizations	37	8.4

Table 1. *(continued)*

	n	%[a]
Currently up to date on immunizations	436	92.4
Hurricane-related experiences		
Evacuated from home due to hurricane	430	81.0
Became dehydrated or experienced heat exhaustion	17	3.9
Living environment (at the time of survey completion) with one or more adverse conditions:	424	78.4
Flood damage	73	14.0
Mold	99	18.9
Roof, glass, or storm damage	252	48.0

[a]Percentages may not add up to 100 due to rounding.
[b]Respondents could indicate more than one condition. This proportion represents participants with one or more conditions. Proportions are of the total sample (N=531).

the hurricane. Unlike the previous question that inquired about "chronic conditions" prior to the hurricane, the symptom panel data were collected based on experience of symptoms provided to the respondent in lay language and not in association with named diagnoses or current medications (Table 2). Children with pre-existing conditions were significantly ($p<.05$) more likely to develop respiratory symptoms (asthma, shortness of breath, and difficulty breathing), headache, and blurred vision. Children without pre-existing conditions were significantly ($p<.05$) more likely to report having bloody diarrhea and household accidents. Irrespective of prior conditions, participants were otherwise similar ($p>.95$), with nearly three-quarters (74.2%) of all children developing at least one new symptom.

There were significant differences between those with and without pre-existing conditions in the psychological reactions and frightening experiences of children (Table 3). Children with chronic conditions were more likely than those children without chronic conditions to exhibit negative psychological consequences of the hurricane, overall sadness and withdrawal, and behavioral changes. Responses to each question indicated significantly higher negative reaction on every question, ranging from a difference of 2.5% to 12.9% (all $p<.05$).

Discussion

This study suggests that following a natural disaster such as Hurricane Katrina, children and adolescents with pre-existing chronic conditions are significantly more likely to experience negative health outcomes than those without. Chronically ill children and adolescents experienced more disruption in care and developed more new symptoms than those without. Children with diseases (including diabetes, asthma, other chronic

Table 2.

SIGNIFICANT DIFFERENCES BETWEEN CHILDREN AND ADOLESCENTS WITH AND WITHOUT CHRONIC CONDITIONS IN THE DEVELOPMENT OF NEW SYMPTOMS FOLLOWING HURRICANE KATRINA (N=531)

Symptom	Participants with pre-existing chronic conditions (n=209) %	Participants without pre-existing chronic conditions (n=260) %
Asthma***	12.4	1.5
Shortness of breath***	16.3	4.2
Difficulty breathing*	12.9	5.2
Headache*	8.6	3.5
Blurred vision*	2.87	.4
Bloody diarrhea*	.0	1.9
Household accidents*	.0	2.3

*p<.05, **p<.01, ***p<.001.
No significant difference with respect to remainder of symptom panel, which includes all body systems.

lung disease, allergies, HIV/AIDS, other immune disease, heart defect/disease, cystic fibrosis, mental retardation, ADHD, autism, depression, other mental health or behavior problems, seizure disorder, sickle cell disease, kidney failure/dialysis, or liver failure) prior to Hurricane Katrina were also significantly more likely than those without them to experience negative reactions to hurricane-related stressors. These reactions included increased fear, depression, post-traumatic stress symptoms, and behavioral alteration.

This study has several limitations. Participants were selected *via* convenience rather than by means of a random sampling method, and these findings are unlikely to be representative of the general population in New Orleans, either before or after the storm. Because this survey was anonymous, it was not possible to evaluate medical records for actual status regarding chronic conditions or current medical or psychological states and measures of interest are entirely based on self-report. Due to the cross-sectional nature of the design, it is difficult to determine temporality of events.

Furthermore, given that individuals with chronic conditions generally seek care more frequently due to their underlying health conditions, we cannot draw direct conclusions from the present study about the extent to which the disaster led to adverse outcomes and/or care-seeking by children and adolescents with chronic conditions. To draw such conclusions, we would have had to compare children and adolescents with chronic conditions who had experienced the hurricane with such children and adolescents who had not. Given the vast geographical region affected by Hurricane

Table 3.

POSITIVE RESPONSES TO STRESS QUESTIONS (N=531)

	Children with pre-existing chronic conditions (n=209) %	Children without pre-existing chronic conditions (n=260) %
For the child[a]:		
"Did a family member or friend get injured or killed?"**	12.3	4.0
"Did you/your child see people getting hurt or killed?"*	13.3	8.9
"Did you see any violence or looting?"*	15.6	8.5
"Do you get upset, afraid, or sad when something makes you think of the hurricane/flooding/evacuation?"*	24.9	15.8
"Do you have upsetting thoughts or pictures that come to your mind about what happened?"**	19.1	10.4
"Do you have difficulty falling asleep at night or find that you wake up in the middle of the night because of what happened?"*	13.4	7.3
"Do you often feel jumpy or nervous?"*	12.9	6.5
"Do you find it harder to concentrate or pay attention to things than you usually do?"**	16.3	7.3
"Do you often feel irritable or grouchy?"*	20.1	12.7
"Do you often feel sad, down, or depressed?"*	13.9	8.1
"Do you have less energy than usual?"*	13.4	7.8
"Do you find it harder to get your schoolwork done?"* (To those in school only.)	11.0	5.0
"Do you worry about something else bad happening to you/family/friends?"*	15.3	8.1
"Are you having a harder time getting along with family or friends?"**	10.1	3.5
"Have you used drugs or alcohol since the hurricane/flooding/evacuation?"*	2.9	.4

Table 3. *(continued)*

	Children with pre-existing chronic conditions (n=209) %	Children without pre-existing chronic conditions (n=260) %
For the parent:		
"Has your child talked repeatedly about or asked questions about the hurricane/flooding/evacuation?"***	22.5	9.6
"Has your child been more quiet or withdrawn?"*	5.7	1.5
"Has your child's play been about the hurricane/flooding/evacuation?"*	5.3	.8
"Do you have other concerns about your child since the hurricane/flooding/evacuation?"*	13.4	7.3

[a]Agreement indicated as "much" or "most" during the last month, except for first three, which are yes/no.
*p<.05, **p<.01, ***p<.001.
No significant difference with respect to remainder of questions.

Katrina and the lack of appropriate controls, this comparison is not possible. Instead, the conclusions that we draw concern differences after a disaster between children with pre-existing conditions and children without such conditions, where both groups experienced the hurricane. While we might have expected differences between these two groups with respect to condition-related experiences such as taking asthma medication, having asthma worsen, or having negative psychological consequences, we believe that the narrow time frame of the study (the first four months after the hurricane and evacuation) makes is unlikely that the observed changes were due to natural progression of chronic illness alone. It is also important to have established that children and adolescents with pre-existing chronic conditions were more likely than those without to miss a visit, to run out of medications, to live with flood damage or mold, and to experience disruption in care.

Additionally, given that individuals with chronic conditions generally seek care more frequently due to their conditions, there may be a bias towards inclusion of participants with chronic conditions. However, just over a third of the sample fell into this category, suggesting that the circularity of exposure and disruption of care may not bias these findings. The prevalence and severity of some chronic diseases such as HIV/AIDS and asthma have been linked to disparities in socioeconomic status,[25-28] which may coincide with stress during times of natural disaster and displacement.[21-24]

Thus, those with chronic health conditions may be exposed to more stressful situations than their counterparts. Several studies suggest, however, that families with the least resources and social status were the last to evacuate, but also the least likely to have returned to New Orleans within the first months after the storm;[29–32] such participants would therefore have been less likely to have been sampled in this study. Finally, the survey was developed following the hurricane, and similar measures are not available to estimate the pre-disaster differences. It may be that these findings are attributable in part to the chronic conditions themselves and not the interaction with the hurricane/evacuation. Future studies will be in a superior position to address this important research question.

This study has several strengths. It is one of the first to evaluate pediatric health outcomes following one of the largest natural disasters to hit the U.S., and to investigate the important role of pre-existing conditions in the care of children and adolescents. The anonymous nature of the study increases the likelihood of candor in response. The multi-faceted nature of the questionnaire allows investigation into a variety of exposures and outcomes. This analysis included data collected through December 2005; as more data become available to describe phenomena longitudinally, the question of whether the discrepancies between children and adolescents with and without chronic conditions attenuate will be examined.

This study suggests that children and adolescents with chronic conditions are at increased risk of adverse outcomes following natural disasters such as Hurricane Katrina. Providers may be able to reduce the negative effects on this population by developing condition-specific continuity of care mechanisms.[33,34] Preparedness measures (such as evacuation medication packs, immunization registries that are readily transferable to other locations, and paperless medical records) may have helped to limit negative health outcomes at the time of simultaneous displacement of chronically ill patients, their families, and their regular health care providers. Clearly defined disaster preparedness plans for children and adolescents with chronic conditions may be able to reduce disruptions of care during disaster. Reductions in disruptions of care may also help reduce stress experienced by children and adolescents, resulting in improvements in health outcomes.

Acknowledgments

The authors kindly acknowledge the hard work of Shuchin Shukla and Mathew Strickland and the clerical and nursing staff at the respective study sites in administering the survey, as well as the patients and their families who volunteered to participate in this project. We also thank Stacy Horn Koch, Kathryn Wheat, and Lakresha Peters at Covenant House New Orleans, as well as Edward Bonin at the Drop-in Center, for their advocacy and encouragement. Many thanks to Drs. Margaret Silio, Patricia Sirois, Sue-Ellen Abdalian, Rodolfo Begue, James Robinson and Richard Oberhelman for critically reviewing the study protocol. We also thank Dr. Edward Morse and Dr. Patricia Morse at Louisiana State University and the National Child Traumatic Stress Network for providing us with the validated PTSD questionnaire as part of our survey project.

Notes

1. Centers for Disease Control and Prevention (CDC). Public health response to Hurricanes Katrina and Rita—United States, 2005. MMWR Morb Mortal Wkly Rep. 2006 Mar 10;55(9):229–31.

2. Centers for Disease Control and Prevention (CDC). Assessment of health-related needs after hurricanes Katrina and Rita—Orleans and Jefferson Parishes, New Orleans Area, Louisiana, October 17–22, 2005. MMWR Morb Mortal Wkly Rep. 2006 Jan 20;55(2):38–41.

3. Perrin K. A first for this century: closing and reopening of a children's hospital during a disaster. Pediatrics. 2006 May;117(5 Pt 3):S381–5.

4. Baldwin S, Robinson A, Barlow P, et al. Moving hospitalized children all over the southeast: interstate transfer of pediatric patients during Hurricane Katrina. Pediatrics. 2006 May;117(5 Pt 3):S416–20.

5. Mani SD. On call for the duration: code gray: a resident's personal account from Children's Hospital of New Orleans. Pediatrics. 2006 May;117(5 Pt 3):S386–8.

6. Parke S, Parke WK. Hurricane Katrina: nursing in the eye of the storm. RN. 2005 Oct;68(10):55–6, 66, 68.

7. Patsdaugher C. From primary care for the underserved to emergency aid for hurricane evacuees: questions raised and lessons learned. J Cult Divers. 2005 Fall;12(3):75–6.

8. Leder HA, Rivera P. Six days in Charity Hospital: two doctors' ordeal in Hurricane Katrina. Compr Ther. 2006 Spring;32(1):2–9.

9. Ginsberg HG. Sweating it out in a level III regional NICU: disaster preparation and lessons learned at the Ochsner Foundation Hospital. Pediatrics. 2006 May;117(5 Pt 3):S375–80.

10. Barkemeyer BM. Practicing neonatology in a blackout: the University Hospital NICU in the midst of Hurricane Katrina: caring for children without power or water. Pediatrics. 2006 May;117(5 Pt 3):S369–74.

11. Gruich M Jr. Life-changing experiences of a private practicing pediatrician: perspectives from a private pediatric practice. Pediatrics. 2006 May;117(5 Pt 3):S359–64.

12. Centers for Disease Control and Prevention (CDC). Hurricane Katrina response and guidance for health-care providers, relief workers, and shelter operators. MMWR Morb Mortal Wkly Rep. 2005 Sep 9;54(35):877.

13. U.S. Census Bureau. New Orleans (city), Louisiana. Washington, DC: U.S. Census Bureau, State & County QuickFacts, 2007. Available at http://quickfacts.census.gov/qfd/states/22/2255000.html.

14. The National Child Traumatic Stress Network. Hurricane Assessment and Referral Tool for Children and Adolescents. Los Angeles, CA: National Center for Child Traumatic Stress, 2005 Sep 19. Available at http://www.nctsnet.org/nctsn_assets/pdfs/intervention_manuals/referraltool.pdf.

15. Norris FH, MJ Friedman, PJ Watson. 60,000 disaster victims speak: Part II. Summary and implications of the disaster mental health research. Psychiatry. 2002 Fall;65(3):240–60.

16. Vernberg EM, Silverman WK, La Greca AM, et al. Prediction of posttraumatic stress symptoms in children after hurricane Andrew. J Abnorm Psychol. 1996 May;105(2):237–48.

17. Gignac MAM, Cott CA, Badley EM. Living with a chronic disabling illness and then some: data from the 1998 ice storm. Can J Aging. 2004 Fall;22(3):249–63.

18. La Greca AM, Silverman WK, Wasserstein SB. Children's predisaster functioning as a predictor of posttraumatic stress following Hurricane Andrew. J Consult Clin Psychol. 1998 Dec;66(6):883–92.

19. McPherson M, Arango P, Fox H, et al. A new definition of children with special health care needs. Pediatrics. 1998 Jul;102(1 Pt 1):137–40.

20. Dolan MA, Krug SE. Pediatric disaster preparedness in the wake of Katrina: lessons to be learned. Clin Ped Emer Med. 2006 Mar;7(1):59–66.

21. Berggren R. Unexpected necessities—inside Charity Hospital. N Engl J Med. 2005 Oct;353(15):1550–3.

22. Atkins D, Moy EM. Left behind: the legacy of hurricane Katrina. BMJ. 2005 Oct 22;331(7522):916–8.

23. Voelker R. Katrina's impact on mental health likely to last years. JAMA. 2005 Oct 5;294(13):1599–600.

24. Bring New Orleans Back Health and Social Cervices Committee. Report and Recommendations to the Commission. New Orleans, LA: Bring New Orleans Back Fund, 2006 Jan 18. Available at http://www.bringneworleansback.org/Portals/BringNew OrleansBack/Resources/Health%20and%20Social%20Services%20Report%20Attach ment%20E.pdf.

25. Ernst P, Demissie K, Joseph L, et al. Socioeconomic status and indicators of asthma in children. Am J Respir Crit Care Med. 1995 Aug;152(2):570–5.

26. Persky VW, Slezak J, Contreras A, et al. Relationships of race and socioeconomic status with prevalence, severity, and symptoms of asthma in Chicago school children. Ann Allergy Asthma Immunol. 1998 Sep;81(3):266–71.

27. Fiscella K, Franks P, Gold MR, et al. Inequality in quality: addressing socioeconomic, racial, and ethnic disparities in health care. JAMA. 2000 May 17;283:2579–84.

28. Zierler S, Krieger N. Reframing women's risk: social inequalities and HIV infection. Annu Rev Public Health. 1997;18:401–36.

29. Brodie M, Weltzien E, Altman D, et al. Experiences of hurricane Katrina evacuees in Houston shelters: implications for future planning. Am J Public Health. 2006 Aug;96(8);1402–8.

30. Whitehead JC, Edwards B, Van Willigen M, et al. Heading for higher ground: factors affecting real and hypothetical hurricane evacuation behavior. Glob Environ Change, Part B: Environmental Hazards. 2000 Dec;2(4):133–42.

31. Van Willigen M, Edwards B, Lormand S, et al. Comparative assessment of impacts and recovery from Hurricane Floyd among student and community households. Natural Hazards Review. 2005 Nov;6(4):180–90.

32. Zhai G, Ikeda S. Flood risk acceptability and economic value of evacuation. Risk Anal. 2006 Jun;26(3):683–94.

33. American Academy of Pediatrics Council on Children with Disabilities. Care coordination in the medical home: integrating health and related systems of care for children with special health care needs. Pediatrics. 2005 Nov;116(5);1238–44. Available at http://aappolicy.aappublications.org/cgi/content/full/pediatrics;116/5/1238.

34. Johnson CP, Kastner TA, American Academy of Pediatrics Committee/Section on Children with Disabilities. Helping families raise children with special health care needs at home. Pediatrics. 2005 Feb;115(3):507–11. Available at http://aappolicy.aap publications.org/cgi/content/full/pediatrics;115/2/507.

35. Steinberg AM, Brymer MJ, Decker KB, et al. The University of California at Los Angeles Post-traumatic Stress Disorder Reaction Index. Curr Psychiatry Rep. 2004 Apr;6(2):96–100.

Chapter 19
News, Social Capital, and
Health in the Context of Katrina

Christopher E. Beaudoin, PhD

Natural disasters place a great burden on an affected region and its population, fracturing social, informational, and physical infrastructure[1-4] and causing death and injury,[2] as well as stress, depression, and vulnerability.[1,5-9] Because disasters exacerbate preexisting social inequalities,[10] these negative outcomes are worse among poor and underserved groups, often best characterized in terms of class, income, race, ethnicity, gender, and age.[11]

By many standards, Hurricane Katrina was the worst natural disaster in U.S. history. The storm surge breached several New Orleans levees, leading to the greatest displacement of a U.S. population ever, the flooding of 80% of the city, the deaths of more than a thousand people in New Orleans alone, and an estimated $100 billion in damages.[12,13] Although a mandatory evacuation was ordered, 120,000 residents remained in New Orleans during the hurricane, in homes, hotels, and several "shelters of last resort."[14] An estimated 27,000 people stayed at the Superdome, with another 20,000 at the New Orleans Convention Center.[14] In the days and weeks that followed, New Orleans residents moved across the country, with many staying in hurricane shelters in other cities and states.

With local, state, and federal governments providing little assistance, the New Orleans public was left, in many ways, to fend for itself. In such an environment, people had to create and adapt to makeshift social and informational resources. As a consequence, Hurricane Katrina affords a unique opportunity to study the public health functions of news information and social capital in the context of a natural catastrophe.

News information and social capital are critical to how people adapt to new situations; construct, manage, and resolve uncertainty; and confront adversity, including threats to physical and mental health. To deal with such challenges, many people rely on the news media.[15,16] News information has been shown to be important in various disaster settings, including reports of a disaster in the aftermath and recommendations related to public safety.[17,18] Conversely, exposure to graphic television depictions of disasters has been associated with the development of psychological illness.[19,20] Concerning Hurricane Katrina, it would be expected that news coverage and its effects would vary according to time period. For example, prior to the hurricane, news information would be critical to survival and safety, in the form of weather predictions and suggested evacuation routes

CHRISTOPHER E. BEAUDOIN is the Usdin Family Professor of Community Health Sciences at the Tulane University School of Public Health and Tropical Medicine.

and other safety strategies. Following a hurricane, news information is also important, taking the form of updates on hurricane-damaged regions, recommendations related to living accommodations and planned returns to damaged regions, and safety tips for reentering such areas. News following a hurricane, however, could well also include graphic and disturbing images.

Also critical to a public's disaster response is *social capital*, which can be defined as resources embedded in social networks that can be accessed and mobilized in purposive action.[21] These social resources result from the social connections and interactions of people.[22] Social capital is defined in terms of its function,[23] with social connections necessary for the achievement of various outcomes. Previous research has considered social capital to be a resource of groups of people and/or of individual people.[24] The current study takes the view that, while social capital exists in links between people, it is individuals who have actual access to the social resources. It should be noted that, with information channels as an integral component,[23] social capital is consistent with the flow of news information during disasters.

Social capital is important because of its connection to positive public health outcomes.[25,26] This carries over to disaster settings, where disaster preparedness and recovery are better for people and groups who have high levels of trust, community participation, and social networking.[4,27-29] Similarly, social support is linked to improved post-disaster health and development,[30,31] including decreased stress and depression.[1,2,5-7] Conversely, social capital can have adverse public health outcomes,[32] such as that evidenced by the link between organization membership and HIV infection in South Africa.[33] In disaster settings, social capital, as measured in terms of social connections and informal groupings, is consistent with illegal activities such as raiding of relief supplies and looting.[34,35]

The current study assesses the public health functions of news information and social capital in a vulnerable population before, during, and after Hurricane Katrina. The current study aims to address two related questions. First, what types of news information and social capital do people rely on before, during, and after a catastrophic natural disaster? Second, what are the relationships between health outcomes and the reliance on news information and social capital?

Methods

In-depth interviews were conducted with 57 adults who were hurricane shelter residents in the state of Louisiana. The randomly selected participants were residents of New Orleans who had left the city as a result of Hurricane Katrina. The in-depth interviews were completed during the first two weeks of October 2005, between 4 and 6 weeks after the hurricane. Each interview lasted between 20 and 60 minutes. The interviews were conducted inside the four most-populated Red Cross shelters in the state: Alexandria, Baton Rouge, Lafayette, and Monroe. Institutional Review Board approval for this study was provided by Tulane University. Participants signed a related consent form prior to the interviews.

Participants were randomly selected, with every 10th shelter resident approached for this study. The study was explained individually to 75 such residents. Among the

75 individuals, 11 expressed a lack of interest during the explanation of the study. The remaining 64 people were asked to participate in the study. Of these, 89% (n=57) agreed and were subsequently interviewed, resulting in an overall cooperation rate of 76%.

The interviews were semi-structured, allowing participants to answer specific questions, as well as provide anecdotal information and tangential ideas. There were both quantitative and qualitative questions. Topics were addressed in chronological order, beginning with the days before the hurricane, moving on to the hurricane itself, and then to the weeks that followed. Each place a participant had stayed was assessed. Questions related to demographics were asked at the end of the interviews.

The aim of the qualitative interview component was to draw comparisons and contrasts with the findings of the quantitative interview component and to provide examples of experiences reported during the interviews. The interviews were audio recorded and then transcribed and entered, in quantitative and qualitative forms, into Microsoft Excel. Excel was used as a step toward further quantitative analysis with Stata 9 (StataCorp, College Station, Texas, USA); its use made the qualitative data more manageable in terms of both categorization and presentation. The qualitative data analysis focused on the content of participant statements. Because of the broad nature of the qualitative data, a sorting process followed, with segments of each interview placed in various content categories. This involved categorization according to grounded theory, including open and selective coding, comparison and categorization, and re-reading and modification.[36]

Quantitative measurement included psychological and physical health problems, news reliance, positive social capital, negative social capital, and demographics. Psychological problems were assessed in terms of depression. The six items involved restless sleeping, sadness, enjoyment of life, crying, feeling disliked by others, and feeling depressed.[37] The timeframe for the questions was the previous week. This specific subscale,[9] as well as other similar subscales,[38,39] have been validated by previous research. Responses to each item were yes (1) and no (0). Responses were added to create a seven-point index of depression (K-R 20=.85; range=0–6; M=2.97; SD=1.81). The index was split to distinguish between participants who met the criteria for depression (4 to 6 symptoms) and those who did not (0 to 3 symptoms). Those respondents with the criteria for depression were scored 1, while those without the criteria were scored 0. By having four, five, or six of the symptoms, 46% of the participants screened positively for depression. Physical health problems were assessed specific to illness and injury. There were two items: 1) one specific to physical illness, including diarrhea, colds, and respiratory problems; and 2) one specific to physical injury, including cuts, bruises, staph infection, and rashes. The timeframe for these measures was from the point of the hurricane making landfall until the time of the interview. Thirteen percent reported physical illness, while 6% reported physical injury. Subsequently, an overall index was created for illness and injury (M=.16, SD=.37).

Use of news information was assessed in terms of news reliance before and after the hurricane. This measure indexed participant reliance on different media (radio, television, newspaper, and Internet) for news information about the hurricane. Participants were asked if they had relied on each of these media for news about the hurricane.[40] For example, for television news reliance after the hurricane, the following item was used: "Did you rely on television news to stay informed about the hurricane and its aftermath?" For hurricane-related information leading up to the hurricane, 54% of the participants relied on television, followed by radio (25%) and newspapers (2%). After the hurricane, television was the most widely relied upon source of news information in the shelters (49%), compared with radio (21%), the Internet (7%), and newspapers (5%). Responses to the four medium-specific items were added to create news reliance indices for before the hurricane (M=.81, SD=.69) and after the hurricane (M=.83, SD=.81). Thus, participants, on average, relied on .81 media outlets before the hurricane and .83 media outlets after the hurricane. As for plans for future news information related to the hurricane, 60% said they expected to rely on radio, followed by television (46%) and newspapers (2%).

Social capital was measured in terms of social interactions before and after the hurricane. The assessment at both time periods had two steps. First, for each place the participants stayed, they were asked how often they interacted with neighbors and other non-familial people.[38,39] Responses were as follows: *never, rarely, sometimes*, and *often*. Second, the valence of these social interactions was assessed, with participants asked if these social interactions were positive or negative in nature. Although previous research makes the distinction between positive and negative forms of social capital, no quantitative measurement could be located for the negative representations of social capital. Participants who responded *sometimes* or *often* to the aforementioned social interaction question were then asked two follow-up questions: 1) *Were the social interactions positive, such as borrowing and lending food and household items and offering and receiving support?*; and 2) *Were the social interactions negative, such as in relation to intimidation, crime, and violence?*[41] Thus, if respondents had interacted sometimes or often with neighbors and other non-familial people *and* indicated that the interactions were positive, they received a score of 1. If not, they received a score of 0. Via this approach, the mean for pre-hurricane positive social interactions was .42 (SD=.50), while the mean for pre-hurricane negative social interactions was .28 (SD=.45).

The approach was more complex for the post-hurricane period. The post-hurricane assessments involved social interactions in each place a participant had stayed after the hurricane. Because the number of places stayed varied, the responses were divided by the total number of places a participant had stayed. This process resulted in two social capital indices: post-hurricane positive social interactions (M=.29, SD=.33) and post-hurricane negative social interactions (M=.15, SD=.28).

Results

Demographics. Of the sample, 25% were Caucasian and 75% African American; 49% were male. The mean age was 47.80 years (SD=16.23). The mean education level was 11.52 years (SD=2.26), with 57% having a high school degree. As for annual household income, 87% reported less than $25,000, and the remaining 13% reported less than $50,000.

Hurricane experiences. When the hurricane hit, 56% of the participants were at a home in New Orleans, with the rest having evacuated to shelters, hotels, and homes elsewhere. As a result of the hurricane, the participants had traveled *via* car, bus, airplane, helicopter, ferry, canoe, and other types of boats. About 82% of the participants did not have personal access to a vehicle for evacuation; among those with access, several reported car problems that prevented a timely evacuation. The participants had stayed in churches, on bridges, overpasses, off-ramps, airports, schools, universities, and homes of friends and relatives; shelters such as the Superdome, the Convention Center and the Astrodome; and even a donut shop. The mean number of places stayed was 2.67 ($SD = 1.43$), with one participant having stayed in 9 different places since the hurricane.

Quantitative findings. Binary logistic regression was employed to test the predictors of the two health outcomes measures: 1) depression; and 2) illness and injury. Control variables included sex, age, income, race/ethnicity, and education. The critical predictors were positive social interactions, negative social interactions, and news reliance, with specific measures representing before the hurricane and after the hurricane. Findings are shown in Table 1. Adjusted odds ratios (AOR) and 95% confidence intervals (CI) are reported.

The first logistic regression model explained 35% of variance in depression, as indicated by the R^2. As depicted in Table 1, there are four significant predictors of depression. An AOR of less than 1 indicates that an increase in a predictor is consistent with the decreased likelihood of an outcome variable. In contrast, an AOR of more than 1 indicates that an increase in a predictor is consistent with the increased likelihood of an outcome variable. Thus, it can be inferred that increases in pre-hurricane positive social interactions and post-hurricane positive social interactions were consistent with not having depression. In contrast, increases in post-hurricane negative social interactions and post-hurricane news reliance were consistent with having depression.

The second logistic regression model accounted for 15% of variance in illness and injury, as indicated by the R^2. As depicted in Table 1, there is only one significant predictor of illness and injury. The AOR indicates that an increase in post-hurricane news reliance was consistent with experiencing illness and injury.

Qualitative findings. News information was critical at various stages of the disaster. For example, in a shelter several days after the hurricane, a woman reported that the absence of information led shelter residents to become frustrated and then hostile. Other participants offered examples of news information being important for their sense of stability.

> In [another] shelter, the news was there. I could see the city and what happened. Here, I don't know nothin.' I don't know if my house is OK. I don't know if my neighbors are OK. It can really bring you down. (Man, 67, African American)

> Not knowin' is the worst thing. I wouldn't feel so bad if I could see my house and know if I could move back. I can't, so things are tough. (Woman, 80, African American)

Satisfaction with news information related to the hurricane varied, with 32% of the participants reporting information satisfaction and 49% reporting information dissatisfaction. Of those who were dissatisfied with information, 29% complained of the lack of information specific to their own neighborhoods. Furthermore, there were numerous

Table 1.

ADJUSTED ODDS RATIOS[a] AND CONFIDENCE INTERVALS FOR PREDICTORS OF HEALTH OUTCOME VARIABLES

	Depression		Illness and injury	
	AOR (95% CI)	p-value	AOR (95% CI)	p-value
Pre-hurricane positive social interactions	.16 (.02, 1.83)	.046	1.60 (.17, 15.22)	.684
Pre-hurricane negative social interactions	.54 (.08, 3.89)	.541	.95 (.13, 7.20)	.962
Post-hurricane positive social interactions	.02 (.00, .74)	.033	.71 (.06, 8.70)	.791
Post-hurricane negative social interactions	17.05 (.92, 315.64)	.047	1.86 (.12, 29.03)	.657
Pre-hurricane news reliance	.59 (.14, 2.50)	.470	.45 (.09, 2.16)	.319
Post-hurricane news reliance	5.49 (1.29, 23.35)	.021	1.13 (1.02, 2.77)	.046
R^2	.35		.15	

[a] Adjusted for race/ethnicity, sex, age, income, and education.
AOR = adjusted odds ratio
CI = confidence interval

cases of mixed messages at different times throughout the disaster. For example, a man reported receiving conflicting messages from the National Guard and television news about whether or not he had to evacuate.

When asked about social connections in New Orleans before the hurricane, 42% of the participants provided examples of the positive forms of social capital.

> We had a beautiful community. Neighbors got along wonderful. It was a no-crime area. (Woman, 67, African American)

> They was cleaning up the streets, the drug activities. People worked together to do good things. We had a neighborhood watch. (Woman, 21, African American)

In contrast, 28% provided examples of the negative forms of social capital.

> Youth were together and doin' bad things. They were killin' like crazy. Everyday killin'. Moms were out there smokin' dope all their life. Kids didn't have no daddy. (Woman, 39, African American)

When people were together, there was a lot of not good. We had a few killings and things like that. It was pretty violent really. (Man, 44, African American)

Other participants offered a mixed picture:

It was kinda nice and kinda violent. People workin' in a good way in some neighborhoods. In other neighborhoods, people were different. People can come together and stick together like family. Other people get together and cause crime. (Man, 25, African American)

When asked about social interactions during and following the hurricane, 50% of the participants provided examples of the positive forms of social capital. For example, one participant, who was caring for an autistic child and two diabetic relatives, referred to being on an Interstate overpass for three days following the hurricane. Another participant agreed:

Where you gonna get your next drink of water the next day and where you gonna get your next food the next day? People worked together. We shared everything, any water, any food. (Man, 53, White)

There were also examples specific to the hurricane shelters:

I got lotta homeboys I knew from New Orleans here. I knew 'em from before. I know 'em again. It brought people closer. People helpin' people. (Man, 25, African American)

We laughed and talked, we created a little group as a family, we just tried to look out for one another, we was a crutch for each other. (Woman, 58, African American)

In addition, one diabetic, who needed regular insulin shots, had lost his medication during evacuation. He reported that another resident, who uses the same type, gave him insulin. Another participant spoke of social support during the hurricane:

I was alone, but in contact with a neighbor. Water coming in, roof collapsing, a skylight created, the wall came down. I was working with a neighbor. The neighbor came over cuz his place was worse. We were holdin' the window in place against the storm. The house was dancin.' Water was leakin' in the kitchen. (Man, 54, African American)

Yet another participant offered an example of how a community helped people in a previous hurricane shelter:

The community reached out with nothin' but love from outside. They came in from the moment we were there. People gave us food, buy us clothes, bring us to their church. They helped us when we weren't feelin' good. (Man, 56, White)

In contrast, 26% offered examples of the negative forms of social capital:

Some young men get together and aren't doing anything. They sit outside, smoke, talk trash, listen to music. And they doin' this and that. You got people stealing things left and right, my money, my cell phone, my medicine. (Woman, 51, African American)

In fact, about 12% of the participants had been victims of theft in the hurricane shelters. In addition, 11% witnessed looting in New Orleans, with about 4% reporting participation in such looting activities (where that term includes taking essentials such as water and foodstuffs). Relevant examples include the following:

Some people doin' bad things. Everybody was mixed up: bad animals and the good animals. The bad animals lootin' stores. (Man, 53, White)

Everyone went [into Sav-A-Center]. They got everything, with buggies, food, beer everything. (Man, 44, White)

The looters started arriving. They're goin' in. They coming down the street in canoes. They were every age. They had their children out there lootin'. There were families lootin'. They're comin' back with hair driers, anything. The looters were lootin' each other. (Man, 54, African American)

Discussion

It is important to note that the hurricane shelter populations were primarily African American, with low incomes and little education. This suggests that the population that ended up in the hurricane shelters was vulnerable even before the hurricane hit. These residents of New Orleans had little access to transportation to evacuate the city and few options when it came to short-term lodging after the hurricane.

Shelter residents sought out news information as a means of dealing with the disaster and related uncertainty and health threats.[15,16] The residents relied primarily on television leading up to the hurricane and in the hurricane shelters thereafter, but expected to rely even more on radio in the weeks and months ahead. In general, however, news reliance was not common, with participants, on average, relying on less than one media outlet both before and after the hurricane. That post-hurricane news reliance was associated with greater likelihood of psychological and physical health problems is inconsistent with research that has suggested the importance of news information in disaster scenarios,[17,18] but consistent with other research that has linked viewing of graphic television images to psychological illness.[19,20] These associations, as well as the low levels of news reliance, may also be explained in terms of information dissatisfaction. As suggested by the qualitative data, misinformation and mixed information were frequent, and such information is likely to foster uncertainty rather than resolve it.[16] Also, media access and user control in the shelters were much more limited than they normally were, which would likely constrain media learning.[43] Finally, the most common stimulus to information dissatisfaction was the lack of information about specific affected neighborhoods. This suggests a first paradox. The Internet appears to have been the best medium for accessing information about specific neighborhoods, including flood levels, but only 4 of the 57 participants reported using the medium for hurricane-related information, and 2 of these required assistance to do so. (There were a limited number of open-access Internet terminals in the hurricane shelters, but they were not widely used.)

There are two other potential reasons for the associations between news reliance and health outcomes. First, it could be that people who faced psychological and physical health problems related to the hurricane subsequently relied more than others on the news media. Perhaps, these people turned to the news media as a potential solution to, or buffer from, their problems. Second, it could be that the news media stimulated increases in psychological problems as a result of the nature of news coverage of the hurricane. Such news coverage included extensive detailed and graphic depictions of the effects of the hurricane, including crowded shelters of last resort, flooded streets and homes, and drowned bodies.

It is important to note that the relationships between news reliance and health outcomes were not clearly borne out by the qualitative data. As noted above, some shelter residents viewed news information as a bridge to understanding and stability, not one to psychological and physical suffering.

The quantitative analysis above was designed in part to identify the social capital predictors of health outcomes. Depression was more common among participants with low levels of pre- and post-hurricane positive social interactions, but high levels of post-hurricane negative social interactions. These findings support research indicating that social capital in positive forms can result in positive health outcomes,[25,26] while social capital in negative forms worsens health outcomes.[32,33] It could be that people who were less depressed were able to develop and rely upon more social connections or that people's mobilization of social connections and related social resources helped them fight off depression.

The qualitative data imply the same relationships. For example, shelter residents provided examples of positive forms of social capital, as well as positive outcomes that followed. Specifically, shelter residents received emotional support from loved ones, information from acquaintances they had known before the hurricane, and insulin from people whom they had just met. These findings support previous research,[25,26] including some specific to disaster response.[4,27,29] Social capital took on negative forms, as well.[32] For example, participants reported looting in New Orleans and theft in the hurricane shelters, which are consistent with the criminal and antisocial behaviors noted by previous research.[34,35] These negative outcomes of social capital appear to have a basis in two rationales: the exclusion of outsiders and downward leveling norms.[32]

It is interesting that there were no significant correlations between the social capital measures and physical health problems related to the hurricane. This could indicate one of three things. It could mean that social capital and related social connections and social support are not effectual determinants of health in the context of a major natural disaster except in the case of psychological problems. Second, it could be that social capital plays a more complex role than that tested in this study. For example, one previous study indicated that social capital's role in these scenarios is one of statistical moderation, not one of correlation, which is what was tested in this study.[27] Third, it could be that the effects of Hurricane Katrina, because of the disaster's enormity, were beyond any control by residents of New Orleans. Thus, social capital was insufficient for avoiding illness and injury.

A second paradox appears in relation to social capital and the shelter population. Social capital is especially important to African Americans in poor urban communities as a means to the attainment of social and economic well-being and advancement.[44,45] Nevertheless, social capital in such environments is limited in its extent and primarily involves bonding. *Bonding social capital* involves social connections that reinforce exclusive identities and homogeneous groups,[46] such as people of the same ethnicity or same socioeconomic status (SES). In contrast, *bridging social capital*, which forms in the presence of weak ties, involves inclusive social connections with people from different social groups.[21,47] In comparison with bridging social capital, bonding social capital allows for only a limited expansion of access to information and social resources. The benefits and detriments of bonding social capital can be seen in the context of the current study. Before, during, and after Hurricane Katrina, kin and friends provided one another with myriad forms of support. Among the shelter population, however, these bonding ties were with people who were also of low SES and, importantly, also residents of New Orleans. The presence of SES-bridging ties, especially to wealthier New Orleans residents, could have facilitated transportation for evacuation. In addition, the presence of geographic-bridging ties, to people who lived outside of the area threatened by the hurricane, could have yielded better places to stay during and following the hurricane.

The current study has two limitations that should be noted. First, generalization of the current findings is limited to residents in Red Cross shelters in Louisiana following Hurricane Katrina. Participants were randomly selected, but it is expected that the functions and uses of news information and social capital may vary by disaster and by geographic region. Second, the sample size has a sampling error that is larger than ideal, which could lead to instances of Type I error, with the null hypothesis rejected even though it is true.[48] Although a bigger sample was considered, the final sample size was decided upon as a result of funding limitations and the fact that later interviews generated redundant qualitative data.

Conclusion

The results of the current study help elucidate the roles of news information and social capital in a time rife with chaos and uncertainty. When Hurricane Katrina hit, a low-income, low-education population was left on its own. It faced the considerable obstacles imposed by evacuation and subsequent lodging. Although a lack of financial resources and bridging social resources landed the participants in hurricane shelters, the participants did not give up when confronted by the hurricane and its aftermath. They traveled by myriad types of vehicle, stayed in myriad places, some makeshift, and developed and redeveloped means of access to news information and social capital that allowed them to confront uncertainty and public health threats in a time in which social support greatly outweighed governmental support.

An avenue for improvement in information following a natural disaster is the Internet. The Internet, after all, would have been the best source of specific types of information, while more traditional mass media provided more general information. For example, the Internet could provide hurricane evacuees with access to neighborhood-specific information, including damage estimates and online entries of neighbors, some of whom had revisited the area. The problem, as noted above, is that the hurricane shelter population was ill prepared to employ this new medium as an informational tool following Hurricane Katrina. Although there were a limited number of open-access Internet terminals in the hurricane shelters, few of the shelter residents availed themselves of this resource. Social capital is important, as well. It is a social resource that anyone, rich or poor, highly educated or not, can develop and mobilize, providing benefits to psychological health, even in the context of the United States' worst-ever natural disaster.

Acknowledgments

Special thanks go out to the hurricane shelter residents who took part in this study. Funding for the study was provided through a grant from the Natural Hazards Center at the University of Colorado at Boulder.

Notes

1. Kaniasty K, Norris FH. Social support dynamics in adjustment to disasters. In: Duck S, ed. Handbook on personal relationships. 2nd Ed. London: Wiley, 1997;595–619.
2. Kaniasty K, Norris FH. Mobilization and deterioration of social support following natural disasters. Current Directions in Psychological Science. 1995;4(3):94–8.
3. Parker G. Cyclone Tracy and Darwin evacuees: on the restoration of the species. Br J Psychiatry. 1977 Jun;130:548–55.
4. Allen KM. Community-based disaster preparedness and climate adaptation: local capacity-building in the Philippines. Disasters. 2006 Mar;30(1):81–101.
5. Norris FH, Kaniasty K. Received and perceived social support in times of stress: a test of the social support deterioration deterrence model. J Pers Soc Psychol. 1996 Sep;71(3):498–511.
6. Watanabe C, Okumura J, Chiu T-Y, et al. Social support and depressive symptoms among displaced older adults following the 1999 Taiwan earthquake. J Trauma Stress. 2004 Feb;17(1):63–7.
7. Kaniasty K, Norris FH. A test of the social deterioration model in the context of natural disaster. J Pers Soc Psychol. 1993 Mar;64(3):395–408.
8. Kaniasty K, Norris FH. Help-seeking comfort and receiving social support: the role ethnicity and context of need. Am J Community Psychol. 2000 Aug;28(4):545–81.
9. Ginexi EM, Weihs K, Simmens SJ, et al. Natural disaster and depression: a prospective investigation of reactions to the 1993 midwest floods. Am J Community Psychol. 2000 Aug;28(4):495–518.
10. Bolin R, Stanford L. The Northridge earthquake: community-based approaches to unmet recovery needs. Disasters. 1998 Mar;22(1):21–38.
11. Blaikie PM, Cannon T, Davis I, et al. At risk: natural hazards, people's vulnerability, and disasters. New York: Routledge, 1994.

12. Graumann A, Houston T, Lawrimore J, et al. Hurricane Katrina: A climatological perspective. Asheville, NC: National Oceanic and Atmospheric Administration; 2005.

13. Greenough PG, Kirsch TD. Hurricane Katrina. Public health response—assessing needs. New Engl J Med. 2005 Oct;353(15):1544-6.

14. Nigg JM, Barnshaw J, Torres MR. Hurricane Katrina and the flooding of New Orleans: emergent issues in sheltering and temporary housing. Ann Am Acad Polit Soc Sci. 2006;604:113-28.

15. Hines SC, Babrow AS, Badzek L, et al. From coping with life to coping with death: problematic integration for the seriously ill elderly. Health Commun. 2001;13(3):327-42.

16. Babrow AS, Kasch CR, Ford LA. The many meanings of uncertainty in illness: toward a systematic accounting. Health Commun. 1998;10(1):1-23.

17. Carey J. Media use during a crisis. Prometheus. 2002 Sep 1;20(3):201-7.

18. Bucy EP. Emotion, presidential communication, and traumatic news: processing the World Trade Center attacks. The Harvard International Journal of Press/Politics. 2003;8(4):76-96.

19. Pfefferbaum B, Nixon SJ, Tivis RD, et al. Television exposure in children after a terrorist incident. Psychiatry. 2001 Fall;64(3):202-11.

20. Ahern J, Galea S, Resnick H, et al. Television images and psychological symptoms after the September 11 terrorist attacks. Psychiatry. 2002 Winter;65(4):289-300.

21. Lin N. Social capital: a theory of social structure and action. Cambridge: Cambridge University Press, 2001.

22. Bourdieu P. The forms of capital. In: Richardson JG, ed. Handbook of theory and research for the sociology of education. New York: Greenwood Press, 1986;241-58.

23. Coleman JS. Social capital in the creation of human capital. Am J Sociol. 1998;94 Suppl:S95-S120.

24. Grootaert C, van Bastelaer T. Understanding and measuring social capital: a synthesis of findings and recommendations from the Social Capital Initiative. (Social Capital Working Paper No. 24.) Washington, DC: World Bank, 2001 Apr.

25. Kawachi I, Kennedy BP, Glass R. Social capital and self-rated health: a contextual analysis. Am J Public Health. 1999 Aug;89(9):1187-93.

26. Beaudoin CE. The impact of news use and social capital on youth wellbeing: A community-level analysis. J Commun Psychology. (In press.)

27. Moore S, Daniel M, Linnan L, et al. After Hurricane Floyd passed: investigating the social determinants of disaster preparedness and recovery. Family and Community Health. 2004;27(3):204-217.

28. Rocha JL, Christoplos I. Disaster mitigation and preparedness on the Nicaraguan post-Mitch agenda. Disasters. 2001 Sep;25(3):240-50.

29. Nakagawa Y, Shaw R. Social capital: A missing link to disaster recovery. Int J Mass Emerg Disasters. 2004 Mar;22(1):5-34.

30. Barton AH. Communities in disaster: a sociological analysis of collective stress situations. Garden City, NJ: Doubleday, 1969.

31. Ibanez GE, Khatchikian N, Buck CA, et al. Qualitative analysis of social support and conflict among Mexican and Mexican-American disaster survivors. J Commun Psychol. 2003 Jan;31(1):1-23.

32. Portes A. Social capital: its origins and applications in modern sociology. Annu Rev Sociol. 1998;24:1-24.

33. Campbell C, Williams B, Gilgen D. Is social capital a useful conceptual tool for exploring community level influences on HIV infection? An exploratory case study from South Africa. AIDS Care. 2002 Feb;14(1):41–54.

34. Quarantelli EL. Disaster research. In: Borgatta EF, Borgatta ML, eds. Encyclopedia of sociology. New York: Plenum Press; 1992.

35. Rodriguez H, Trainor J, Quarantelli EL. Rising to the challenges of a catastrophe: The emergent and prosocial behavior following Hurricane Katrina. Ann American Acad Polit Soc Sci. 2006;604(1):82–101.

36. Strauss AL, Corbim J. Basics of qualitative research: Grounded theory procedures and techniques. Newbury Park, CA: Sage, 1990.

37. Radloff LS. The CES-D scale: a self-report depression scale for research in the general population. Appl Psychological Measurement. 1977;1:385–401.

38. Beaudoin CE, Tao CC. The impact of online cancer resources on the supporters of cancer patients. New Media & Society. (In press.)

39. Beaudoin CE, Tao CC. Benefiting from social capital in online support groups: An empirical study of cancer patients. CyberPsychology & Behavior. (In press.)

40. Beaudoin CE, Thorson E. Testing the cognitive mediation model: the roles of news reliance and three gratifications sought. Communic Res. 2004;31(4):446–71.

41. Beaudoin CE, Thorson E. Social capital in rural and urban communities: testing differences in media effects and models. Journalism & Mass Communication Quarterly. 2004;81(2):378–99.

42. U.S. Census Bureau. Poverty thresholds 2004. Washington, DC: U.S. Census Bureau, 2005. Available at http://www.census.gov/hhes/poverty/threshld/thresh04.html.

43. Eveland WP Jr. A "mix of attributes" approach to the study of media effects and new communication technologies. J Commun. 2003 Sep;53(3):395–410.

44. Musick MA, Wilson J, Bynum WBJ. Race and formal volunteering: the differential effects of class and religion. Soc Forces. 2000 Jun;78(4):1539–70.

45. Stack CB. All our kin: strategies for survival in a Black community. New York: Harper & Row, 1974.

46. Putnam R. Bowling alone: the collapse and revival of American community. New York: Simon and Schuster, 2000.

47. Granovetter MS. The strength of weak ties. Am J Sociol. 1973 May;78(6):1360–80.

48. Agresti A, Finlay B. Statistical methods for the social sciences. 3 Ed. Upper Saddle River, NJ: Prentice Hall, 1997.

PART III: Looking to the Future

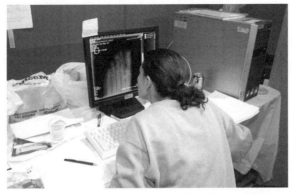

Figure 8. Injuries were among the conditions treated.
Photograph courtesy of Baylor College of Medicine Office
of Public Affairs.

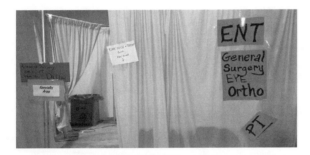

Figure 9. General Surgery, Eye Care, Orthopedic Care.
Photograph courtesy of Baylor College of Medicine Office
of Public Affairs.

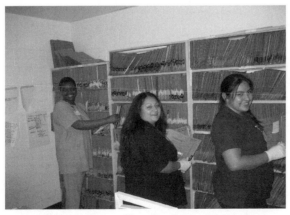

Figure 10. Medical record keeping during the emergency.
Photograph courtesy of the Baylor College of Medicine
Office of Public Affairs.

Chapter 20
Mitigating the Health Effects of Disasters for Medically Underserved Populations: Electronic Health Records, Telemedicine, Research, Screening, and Surveillance

Dominic Mack, MD, MBA
Katrina M. Brantley, MPH
Kimberly G. Bell, MHA, FACHE

Overview of Region

Hurricanes Katrina and Rita had a devastating impact on health care in the Southeastern and South Central United States. According to the Department of Homeland Security, Katrina displaced an estimated 248,431 people who were evacuated to shelters in 22 states and the District of Columbia.[1] A total of 48,500 people were rescued, with more than 23,000 of them saved by the United States Coast Guard.[2,3] Katrina induced a breach in the levee system surrounding New Orleans, flooding nearly 80% of the city.[4] The storms and flooding destroyed homes, businesses, and health infrastructure over 90,000 square miles of Louisiana, Alabama, Mississippi, and the Florida Panhandle.[5]

The region's health care system was disrupted and remains greatly challenged by the massive destruction. For example, the Louisiana Department of Health and Hospitals reports that New Orleans has 77 psychiatric inpatient beds today in all hospitals other than those run by the United States Department of Veterans Affairs, compared with 460 before Katrina.[6] A quarter million evacuees in various shelters in the region needed medical attention and were separated from their health records at some time. The damage of the storm resulted in more than 1,800 lives lost, 780,000 people displaced, 850 schools damaged, 200,000 homes destroyed, 18,700 businesses destroyed, and 220,000 jobs lost.[7] Staving off major disease outbreaks among the evacuees and those remaining in affected areas represents a formidable public health challenge throughout the Southeastern and South Central region of the United States.

The cost of the devastation on the Gulf Coast caused by Hurricane Katrina is estimated to exceed $100 billion. There have been more than 1,800 deaths (1,577 in Louisiana and 238 in Mississippi), making Katrina the costliest and deadliest hurricane in U.S.

DOMINIC MACK is the Project Director of the Regional Coordinating Center for Hurricane Response (RCCHR) at the National Center for Primary Care at Morehouse School of Medicine. **KATRINA BRANTLEY** is the Research Coordinator at the RCCHR and **KIMBERLY BELL** is the Assistant Project Director.

history.[8] The full extent of its impact on the health system of the Gulf Coast remains undetermined. However, it is evident that this disaster will complicate the delivery of care in a region and among populations that suffered from major health disparities even before Katrina.

Before the hurricanes, the states of Mississippi and Louisiana had the highest poverty levels and age-adjusted mortality patterns for African Americans in the U.S.[7] Nearly half (48%) of Orleans Parish residents and a third (32%) of Jefferson Parish residents had low incomes (below the federal poverty level).[7] In New Orleans, 67.5% of the 450,000 residents were Black and 25% were living in poverty.[1] Within the city itself, the impoverished tended to live in the flooded areas. Bayou La Batre, the hardest hit area in Alabama, was 52% White, 33% Asian and 10% African American, with 28% of the population living below the poverty line.[9]

The hurricanes' devastation affected people of all colors and economic statuses, but especially the poor and underserved, who are historically disproportionately affected by disasters as well as by persistent health disparities between socioeconomic groups and between racial/ethnic groups. Disparities in health care have been linked to multiple factors, including poverty, race, ethnicity, the environment, education, access to health care, geography, and quality of service.[10] Evidence also shows that people who were traumatized by the hurricanes will most likely have a higher incidence of psychiatric disorders, including depression, which is also linked to higher risk for hypertension, diabetes, and heart disease.[10]

Health System Status

In March of 2006, the United States Government Accountability Office (GAO) reported that, 6 months after Hurricane Katrina, New Orleans had lost 80% of its hospital beds and 75% of its safety net clinics. At that time, 68% of the population was displaced from the city.[11] Since then, the city has returned to an estimated 50% of hospital capacity; 40% of its population remains displaced.[7] Charity Hospital, the major safety net hospital, and other safety net outpatient services for the uninsured and underserved population remain closed.[5,7,11-14] Charity, a principal source of health care and the only Level 1 trauma center for the entire Gulf Coast region, was left devastated and dysfunctional, furloughing nearly 2,600 employees as of November 7, 2005.[5] Recent estimates project that only 140 of 617 primary care physicians returned to practice in New Orleans after Katrina and that only 22 of 196 psychiatrists did so.[8]

According to a Columbia University School of Public Health Study, 44% of children in New Orleans had symptoms of new mental health problems such as depression, anxiety, and sleep disorders since Hurricane Katrina.[8] Similar troubles affected children in Alabama and Mississippi.

Recent studies of the tsunami-affected areas in southern Thailand showed that children affected by that disaster had an increased prevalence of post-traumatic stress disorder (PTSD) and depression. Prevalence rates of PTSD symptoms were 13% of children displaced from villages and staying in camps, 11% of children in affected villages, and 6% in unaffected villages. The study showed that the delayed evacuations, the experience of extreme panic and fear, and experiencing feelings that a family member's life was in danger were independent risk factors for PTSD.[15]

A study of adult tsunami survivors by Griensven showed a PTSD prevalence of 7–12% at 8 weeks after the tsunami. The prominent risk factors for the development of PTSD and depression for adults was the loss of livelihoods after the tsunami.[16] These culturally sensitive studies concluded that children may benefit from therapeutic interventions whereas adults may benefit more from a restoration of their livelihoods. In a 9-month follow up study, the prevalence of PTSD and depression among the children in one town had not declined. However, in the study by Griensven, 50% of the adults showed decreased rates of symptoms of PTSD and depression after the same period of time.

Although loss of life was much greater during the tsunami, these data may aid in developing a scientific perspective concerning the events of Hurricanes Katrina and Rita. A study prepared for the Louisiana Office of Mental Health showed that 45% of individuals interviewed scored high enough on a rating scale for PTSD that they would be referred for mental health services.[17] Based on existing studies of mental health repercussions after major floods and hurricanes, the federal Substance Abuse and Mental Health Services Administration (SAMHSA) has estimated that 25% to 30% of individuals living in areas hit hard by Katrina will have clinically significant mental health needs and another 10% to 20% will have important, subclinical mental health needs.[17,18]

Overview of Project

In October of 2005, the National Center for Minority Health and Health Disparities (NCMHD) of the National Institutes of Health (NIH) and the Office of Minority Health (OMH) joined with Morehouse School of Medicine's (MSM) National Center for Primary Care to establish the Regional Coordinating Center for Hurricane Response (RCC). The RCC's mission is to work with the National Institutes of Health's (NIH's) Centers of Excellence in Partnerships for Community Outreach, Research on Health Disparities and Training (EXPORT Centers) to aid in the revitalization and rebuilding of the health systems in the Gulf Coast states that were damaged by Hurricanes Katrina and Rita. Specific aims include expansion of systems' capabilities through medical technology, which includes electronic health records (EHRs) and telepsychiatry.

The RCC also aims to collaborate with the EXPORT Centers in the Gulf region to perform screening and surveillance projects within the communities and to develop research projects focused on the health problems affecting the underserved populations in the region. Another goal of the RCC is to establish an effective communications and strategic response infrastructure connecting EXPORT Centers in the Southeast and South Central regions of the United States with front-line community health centers and other essential primary care practices in hurricane-ravaged communities. This infrastructure should help rebuilding efforts and build a cadre of academic health centers to serve as resources for responding to future catastrophic events and on-going health disparities. It also creates a pipeline for the translation/diffusion of research discoveries, not only from the bench to the bedside, but out to the curbside and the countryside.

Long-term, the RCC aims to contribute to a balanced health care system that allows for equality in the provision of care to all patients in the community.

Electronic Health Records Initiative

Katrina left more than one million people without medical records.[19] This loss of patient information suggests the importance of storing patient data on EHRs that can be protected from local disasters. Electronic Health Records can also reduce medical errors, improve quality of care, lower long term costs, eliminate paperwork hassles, and offer an alternative to local storage of paper records.[19] According to a cost benefit analysis prepared by researchers in Santa Monica, California, 256 studies were reviewed and the findings indicated that EHRs improved the quality of care in ambulatory care settings and demonstrated improvements in provider performance when clinical information management and decision support tools were made available within the system.[19,20] According to Dr. Stephen Waldren of the American Academy of Family Physicians (AAFP), "EHRs have the potential to create a community network across community health centers . . . potentially enabling physicians who practice evidence-based medicine to aggregate data to provide better care and anticipate the needs of the population more effectively and on demand" (p. 16).[19]

The Regional Coordinating Center's EHR initiative is intended to re-populate and upgrade medical record systems in medical practices that were damaged and to serve those communities that were affected by the hurricanes. The centers contracted through the RCC initiative lost the majority of their paper records and did not have an electronic health system in place before Hurricanes Katrina and Rita. This will include the utilization of the Continuity of Care Record (CCR), which is a new XML (computer language) standard for clinical and administrative health information exchange and interoperability. This format of information can be used for information-sharing between health care facilities through a medium such as thumb drives or compact discs. This information can also be put into the hands of patients and can become a valuable resource during emergency situations.

The RCC began its CCR initiative at the New Orleans Health Recovery week held at the Audubon Zoo in New Orleans on February 6th–12th, 2006. The New Orleans Health Department (NOHD) and the City of New Orleans sponsored this seven-day health care event. The community response was overwhelming. An estimated 6,000 participants generated over 18,000 encounters (see Table 1). The patients seen during this event were referred to available medical services in the area.

The RCC was involved with the planning and management of the operations of this event, which required months of planning with NOHD, Solventus software company, Remote Area Medical, Inc. (RAM), the American Academy of Family Physicians (AAFP), and the Intel Corp. Many other organizations participated by providing health care screenings, mental health services, and health education. This initiative met the basic needs of the population within 6 months of the storm. Due to the large number of displaced physicians, loss of medical insurances, and the closing of New Orleans's major safety net hospital (Charity) these services were necessary to meet the immediate needs of the residents of the Gulf Coast. This initiative allowed the RCC to pilot the process of passing out CCRs to people who really need a snapshot of their medical records in their hands at all times. The RAM volunteer organization provided equipment and volunteer services for the medical, dental, and optical areas. Volunteers from the Association of Black Cardiologists, REACH 2010 of New Orleans, Tulane University, Louisiana State University, University of Tennessee, Medical College of Virginia in Richmond, Virginia, and many other local and regional organizations also participated.

There were over 4,500 CCRs created during the seven-day event and some patients received their CCRs on compact disc or thumb drive. All patients' consents were obtained before entering their personal health information and the data is housed in a secure location accessed only by password-protected individuals. All procedures were in keeping with Health Insurance Portability and Accountability Act (HIPAA)-mandated policies and procedures. The RCC continues to work with public health departments, community health centers (CHCs), and private physicians in Florida, Alabama, Mississippi, Louisiana, and Texas to either install full electronic health record systems or to create CCR systems for portable health information and emergency preparedness.

The RCC has also worked with the Primary Care Associations (PCAs) in the states of Louisiana, Mississippi, and Alabama collaboratively to develop projects around the propagation of EHRs in the CHCs in those states. The RCC has identified three multi-site CHCs for the implementation of EHR initiatives. The RCC has provided EHR training to over 200 individuals in Mississippi and Alabama. Further training was anticipated during the PCA statewide conferences in Mississippi and Alabama in late 2006. Its PCA partners have informed the RCC that EHR education is what is needed most. There are examples of physician groups who have purchased EHR systems that were not a good fit for their organizations. Valuable time and resources were wasted in these cases, which makes it all the more important to focus on proper education and training before implementation of any EHR system. The RCC has contracted to place 50 EHR systems in community health centers by the beginning months of 2007.

Telemedicine Initiative

The RCC also aims to develop and test reproducible age-appropriate and culturally-relevant telepsychiatry models that respond to the disparities in the area of mental health affecting the targeted communities. The goal is to place video-conferencing units and facilitators in health care facilities that serve communities in need and link them to similar units staffed by mental health experts trained to treat both PTSD and chronic mental illness. To date, no active telemedical psychiatric services have been provided to the CHCs in the New Orleans parish areas that we are contracted to serve. The RCC is working with several local New Orleans parish community leaders and interstate agencies to provide this initiative beginning in the first months of 2007.

The telemedicine component of this initiative is focused on delivering mental health services to those underserved communities that have limited access to mental health providers. In the case of areas affected by the hurricanes, this limited access is in part due to the displacement of mental health providers. The RCC is not providing this service to replace the traditional face-to-face mental health services but offer it as a complement to assist the massive numbers of patients that may be in need of

Table 1.

NEW ORLEANS HEALTH RECOVERY WEEK AT THE AUDOBON ZOO: STATISTICS FOR PATIENT SERVICES[a]

		GYN[b]	General medicine	Eye testing	Eye test & glasses	Dentistry service	Total patients
6 Feb	Daily	1	1,225	14	170	448	1,858
7 Feb	Daily	44	1,200	61	222	427	1,954
8 Feb	Daily	9	3,191	31	247	828	4,306
9 Feb	Daily	78	2,236	77	196	495	3,082
10 Feb	Daily	5	2,881	96	225	588	3,795
11 Feb	Daily	0	2,500	67	189	464	3,220
12 Feb	Daily	0	190	55	84	0	329
TOTAL		137	13,423	401	1,333	3,250	18,544

[a]Data provided by Remote Area Medical Inc. (RAM). This data includes both adults and children.
[b]GYN = Gynecology

mental health services due to catastrophic events. The development and delivery of telemedical (i.e., telepsychiatric) services entails coordinating and working through: (1) local patient sites; (2) remote provider sites; (3) technology partner, wiring solution, hardware; (4) administrative, legislative, economic, and collaborative matters; and (5) assessment and research.

Progress was and is achieved through cultivating relationships with the communities and relevant individuals through phone calls, teleconference calls, emails, and site visits. The EXPORT Centers have been instrumental in providing information technology expertise and infrastructure for the proposed telemedicine sites. To date, six sites in four Gulf Coast States (Alabama, Mississippi, Louisiana, and Texas) have been identified to develop and deliver telepsychiatric services from within primary care environments. Efforts to date have focused on identifying existing clinician resources within the communities and states targeted for assistance. In the wake of Katrina, staffing resources are difficult to quantify in most of the target sites and are expected to be insufficient to meet current demands. Concentrated clinician sources beyond the target communities include academic centers; efforts have been made to discuss telepsychiatric staffing solutions with personnel there. The RCC is working with local providers and community members to develop a clinician network to provide culturally appropriate telepsychiatry services.

Current licensure standards dictate that telemedicine physicians obtain unrestricted licenses in any state in which they practice. For clinicians outside the Gulf region it is cost prohibitive to become licensed in the Gulf Coast states where they seek to counsel disaster victims. In cases such as the devastation caused by Hurricanes Katrina and Rita, the costs for tele-clinicians undercut the potential benefits. This is a legislative issue that requires policymakers' assistance in the creation of a reasonably priced special purpose or national license. Another challenge the RCC has encountered in providing telepsychiatry health services in the Gulf region is reimbursement. Reimbursement for services is necessary to ensure long-term sustainability, but income sources to support it remain in their infancy. Only 18 states offer Medicaid/Medicare reimbursement for telemedical services. Discussions of the issues recurrently involve sustainability and resource management. Allowances can be made to offer up clinical time without compensation, but the risk is that a 'musical chairs' phenomenon will occur, pulling clinicians away from their local clinical duties and therefore yielding no net benefit. Compensation for physicians and insurance reimbursement will be key issues for future planning. The RCC recognizes how lengthy the processes behind policy and procedural changes are, but we suggest that the best short-term solution is to retain in-state providers or out-of-state providers with a current state license.

Screening and Surveillance Initiative

The RCC also works with the EXPORT Centers to assist with the development of effective community-based screening and surveillance systems to monitor health needs of individuals evacuated from hurricane-ravaged communities, as well as those returning to communities as they are re-built, with a special focus on exacerbations of existing health disparities. An RCC assumption is that the Centers for Disease Control and Prevention and state/local public health officials will put into place appropriate monitoring and surveillance systems for tracking infectious disease, birth outcomes, mortality, and other traditional public health indices and measures. They may also monitor for environmental exposures to toxic chemicals, or assess signs of on-going mental health impact such as suicides and PTSD.

However, it is not clear that there will be effective monitoring to ensure that health disparities are not widening as a result of the hurricanes' disproportionate impact on low-income populations. The poor have been disproportionately affected by the hurricanes, in part because health care providers who serve the poor have also been disproportionately affected, raising the likelihood of negative force-multiplier effects on vulnerable populations.

The RCC has begun subcontracting with EXPORT Centers in each of the states of Alabama, Mississippi, and Texas. At present, Louisiana does not have an EXPORT Center, but the RCC intends to work with the academic centers of Louisiana to develop a new center. Additionally, the RCC will work with the EXPORT Centers to form an External Advisory Committee comprising key stakeholders of the devastated areas. The function of this Committee will be to survey the needs of the hurricane-ravaged community and match those needs with research-based practices that will focus on existing health disparities.

Three research subcontracted projects have begun at Jackson State University (JSU), the University of South Alabama (USA), and the University of Texas MD Anderson Cancer Center (UTMD). Each institution's research objectives are summarized below.

- Jackson State University's objective is to serve as a clearinghouse and temporary repository of data on health services utilized by populations whose health is most negatively affected by health disparities. Memoranda of Understanding for data sharing are being established with key health care organizations serving Mississippi and Louisiana. Further, they will create a database with common elements to be used to report data to the RCC. The project will provide comprehensive reports on health care access, utilization and delivery by medical institutions located in areas affected by Hurricane Katrina.

- University of South Alabama's objective is to survey the health care needs of underserved people displaced to Mobile and Baldwin counties and to ascertain how their health care needs were met so that health care entities can adequately serve their constituents. The survey will identify health providers' perceptions of disruption of chronic disease management due to a disaster and how best to deal with those disruptions. It will also identify patient perceptions of disruption of disease management and how they dealt with those disruptions. Finally, it will list resources needed to sustain the critical components used to track patients and facilitate continuity of care.
- University of Texas MD Anderson's objective is to review and compile data from medical records of Asian evacuees to identify major health needs of this population. They will use this information to develop programs that could address the health needs of this population. The patients' demographic information will be extracted without identification and the frequency of common chief complaints and priority health needs will be used to design health education or screening programs.

These research projects will begin to provide vital data concerning the communities affected by Hurricanes Katrina and Rita. The projects are using various methods to extract this information (i.e., survey, medical record extraction and data-sharing from health organizations). Collectively, the EXPORT Centers and the RCC will be able to use these data in an effort to effect a positive change in the health status of the population.

Discussion of Lessons Learned through RCC Initiatives

The mission of the RCC initiative is ambitious. Carrying out the objectives depends on the participants' ability to work in conjunction with the EXPORT Centers to develop new partnerships within the targeted health care systems of the Gulf Coast. The actualization of anticipated partnerships and collaborative efforts has been challenging. After identifying key organizations and their leadership, it has been sometimes difficult to gain a sense of trust among these representatives. Paradoxically, this sometimes reflects an overwhelming bombardment of organizations offering support and aid. There are also internal limitations that contribute to slow delivery of funds. Together, these factors contribute to skepticism from leadership and add to the complexity of developing sustainable relationships with communities.

This cumbersome process of partnership building is also influenced by what is known and what is not known about targeted communities and their health care systems. Furthermore, there are cultural differences among and within ethnic groups that must be considered. In a related vein, the various existing organizations are structured differently and have different organizational cultures that must be considered. Some organizations are familiar with and friendly to medical technology advancements, such as telemedicine and EHR, whereas other groups are unfamiliar and resistant. With the more resistant organizations, the RCC has found it very important to exhibit patience and to nurture the relationship by means of extensive dialog and formal meetings, which can lead to the growth of mutual understanding and trust. This lays the groundwork for a fairly open relationship and allows for effective education and understanding of the new concepts, whether they concern technology or basic health care initiatives.

It is also important to understand state policies and laws, and the state's mechanism for providing care to the underserved. For instance, the way services are provided to the underserved in Louisiana is very different from the way it is done in Mississippi and Alabama. The funding of health services is also different and an understanding of these differences can aid in navigating the health care terrain and determining the hierarchy for decision making in the states. Recognizing these parameters is essential for making effective approaches to influential organizations without causing conflict or, as it were, butting heads. The RCC understands that even when one intends to do good, offending people in the existing system can lead to ostracism and inability to reach goals. Ultimately, the community suffers from such lack of communication and implementation.

Conclusion

Overall, the RCC's goal is to develop models of balanced community health systems in specific hurricane-ravaged communities as they rebuild. The RCC seeks to establish local and regional partnerships between public health programs, primary care practices, community-based health promotion programs, hospital/emergency departments, sub-specialty practices, pharmacies, local business partners, and academic health centers to ensure that every person in the community has equitable access to resources for healthy living. This will also require comprehensive and culturally appropriate primary health care, mental health services, preventive care, healthy behavior change, and integrated referrals to specialty care and academic health centers within the region. The intended outcome is to leverage the social upheaval created by Hurricanes Katrina and Rita by creating rapid-cycle change and seizing opportunities for transformation and expansion rather than just re-building a health system.

The assumption is that any disaster such as Hurricane Katrina that worsens the economic and health care infrastructure of our nation will disproportionately affect the poor and underserved. Through partnerships with the academic health centers, the RCC endeavors to develop the surveillance and research projects to investigate and produce data that will lead to solutions that will ultimately contribute to the elimination of health disparities. While lofty, this goal is attainable. Through efforts to transform health care systems, what may emerge from Katrina are new policies that may also help to improve care for other poor and underserved populations throughout the United States.

Acknowledgments

This project is made possible through grant number US2MP02001 from the U.S. Dept. of Health and Human Services, Office of Minority Health, with support from the National Institutes of Health, National Center on Minority Health and Health Disparities to Dr. David Satcher, Former Principal Investigator, Drs. Sandra Harris-Hooker and George Rust, Co-Principal Investigators.

Notes

1. Centers for Disease Control and Prevention (CDC). Morbidity surveillance after Hurricane Katrina—Arkansas, Louisiana, Mississippi, and Texas, September 2005. MMWR. Morb Mortal Wkly Rep. 2006 Jul 7;55(26):727–31.

2. U.S. Coast Guard. Coast Guard response to Hurricane Katrina. Washington, DC: U.S. Coast Guard, U.S. Department of Homeland Security, 2005 Nov. Available at http://www.uscg.mil/hq/g-cp/comrel/factfile/Factcards/Hurricane_Katrina.htm.

3. Caldwell SL, U.S. Government Accountability Office (GAO). Coast Guard: Observations of the preparation, response, and recovery missions related to Hurricane Katrina. Washington, DC: GAO, 2006 Jul.

4. Centers for Disease Control and Prevention (CDC). Public health response to Hurricanes Katrina and Rita—United States, 2005. MMWR. Morb Mortal Wkly Rep. 2006 Mar 10;55(9):229–31.

5. Rosenbaum S. U.S. health policy in the aftermath of Hurricane Katrina. JAMA. 2006 Jan 25;295(4):437–40.

6. Lamberg L. Katrina survivors strive to reclaim their lives. JAMA. 2006 Aug 26;296(5): 499–502.

7. Rudowitz R, Rowland D, Shartzer A. Health care in New Orleans before and after Hurricane Katrina. Health Aff (Millwood). 2006 Sep–Oct;25(5):w393–406.

8. Weisler RH, Barbee JG 4th, Townsend MH. Mental health and recovery in the Gulf Coast after Hurricanes Katrina and Rita. JAMA. 2006 Aug 2;296(5):585–8.

9. Encyclopedia W. Hurricane Katrina. In; 2006. Available at http://en.wikipedia.org/wiki/Bayou_la_Batre%2C_Alabama

10. Satcher D, Rubens JP, eds. Multicultural medcine and health disparities. New York: McGraw-Hill Companies, Inc., 2006.

11. Bascetta C, Siggerud K, U.S. Government Accountability Office. Hurricane Katrina: status of the health care system in New Orleans and difficult decisions related to efforts to rebuild it approximately 6 months after Hurricane Katrina. Washington, DC: GAO, 2006 Mar 28.

12. Frank IC. Emergency response to the Gulf Coast devastation by Hurricane Katrina and Rita: experiences and impressions. J Emerg Nurs. 2005 Dec;31(6):526–47.

13. Brodie M, Weltzien E, Altman D, et al. Experiences of Hurricane Katrina evacueees in Houston shelters: implications for future planning. Am J Public Health. 2006 Aug; 96(5):1402–8.

14. Berggren RE, Curiel TJ. After the storm—health care infrastructure in post-Katrina New Orleans. N Engl J Med. 2006 Apr 13;354(15):1549–52.

15. Thienkrua W, Cardozo BL, Chakkraband ML, et al. Symptoms of posttraumatic stress disorder and depression among children in tsunami-affected areas in southern Thailand. JAMA. 2006 Aug 2;296(5):549–59.

16. van Griensven F, Chakkraband ML, Thienkrua W, et al. Mental health problems among adults in tsunami-affected areas in southern Thailand. JAMA. 2006 Aug 2; 296(5):537–48.

17. Voelker R. Post-Katrina mental health needs prompt group to compile disaster medicine guide. JAMA. 2006 Jan 18;295(3):259–60.

18. Coker AL, Hanks JS, Eggleston KS, et al. Social and mental health needs assessment of Katrina evacuees. Disaster Manag Response. 2006 Jul–Sep;4(3):88–94.

19. Gooden RA. After the storm: visions of a revitalized health care system. Atlanta: Morehouse School of Medicine, 2006 April.

20. Southern California Evidence-based Practice Center. Costs and benefits of health information technology. (AHRQ Publication No. 06-E006.) Rockville, MD: Agency for Healthcare Research and Quality, 2006 Apr.

Chapter 21
Katrina-Related Health Concerns of Latino Survivors and Evacuees

DeAnne K. Hilfinger Messias, PhD, RN
Elaine Lacy, PhD

The experiences of hundreds of thousands of Latino residents of the Gulf Coast during and after Hurricane Katrina are among the stories untold in both the mainstream media and the professional literature. Compared with members of other racial/ethnic groups, very little systematic information has emerged regarding how Latino residents fared during and after the storm or about the disaster's effects on their physical and emotional well being. Like other residents of the region, Latinos found themselves uprooted, homeless, jobless, and without resources as a result of the hurricane and ensuing flooding. At the time of the initial disaster, however, Latinos' stories rarely appeared in the national media. In the weeks after the storm, the few reports that surfaced suggested language and cultural barriers prevented many Latinos from evacuating, that rescuers were ignoring Latinos and African Americans while helping White people, and that Latinos were largely absent from shelters and other relief sites.[1-6] In the ensuing year, although researchers have focused on the social, environmental, and political implications of Katrina, the disaster's impact on the Latino population has largely been ignored.

In this chapter we present an analysis of the health-related concerns identified by Latinos living in the path of Hurricane Katrina. Research that includes the voices of those marginalized by language, culture, immigration status, and other axes of inequality is needed in order to further develop knowledge and theoretical frameworks about the health implications of disasters. An examination of the health and health care experiences of Latino survivors and evacuees of the Katrina disaster also can contribute to public health policy development and the provision of disaster-related health care among minority and underserved populations.

Background and Context

The pre-Katrina Latino population in the Gulf Coast region. Latin American consulates estimated that 300,000 Latinos in the Gulf Coast region were affected by Hurricane

DEANNE HILFINGER MESSIAS is an Associate Professor in the College of Nursing and Graduate Director of the Women's Studies Program at the University of South Carolina (USC). **ELAINE LACY** is a Professor in the Department of History and Aiken Director of Research Initiatives for the Consortium for Latino Immigration Studies at the USC.

Katrina.[7] The distribution of the Latino population in the region varied by country of origin. Central Americans predominated in the New Orleans area and Mexicans constituted the majority in communities along the Mississippi coast. Migrants from Honduras accounted for a large portion of the Central Americans in New Orleans, largely due to connections between New Orleans-based Standard Fruit Company and Honduran banana producers.[8] New Orleans was also a prime destination of thousands of Nicaraguans and Salvadorians who immigrated following Hurricane Mitch in 1998. The Honduran population in New Orleans grew from 6.7% of Louisiana's foreign-born population in 1980 to 9.7% in 2000.[8] By August of 2005, an estimated 150,000 Hondurans lived in New Orleans, constituting the largest Honduran population in the country.[8] Mexicans constituted 10% and Puerto Ricans 5% of the city's Latino population.[9]

Language and information barriers. Language barriers and lack of access to storm information and personal safety advisories were among the many challenges Latinos experienced as Katrina approached. According to 2005 data from the U.S. Census Bureau,[10] nearly a third of Spanish-speaking residents of New Orleans spoke English "less than very well." Language barriers contributed to delays in learning about the storm's path, difficulties in interpreting the potential severity of the storm, and lack of access to and comprehension of local officials' plans and warnings. Provision of weather information in languages other than English depends upon both the availability of ethnic media outlets and the willingness and ability of local forecasting services to work with these outlets to keep them up to date.[11] In Louisiana and Mississippi, no television channels provided local weather information in Spanish; in New Orleans, one Spanish-language radio station offered local weather updates, but none did so in Mississippi.[11]

Immigration status as a barrier to assistance. Immigration status posed another major challenge for many Latinos in Katrina's path. Undocumented immigrants do not qualify for most types of federal assistance in times of emergency. According to the Federal Emergency Management Agency (FEMA), undocumented immigrants could receive temporary assistance but not financial or housing aid. The practical implication was that undocumented immigrants could stay in shelters, but data collected from them would not be considered confidential.[11,12] Contrary to precedents (e.g., Hurricane Andrew and the terrorist attacks of September 11, 2001), the federal government decided not to waive federal guidelines regarding immigration status, which kept many undocumented Latinos from seeking and gaining assistance, and meant that some who did paid a price. After the hurricane, officials in the Department of Homeland Security urged (in both English and Spanish) anyone needing assistance to seek it from all agencies, but undocumented immigrant evacuees who sought shelter in Texas were told to appear for deportation hearings.[12,13] Even undocumented immigrants who applied for aid for their documented children risked deportation.[14] In some areas of Mississippi, Latinos who sought shelter in Red Cross facilities also had difficulty getting help after the storm, when some were evicted and threatened with deportation by law enforcement personnel. In several documented cases, Latinos with legal residency status were told by law enforcement officials to leave Red Cross shelters or face deportation.[13,15] Not surprisingly, many documented and undocumented Latinos steered clear of shelters and governmental aid centers.[11] The fact that a recently published study of the health needs of evacuees in shelters in Houston (N=680) included no mention of Latinos[16] no doubt reflects this phenomenon, but also is indicative of the invisibility of Latino experiences in both the mainstream media and the professional literature.

Methods

This was a qualitative descriptive study[17] aimed at exploring the experiences of Latino survivors and evacuees of Hurricane Katrina. In the weeks immediately following Katrina's landfall, we formed an interdisciplinary, bilingual, multi-state research team to explore the initial experiences of Latino survivors and evacuees of the storm. The research was approved by university Institutional Review Boards and by local community groups who collaborated in the recruitment process.

Data collection. Data for the analysis presented in this paper were collected between October 2005 and March 2006 through face-to-face interviews with 93 Latino survivors and evacuees. To capture a wide range of survivor and evacuee experiences, we conducted interviews in Atlanta (October 2005), New Orleans (November 2005 through March 2006), and Biloxi and Gulfport, Mississippi (March 2006). Throughout this period we also monitored the media for reports on Latinos affected by Katrina.

The primary recruitment strategy for obtaining this convenience sample was snowball referral. In Atlanta, we contacted a Latino community-based organization that granted permission for us to request interviews with Katrina evacuees coming to the agency's relief site to pick up donated food or clothing. In Louisiana and Mississippi we used a combination of personal and community contacts and posted Spanish-language fliers in apartment complexes, *tiendas*, laundromats, restaurants, and work places in areas where Latinos were known to live, work, or congregate. We also asked participants to refer us to others who might be interested in sharing their experiences.

We trained a team of bilingual interviewers who conducted individual, audiotaped interviews in Spanish. Interviewers obtained oral informed consent from each potential participant prior to collecting demographic information and proceeding with the qualitative data collection. The semi-structured interview guide developed specifically for this study consisted of a series of open-ended questions designed to elicit descriptions of the respondents' Katrina-related experiences (e.g., how they learned of the storm and made the decision to stay or leave; what kind of assistance they received from, or gave to, others; their major concerns and stressors; and their plans for the future). Participants received a $40 gift card at the conclusion of the interview.

Data analysis. Professionals whose native language is Spanish transcribed the audiotaped interviews. Prior to proceeding with the data analysis, members of the research team compared the transcriptions with the audiotapes to ensure their fidelity and corrected discrepancies or errors. The authors are bilingual researchers and conducted the qualitative analysis using the original Spanish-language transcriptions.

For analysis, we employed a variety of descriptive qualitative and narrative techniques.[17,18,19] Initial phases involved line-by-line, open coding of individual transcripts, followed by more focused coding. For this particular analysis, we identified relevant health-related issues, themes, and salient storylines. We used constant comparative techniques to explore specific themes within and across interviews and to identify negative cases.

To illustrate our findings, we present examples of supporting data in two forms: short quotations and more fully developed stories told in the course of the interviews. We personally translated these data directly from the original transcripts in Spanish into English. Two native Spanish-speaking research assistants checked our translations. To improve readability, we utilized elements of structure (e.g., order of presentation, punctuation) and eliminated the repetition that occurs naturally as part of oral speech. Translated quotations are represented in italic font. Words inserted to provide clarification are enclosed in square brackets and omitted material is noted by three spaced ellipsis points. We removed names to protect confidentiality, but did maintain geographical locations for reference and context.

Sample characteristics. Among those interviewed (n=93), the vast majority (78%) was of Central American origin, primarily from Honduras and Guatemala. Others were either of Mexican origin (11%) or from South America or the Caribbean (11%). The sample was predominantly female (61%). Length of time living in the U.S. ranged from less than a year to 65 years, with a median of 13 years. The mean years of formal education was 9.92 (SD=3.99). Self-reported English skills ranged from none to poor (35%), medium (24%), and good-to-excellent (41%). Among males, the predominant areas of employment at the time of the storm were service sector (e.g., restaurants, hotels, and casinos), construction, and manufacturing. The most common occupation among employed women was housekeeping and hotel cleaning.

Results

Health-related concerns. Our findings illustrate the personal, familial, and environmental health and health care access concerns of Latinos directly affected by Hurricane Katrina. Decisions to stay in the path of the storm, evacuate, or return often hinged on personal or family health concerns. Respondents attributed a variety of health problems to the disaster itself or the relocation process. These ranged from physical symptoms (e.g., hunger, headaches, nausea, chest pain, shortness of breath, earaches) and exacerbation of chronic diseases (e.g., hypertension, diabetes, asthma) to sleep disturbances, fear, anxiety, depression, and chronic sadness. Access to health care was a key concern, frequently compounded by being uninsured, language barriers, and undocumented immigration status. Environmental health risks included contaminated water, infectious diseases, and unsanitary, overcrowded living conditions. In the face of extreme adversity, there were examples of selfless heroism in which individuals and families risked their own safety to provide assistance to others in greater need. As Latinos described their Katrina experiences, from unanticipated danger to "total loss," they often expressed their gratitude and thankfulness for being alive and for the assistance they had received.

Unanticipated danger and lack of preparation. Findings from this extensive set of interviews suggest that many Latinos living in the areas affected by Katrina did not anticipate the potential strength of the storm and were not prepared for its impact. This common stance of not having anticipated the storm's destructive capabilities framed the experiences of both survivors and evacuees. Barriers to emergency preparedness and to understanding the impending danger included economic constraints, lack of transportation, language, and culture. Additionally, many Latino interviewees acknowledged they simply had not taken warnings seriously, did not anticipate the storm's strength, or believed "nothing was going to happen."

Although many residents from Nicaragua, Honduras, and Puerto Rico had prior experiences with hurricanes and other natural and man-made disasters, some of the newer immigrants from Mexico had little or no prior experience with hurricanes. More long-term residents of New Orleans had experienced numerous hurricane warnings over time, but most of these storms had changed course and missed the city. Based on previous experiences, some naively assumed they had nothing to worry about:

> I suffered through Hurricane Fifi in Honduras. This was some 32 or 33 years ago. There I lost everything. All my things went flying out of the house, because the little house I lived in was very low. I lived through that very traumatic experience. But here I didn't imagine that it would be like this. Or perhaps I had forgotten the experience that I had lived through so many years ago. But like I said, we thought this [storm] was something that would blow over quickly, that it wouldn't be so strong. (Honduran woman, age 70, 20 years in U.S.)

Latinos with limited-English-proficiency noted difficulties in understanding warnings and instructions in English. Immigrants accustomed to the metric system had difficulty interpreting weather reports that referred to the storm's strength and direction expressed as *miles per hour*. Participants identified family, friends, and coworkers as the primary sources of information about the impending hurricane. Other information sources included Latino radio stations and English language media. Monolingual Spanish speakers tended to get information from English language media second-hand, through bilingual friends or family members:

> [I found out about Katrina] through my friend, who knows how to speak [English], and we always had the television on. So we were aware that the hurricane was coming. But supposedly, we thought that it wasn't going to be very strong, very severe. Because before, when Ivan came, Ivan came and went . . . [After the storm] when my friend called 911, they asked us why we didn't leave . . . she told them we didn't have a car. The truth of the matter was that we didn't believe it was going to be so terrible. (Honduran man, age 28, 6 years in U.S.)

In hindsight, even those who had engaged in some type of hurricane preparations were surprised by the destructive impact of the storm. Yet the words of one relatively recent immigrant also suggested a relationship between low expectations and class/societal position:

> In reality, I had no expectations. I didn't expect anything, because we Latinos are always left in last place. We only thought that we would lose things, our work, our whole lives. (Guatemalan man, age 28, 3 years in U.S.)

Hunger: an immediate health concern. Hunger was the most common immediate physical and emotional health concern. Even those who had stocked up on food and water often found themselves hungry when their food supplies were damaged or lost in the flood. In the case of one family, prior experience with spoiled food as result of electrical outages resulted in inadequate preparation and subsequent hunger:

> We didn't have anything. There was nothing. There wasn't any food at all. We hadn't even bought [extra] food, because I figured that if the electricity went out we would lose all the food we had. And if we had to leave, we would lose the food we left. So we hadn't even bought any food. We went hungry for a week, until some people from Dallas showed up and gave us food. That was the first food we had. (Nicaraguan man, age 46, 19 years in U.S.)

Those who evacuated also suffered from lack of food and water, often as a result of leaving hastily, being unprepared, or getting waylaid or stranded en route from the storm area. An extended Nicaraguan family (grandparents, daughter, son-in-law, and grandchildren) left New Orleans headed for Alabama, where another daughter resided. They started out in two cars but had to abandon one because of gasoline shortages. The grandmother was no stranger to adversity, having survived earthquakes and war in Nicaragua, but she became desperate as food ran out and her grandchild got hungrier:

> By the second day we didn't have any food. We only had some bread and water. My granddaughter is three years old. She said, "I want chocolate milk." I just cried— because where were we going to get chocolate milk? We kept driving until we got to a little town in Mississippi. We stopped and didn't see anything except what looked like an abandoned gas station. Then I saw someone going into a storage shed at the gas station. So I went running over and went in. The woman said to me in English, "I didn't come here to sell anything. I just came to check on my business." So I told her, in English, "I'm sorry. I have children. I need food and drink. I have the money. I pay for something." I picked up two sacks of ice, some chocolate milk, doughnuts; whatever I found that was edible. I paid. I said, "Charge me whatever because we have two children." The nice lady said, "Okay." After that I felt better because I had food with me for my grandchildren. (Nicaraguan woman, age 68, 23 years in U.S.)

Getting by without food or water was physically and emotionally challenging for all concerned. For parents, even more challenging were feelings of impotence and the emotional pain of not being able to provide for children's needs. Hunger was also difficult and potentially more serious for pregnant women:

> Just knowing that you have lost everything and that you have to start all over again, and you don't have a job . . . it's really difficult on my health. Being hungry and pregnant was horrible. In the beginning, I was dying of hunger. What are we going to eat? There was a whole bunch of people in that house and you couldn't eat. When you're pregnant, it's not enough to eat three times a day. You need to eat up to six times. When I went to the pre-natal visit [after the storm], I was anemic. They told me, "You're not eating well." So I'm telling you the truth, I'm eating, but I'm not eat-

ing nutritious food, just whatever food there is to eat. (Honduran woman, age 35, 9 years in U.S.)

In the face of extreme adversity, resourcefulness and ingenuity served to stave off hunger. A man and his neighbors stranded in New Orleans for nearly a week told this story of collective survival strategies:

The day after the storm things were calmer, but the water was rising; the water had almost covered the cars . . . and we were waiting there [for help]. There was no electricity, nothing. So we started looking for pieces of wood so we could build a fire [to cook], because there were children who needed to eat. So we had to find a way to feed everyone that was there. So we built a fire. There wasn't anything to eat so we fried fish that we caught. It was fortunate that we had some lemons, the girls got busy washing [the fish] with the lemons and the little fresh water that we had. We were dying of hunger, because we were there for more than a week. The helicopters just passed over us and shone their lights on us, but most of them flew in the direction of New Orleans, where most of the people were. One day we didn't eat anything, because there wasn't very much and there were children. We older folks didn't eat. We had to give the food to the children, because they needed it more. We could hold out a little longer. (Honduran man, age 28, 6 years in U.S.)

An interesting negative case, in which a Latino family stranded in New Orleans did not suffer from hunger, also demonstrated their resourcefulness. This story contained an interesting touch of cultural commentary on dietary assimilation:

Sincerely, I'll tell you that during and after the hurricane I ate better [than before]. Because there are times when I've been working and running around and only ate at Burger King, McDonald's, Popeye's. During the hurricane we were cooking much better and were not hungry. At least we had food . . . my grandmother always has a stock of canned food in her closet and my aunt also, so that helped a lot. (Honduran man, age 40, 25 years in U.S.)

Risking personal health and safety in the process of providing mutual assistance. All participants, survivors and evacuees alike, had experienced some degree of personal risk and loss. In the face of extraordinary danger, some individuals further risked their own health and safety in order to help others. In relating her experience of surviving the hurricane, a 30-year-old Puerto Rican woman noted her concerns about the disruption of health care services, which put her family's health in jeopardy:

This is the first time I've experienced a hurricane of this category. I lived in Puerto Rico in 1989 when Hurricane Hugo came, but I was young, I was only 15 or 18 years old, and I didn't know as much. Now I'm married, I am a mother; I have children who depend on me, so this one has affected me much more. My husband is diabetic and my son has chronic asthma. We didn't have the therapy machine for the child if he would get asthma. The closest hospital was closed. The only hospital that was open in the whole disaster area was Jefferson.

Despite these immediate health care concerns, the family stayed through the storm to assist others in more dire need. They put themselves in immediate danger and took even greater personal health risks to assist the frail, elderly residents of the nursing home where her husband worked as a janitor:

> At my husband's work, there were only two housekeepers, the manager, and three nurses. My husband felt pity for them. He did not want to leave them alone. They were all women, but he was the only male housekeeper. So he said, "Let's stay here. At least I can offer my help in case we need to move the elderly from one room to another." So we stayed to help people. My brother also stayed with us. While my brother was taking care of my children, I helped [move] the elderly into the hall, because there was no electricity. They were 80, 90 years old. They were really in need.

Such acts of mutual assistance and selfless heroism by Latinos rarely surfaced in the mainstream media. Another example of selfless heroism was the collective mobilization of a neighborhood rescue effort by a group of Latino men in New Orleans:

> The day after [Katrina] another Nicaraguan man said to me, "There are almost 45 people that need to be evacuated in this block . . . pregnant women, old people, children." So the following morning, we decided to look for help. We left the building swimming . . . I swam past a man yelling from the top of a roof, but I don't understand anything anyone says in English, so I just kept swimming . . . We swam almost 12 blocks . . . [to] the Windsor Hotel, [where] there was a friend . . . that would let us stay there. We told her that there were almost 20 of us. She agreed, since the hotel manager knew that they would receive many victims. When we left the hotel, there weren't any boats, any policeman, or any soldiers—no mayor or governor directing the people . . . Earlier we had met the Fire Chief of New Orleans. When we informed him that we needed help [to evacuate the people from our block], he said, "There are 700,000 people that need to be evacuated in New Orleans. Go and try to help them." It was then that I realized that the trouble was too serious for those people to remain alone another day or even another hour [without help]. So, we found a wooden bed that was floating by Charity Avenue and we pulled it [back to the neighborhood]. We arrived where the people were waiting for us. Along the way we informed people we saw what was really happening. The only thing we could do was to go through the neighborhood in groups of three and search for children and elders in each building so that they would not drown . . . There were 12 blocks where we could not touch the ground with our feet. There were 13 of us, all men. We found a 30-foot hose and tied together the wooden bed and some plywood. We pulled it and we started to carry four people [at a time]. We left them and returned to carry four more people and so on . . . Hours passed and more and more people arrived. By that time, they felt more courageous because there were many people that could not swim. Some teenagers drowned because they could not swim . . . During the whole rescue we tried to give people courage, we asked them not to be afraid, we said there were no snakes . . . I spent the whole week helping, helping people.

In telling the story, almost as an after-thought, the narrator noted that as he worked to save others, surrounded by death and horror, he actually did suffer a snakebite:

I got a snakebite in my leg. It was a thin serpent, brown colored. [When the serpent bit me] I felt dizzy but I drank alcohol so as not to suffer from poison problems. Alcohol helped me . . . I estimate that I saw some 400 dead bodies. There were 3 dead people over the Levee. To my horror, a big animal comes out and is devouring one of them. Bum! In 6, 7 minutes the bodies were gone. I will not go back there anymore, it was full of alligators! (Nicaraguan man, age 37, 5 years in U.S.)

Health and health care access concerns, and decisions to stay, leave, or return. An individual or family's decision to evacuate or stay depended on a number of factors. These included availability and sources of information and advice, prior personal experiences, and the availability of transportation and economic resources. In some cases, a personal or family health concern (e.g., pregnancy, chronic illness, acute illness, access to health services) was the pivotal factor in deciding whether to stay, leave, or return. The following case illustrates how access to pregnancy care was the tipping point in a family's decision to leave New Orleans and not return:

[In previous storms] what we did before was to put tape on the windows . . . but this time I didn't do anything [to prepare]. Before I had never decided to leave when there were hurricane warnings; I wouldn't have left this time either . . . But when I saw the route and the form of the hurricane that was coming towards New Orleans, then I decided to move, most of all because of my wife who is seven months pregnant. Other times I stayed. On Saturday at noon I saw the trajectory of the storm that was coming [and I said], "Okay, we're going because this is a really strong one that's coming. We're not running the risk." I have some friends who are not very well informed, and I called them to tell them about the strength of the storm. They didn't believe it. They said, "We are going to stay here. Nothing is going to happen." So I told them, "Listen, this one is strong, this one is coming right here, we need to get out." They said, "No, you go with your wife and your [unborn] child, because we are going to stay." So I came alone, with my wife. We stayed here [in Atlanta] because my wife is pregnant and is getting prenatal care [here]. In New Orleans the hospitals aren't available, they aren't open, there aren't doctors, there aren't hospitals. So for the time being we are staying here so that she and the baby can get medical care. (Honduran man, age 42, 15 years in U.S.)

Illness and the lack of available health care forced some to evacuate. An example was the case of a single mother and her young child stranded in Mississippi at a friend's home for two weeks without potable water. Not surprisingly, the child eventually succumbed to severe diarrhea. While attempting to find medical assistance, a chance encounter with a volunteer of Mexican origin precipitated the trajectory that led to her evacuation to Atlanta:

My son got sick. That's why I left [Mississippi]. Otherwise I would have stayed. My son got really sick with diarrhea, really bad diarrhea. When my son got sick we went to the doctor, but there were no doctors. There were just assistants, who are not the same as doctors . . . All they did was give him something to lower his temperature. Usually when the baby has a temperature it's an infection . . . By chance, when I went [for medical care] I met a Mexican girl who helped me to take him to a hospital, because I needed help to take him to a hospital. She said she came to help people who were sick and so she could help me get out of there with him. [She told me] to go get everything and we would take the baby to the hospital. So I picked up the few things I had there and went with her. I happened to be very lucky in meeting up with that young Mexican woman. She was wonderful; she bought things for me and my son. It was just by chance, because if she hadn't been there, what would have happened to my sick child? (Argentinean woman, age 34, 4 years in U.S.)

As they pondered whether or not to return home, the lack of available and accessible health care services in the New Orleans area was a factor some evacuees took seriously. Others were leery of returning to the devastated areas because of existing health problems. Such was the case of an unemployed, elderly diabetic woman who had evacuated to Atlanta with her daughter and grandson:

I won't go back there because I am a diabetic, so I say to myself, and my daughter told me, "You can't go back." My daughter went back, but she came back in really bad shape after seeing what things were like [in New Orleans]. So I believe I will stay here [in Georgia]. Look, I can't take much, if I walk a lot I get tired, my legs hurt and with the diabetes, I have to be very vigilant about my food. I have to eat every little while. I can't eat a lot at one time. And I need a lot of tranquility; because these things [health problems] make me sick, make me depressed, I can't get around. (Honduran woman, age 70, 20 years in U.S.)

Finding alternate sources of health care and obtaining health insurance were major concerns for both those who stayed and those who evacuated. Loss of their usual sources of health care, particularly for pre-existing chronic health conditions, was an immediate worry among those caught in Katrina's path. A Guatemalan woman afflicted with macular degeneration had survived the storm in New Orleans. However, she was worried about the personal implications of the closing of a health facility where the poor and underserved had received treatment:

I feel very depressed . . . Also, I used to go to Charity Hospital, about my eye, about the stroke I had [in my eye]. In January I'll have to find [another health care provider] because I need to have my eye checked. Even if I have to pay I'm going to find a place . . . because I have a problem that my eye bleeds inside. (Guatemalan woman, age 54, 13 years in U.S.)

Being insured prior to the storm did not guarantee access to care. As exemplified by the concerns voiced by this father, loss of insurance was one of the negative health care implications of evacuating to another state:

One of the problems we had was health insurance. My health insurance doesn't cover me here in Georgia. In other words I have had to look for another way to get health insurance. I've been trying to get health insurance for my children through Medicaid, because financially now I cannot do what I used to do. So I'm trying to at least get medical insurance for them. That has been one of the biggest problems. (Colombian man, age 46, 22 years in U.S.)

Compounded risks of being undocumented and uninsured. For uninsured and/or undocumented Latinos there were additional social and economic costs of accessing health care. Another story told by the Nicaraguan man who participated in the spontaneous rescue efforts (described above) exemplified how being undocumented and uninsured compounded the physical and emotional harm he suffered. Having survived the New Orleans storm and heroically assisted others in the process, he temporarily evacuated to Texas for a few days before returning to New Orleans to look for work in post-Katrina reconstruction efforts. Although the opportunity for employment was welcome, the reconstruction work itself involved significant environmental health risks:

I started to work for the Jefferson Hospital, cleaning and dismantling everything. I stayed only four days because the company's working conditions were not appropriate. The hospital was very polluted and we did not have any kind of protection. Eight dollars an hour was not worth it. The second week I started working [with another company]. They told us that we would work with painting, sheetrock and demolitions. But that was not true . . . we had to demolish a ceiling that has a kind of tile that is picked up and put in. It is not sheetrock. As time goes by it gets really dirty and the insulation drops fibers that make you itch. They gave us a pair of plastic glasses but they were not adequate. So, I worked for two weeks dismantling five stories. By the third week I could not stand it anymore. My vision was injured. I lost 60% of the vision in one eye . . . I wanted to sue the company because I was sure that I was injured on the job. You know what? I blame the water, the food we ate the eight days we were in water. I blame the ceiling because there must have been rats and dust there, where everything gets in your body.

Uninsured and out of cash, he sought treatment for his vision loss at an emergency room. However, he was very dissatisfied with the providers' explanations and diagnoses and the cost and quality of the treatment he received:

The first time I went to the hospital they saw me and sent me a bill for $500 . . . How is it possible that this doctor diagnosed me with conjunctivitis? This was not conjunctivitis. And they sent me a bill, just for having said it was conjunctivitis, without having given me any medicine. The point is that, after going to the hospital and being charged $500, a doctor diagnosed conjunctivitis. How is that possible? I have all my medical documents. After having this [eye] problem for two months, I haven't even been able to get an antibiotic for the infection that I have, because the cost is too high. Here I am with 3 bills for $500 that they have sent me . . . I'm afraid to go back there because I have a bill for $360 for some exams that they had me do. They didn't explain any of them. The same doctor who saw me, he said, "I can't prescribe anything for you because it's not clear [what the problem is] . . . A while later I went for an appointment with two other doctors, one a cornea specialist, and the other a more general physician. They told me it is an infection . . . I now have a total of $1,600 in doctor's bills. That's without spending anything on prescriptions. I don't have insurance; because of my [undocumented] status, I don't have anything. (Nicaraguan man, age 37, 5 years in U.S.)

Language and cultural barriers between patient and provider certainly may have played a part in this man's interpretation of the care he received. It was not clear if this limited-English-proficient Latino had any language assistance (e.g., interpreter, bilingual provider) in his interactions with providers. It is possible the meaning he attached to the diagnosis of "conjunctivitis" was common eye irritation, which he interpreted as not reflective of the severity of his symptoms. But regardless of the health care providers' intentions, the unresolved health problem and mounting bills only left him feeling more vulnerable, marginalized, and dissatisfied with the health care he received.

Environmental health risks. Both survivors and evacuees experienced environmental health risks. *Plague* was a word some used in describing the conditions created by contaminated floodwaters, accumulating debris, and the lack of water, food, and electricity. Health hazards posed by mosquitoes and other insects and fears of contracting disease through contact with contaminated floodwaters were common concerns.

> We couldn't get out of the apartment because of the floodwaters. And the water that came in was very contagious. It was black water. We couldn't walk through it because we could get an infection. They were fishing bodies out of the water. There were dogs that drowned. It was very contaminated. (Honduran man, age 28, 6 years in U.S.)

Stranded survivors devised numerous strategies to protect themselves from exposure to health risks. Such strategies were not always successful or sanctioned, as in the case one group that "built bonfires to keep the mosquitoes away but at night the police and the firemen would come and put out the bonfires." Some survivors lived for weeks in unsanitary conditions before they received any type of assistance:

> We went for days without being able to take a bath. There were huge blue flies . . . I'm telling you, they were huge. There was a swimming pool and we went to take a bath there, trying to clean ourselves up a little. But lots of people were using the pool to bathe, so it got dirty. It was at the point of there being an epidemic. We were there for 15 days without water, without anything. Finally they started bringing us some things, like sacks of ice. The Red Cross sent in a medical crew who vaccinated us one night. They came at 4 o'clock in the morning. (Nicaraguan man, age 46, 19 years in U.S.)

A casino employee in Mississippi initially evacuated with a group of Latino co-workers to Florida. When they returned two days later, she found conditions much worse than she had anticipated:

> [When we returned after the storm] my friend said she would drive me [to my house] to get the food. Knowing that something was coming, I had bought more than $150 worth of food and water. But it was a waste of money because the water and mud ruined everything. The water had covered my apartment. I never expected that. My home was unrecognizable. The mud was up to here and the ceiling had fallen down on all the furniture. I couldn't salvage anything, I only took a photograph and left. I [went back and] stayed with my friend. We didn't have anything but a little bit of water. I stayed there for two weeks. I think my friend is still there, unless someone has

gone to get her out . . . It is very difficult without electricity, without water, without anything, in that heat, my God. (Argentinean woman, age 34, 4 years in U.S.)

Another evacuee returned to New Orleans to check on her family, home, and belongings. She described the physical and emotional trauma of witnessing the tremendous environmental damage from Katrina:

My house was full of mold and there were lots of flies and mosquitoes, lots of them. I came back all bitten up. Luckily the Red Cross had given me a shot, so I was supposedly a little protected. But I'll tell you that even if you think you are prepared for what you are going to see, you're not. The last day, when I was leaving, I just broke down crying. I just gave in. It was so very sad. (Honduran woman, age 50, 25 years in U.S.)

Latino evacuees often ended up in homes of other Latinos. Many were taken in by their own family or friends; others found themselves in the homes of strangers. Both survivors and evacuees reported having to endure crowded living conditions. Evacuees interviewed in Atlanta described the despair of living with 14–15 people in two-bedroom apartments, alluding to the potential social and emotional health risks from overcrowding.

Emotional stressors. Respondents identified various physical health conditions they associated directly or indirectly to the disaster. Yet the vast majority of storm-related stressors were emotional. The extreme environmental conditions themselves also created emotional stress:

It was difficult to sleep at night. I couldn't get to sleep, there were so many mosquitoes; the door was open and we couldn't sleep. There was no water, you couldn't take a bath, no air conditioning—the things you take for granted. I became desperate. It was truly terrible, especially for the children. (Honduran woman, age 40, 25 years in U.S.)

Others who stayed through the storm reported reliving the trauma from the terrifying noise of the devastating hurricane winds. Uncertainty and fear for the safety of family members was another significant source of stress:

My greatest worry was [that my son was dead]. I thought I would go crazy . . . I prayed the rosary, asking God that my son would not be taken away by the wind, because it was terrible. But thank God [my son] managed to get out on Thursday. But we didn't have any word from him. Neither did my family in New Jersey have any news about us, because the cell phones didn't work. (Nicaraguan woman, age 68, 23 years in U.S.)

Crowded conditions and family stressors also increased levels of irritability:

Everything bothers me, everything is irritation. The kids scream and I can't stand it. I don't want any noise, and don't want anything. If I could, I'd go away . . . I'd disappear, I would just disappear. (Colombian woman, age 44, 25 years in U.S.)

In some instances, previously strained family relations were made worse by the stressful conditions resulting from relocation:

> My wife is very nervous . . . she gets upset about this problem, she is always thinking about it, and is always in a really bad mood and is not feeling well. She always causes lots of family problems. It's a pity, morally, these family problems. I wish I could have more tranquility. (Colombian man, age 71, 42 years in U.S.)

Whereas some Latino survivors and evacuees found themselves dealing with the stress of too many people living in small, cramped quarters, social isolation was a significant emotional stressor for others:

> It was like a desert here [in New Orleans]. (Honduran woman, age 56, 22 years in U.S.)

> When we arrived here [in Atlanta] we felt like when you arrive at a lake and don't know anyone and you feel alone, abandoned, that you have lost everything. When the storm passed and we arrived here we felt like we were going to have to start all over without anything. Psychologically, we felt really down but at the same time we felt good because we saved our lives. (Honduran man, age 42, 15 years in U.S.)

The unfamiliarity of a new environment was another source of stress among those who evacuated:

> Worst of all is the stress. I'm not familiar with the city [Atlanta]. I'm confined in the apartment. We try to get out a little, but stay close by so we don't get lost. One day we went past an exit and we got lost and we didn't know where we were. It's been pretty hard. This is a big city, much larger than New Orleans. (Colombian woman, age 44, 25 years in U.S.)

Sleep disturbances. Difficulty sleeping was one of the most common complaints. Reliving the traumatic experience of the hurricane and its aftermath resulted in sleep disturbances in adults and children:

> It's hard to sleep. Especially my little girl, when she goes outside and she sees those trees moving, she says, "Mommy, Katrina, Katrina," because they were awake when the hurricane came, they saw how everything moved [in the wind]. The place where we were holing up the roof was blown away. The children also waded through the water, because we had to get out of where we were. They saw everything; they even saw two dead people. (Puerto Rican woman, age 30)

Underlying sleep disturbances were physical, emotional, financial, and social stresses related to the trauma of recent events and to uncertainty about the future:

> I wake up in the night and can't get back to sleep because I think and think about what is going to happen to us. It's pretty hard. It's almost impossible to sleep . . . We don't have a real place to live yet. Doctors say that if you have lots of stress, lots of

problems, tensions, that affects your ability to reconcile your sleep . . . That's what happened in my case. I had to think a lot about how to establish myself here [Atlanta] . . . This has been hard and I couldn't get to sleep thinking about it all. (Guatemalan man, age 33, 5 years in U.S.)

Respondents also attributed a variety of symptoms indicative of mental health problems (e.g., chronic sadness, anxiety, depression, chest pains) to their Katrina experiences. Being undocumented also contributed to fear and anxiety levels among Latinos:

We didn't feel like going [to get assistance] because we are undocumented. We were afraid that they would arrest us or something . . . They only took us to the Red Cross . . . they gave us a little food and clothing. Being undocumented, you are always fearful of going [to seek help] because you know how much it costs to come here and the money you pay [to get here] . . . it always makes you afraid. (Guatemalan woman, age 22, 7 months in U.S.)

Evacuees and survivors alike were dealing with multiple losses—home and possessions, employment and livelihood, security, social networks. Feelings of insecurity and uncertainly about the future were compounded by these significant losses:

Most of the apartments [where my husband and I worked] were destroyed. All the neighbors are gone . . . even those who stayed, they can't get in [the apartments]. It makes me sad and depressed, seeing my job gone. That's been the main thing. At my age I think it will be difficult to get work, it's not like a younger person who can apply for jobs anywhere . . . I had to go to the doctor because I'm so depressed and anxious about the uncertain future. It's uncertain whether or not the [landlord] is going to fix up the apartments or not, I don't know where we are going to go. We are waiting on God's willingness and other people also that they may show us kindness. (Nicaraguan woman, age 68, 23 years in U.S.)

At the time these interviews were conducted, very few respondents had sought or actually received any formal mental health services. There was little indication as to whether or not they would seek such services, if available. However, there was evidence that participants recognized the impact that compromised mental health status has on one's ability to function in society:

We want to reconstruct our lives but we don't have any financial assistance. We need so much. And besides that, psychologically we have been injured. That is a basic issue, if a person isn't well in his head, he can't work very well. (Honduran man, age 42, 15 years in U.S.)

Personal strategies to ameliorate stress included prayer and working constructively on family and interpersonal relations:

I pray a lot and I have a lot of patience in order to know, understand [others], because we are all going through the same problem. (Nicaraguan woman, age 68, 23 years in U.S.)

Unfortunately, some coping strategies involved further health risks:

> I never smoked in my whole life. But ever since the hurricane until now I've been smoking a pack of cigarettes [a day]. In my 46 years I had never before smoked. It's because of the stress, because it seems that smoking calms me down, something like that. But I'm trying to forget it and I'm trying to quit. (Nicaraguan man, age 46, 19 years in U.S.)

Resilience expressed through simple thankfulness. Given the nature of disruption and loss these Latinos had recently experienced, their expressions of gratitude were particularly noteworthy. Health and access to resources were among the blessings these survivors recognized.

> What I'm going through is normal, after something of this nature. I believe that other people are having more serious difficulties. We are fine. Other than the stress, in other ways, we have good health, thank God. (Honduran woman, age 50, 25 years in U.S.)

Success in obtaining public assistance and access to health care was a major reason for feeling grateful. Not having to worry about access to health care provided this evacuee with a sense of tranquility and security in the midst of ongoing loss and uncertainty:

> As I say, although it has been very hard for me, I am also thankful to be here [Atlanta] because the baby, and the medical care I need was my primary worry. But I went to Grady Hospital—it is a public hospital—and they immediately changed my Medicaid, immediately they gave me [access to] the WIC Program. Immediately, the very same day I went. Sincerely, I have had more medical attention here than [I had] in Louisiana, so I am truly very thankful and that has given me a little more tranquility. (Honduran woman, age 35, 9 years in U.S.)

A self-employed Latino business owner who had lived in New Orleans for 22 years reported how he lost his home to the storm and his business to looters. Despite these overwhelming losses, he felt fortunate to have evacuated successfully and was thankful for the assistance of the Latino Community in Atlanta:

> Well, it has been very difficult. I thank God because here [Atlanta] we received help. The Latino assistance here has been really strong and helped us out a lot. I am truly happy to have my children in a school, a good Catholic school, and to have received so much care from the community. I would say that it has been a very difficult situation for us, but thank God, I believe that we are in better shape than many. For example, the people who didn't get out in time when the hurricane came, the people who had to be saved after the flood, and who perhaps did not have a place to sleep, or who went hungry for two or three days. That said, for us it was difficult, it was frustrating, it was tedious to have to drive so far, and worrying about the children. But overall, I believe that there are others who had it much worse than we did. (Colombian man, age 46, 22 years in U.S.)

Some, like this elderly hotel worker who had hoped to be able to retire, struggled with feelings of resignation of how this unexpected disaster had disrupted his hopes and dreams. Similar to others in the midst of significant disappointment and loss, he expressed his thankfulness for being alive:

> One just has to ask the Lord for resignation . . . because one feels a little cheated . . . In reality, you should not become so attached to the material. But after everything I have suffered through in order to get [what I had] and to lose it all, it certainly is unpleasant. I'm not at all happy about it, as they say. My plans for the future have been affected. I was thinking about retiring, having my own home. I'm 71 years old. So I should be resting and living in the hands of the Lord. What I need to tell you, that I forgot to say, is that we give thanks to the Lord that we are alive. (Columbian man, age 71, 42 years in U.S.)

These attitudes of thankfulness may reflect the strength of these Latino's faith and/or indicate their emotional resiliency. There were many examples of resiliency in the face of ongoing adversity, such as one Guatemalan family living in New Orleans three months after the storm. The couple had lost their employment and belongings and was living in an apartment without electricity, thankful to have a place to stay rent-free:

> My daughter is here [in the U.S.] with us now, but she can't stay here [in this apartment] because she has children. She can't stay here because we don't have electricity, we only have water. This isn't the apartment we used to live in. It's one that the landlord has let us stay in. Some people say, "Get out of here. They [the owners] are responsible. The City doesn't allow you to stay here because there is no electricity." But we have much to be thankful for because he [the landlord] has let us stay here even though there isn't any electricity. But we do have a roof over our head and we can stay here for now. I thank God and the landlord, and also the man who works here. He has helped us out a lot so that we can stay here even though there isn't any electricity. Because you can't find a place to rent anywhere. So this is a very desperate situation. But what can we do? Everything is so expensive, so we are just taking advantage of this opportunity for a place to stay. (Guatemalan woman, age 48, 5 years in U.S.)

A common refrain heard over and over again across this set of interviews was "we lost everything." Yet respondents repeatedly expressed a thankfulness that transcended the trauma—gratitude for being alive, and for the kindness and assistance of family, friends, and strangers. The findings illuminate the depth and breadth of the mostly silent suffering and informal solidarity experienced by Latinos, who were often at the margins of the broader, more public disaster. They suffered greatly, as did others, but they also demonstrated resilience and drew strength from their families, community, and faith.

Discussion

The experiences of individual Latinos who evacuated or survived Katrina do not necessarily depict those of the Latino population in general or other racial/ethnic groups. However, the findings of this qualitative descriptive research do provide important insight into health and health care experiences of those who live on the margin of the dominant society because of language, culture, and immigration status. Our discussion addresses implications for disaster research, policy development, and service provision.

Gender, age, culture, ethnicity, severity of exposure and loss, subsequent life transitions and stressors, and levels of social and emotional support are all factors that can affect health in times of disaster.[20] There is some support for the notion that Latinos are at higher risk than the general population for adverse health effects of disasters. Studies conducted after Hurricane Andrew[20] and the September 11, 2001 terrorist attacks[21] reported higher levels of post-traumatic stress disorder among Hispanics. Our findings reflect the perceptions and experiences of Latino survivors and evacuees at the time of the interviews (i.e., one to seven months post-Katrina), and clearly indicate the prevalence of anxiety, depression, sleep disturbances, and somatization among this sample of Latinos. These findings are limited by the cross-sectional research design and the nature of the data (self-report among a convenience sample). Disaster researchers suggest the long-term effects of disasters may peak during the first year, and that recovery is a long-term process that needs to be monitored over time.[20,22,23] To fully understand the mental and physical health implications of Katrina on Latinos, there is an urgent need for longitudinal studies that take into account levels of disaster exposure and measure changes in depression, anxiety, social and emotional support, and coping strategies over time.

Studies on the impact of disasters on social support networks have produced somewhat inconclusive and conflicting findings but there is research indicating that Latinos tend to seek and receive more assistance and support from informal than from formal sources.[25] In our analysis of health concerns, seeking and obtaining access to formal health care services was a salient theme. There was substantial evidence, however, that these Latinos relied primarily on informal social networks for information, assistance, and support prior, during, and after Katrina. In the course of dealing with the disaster, new informal networks formed, some of which were transitory. The examples of selfless assistance to others in need and the prevalence of expressions of thankfulness in the face of adversity must be noted. Further exploration of the impact of disasters on informal and formal networks and individual and collective assets is warranted. Building on existing research in the areas of help-seeking and social support,[26] an emerging area for disaster research is the exploration of possible associations between resiliency, thankfulness, and actions of seeking, receiving, and giving assistance in the context of different cultures and communities over time.

Another significant finding was the extent to which respondents reported they were not prepared and/or did not anticipate the potential strength of the storm and the implications of staying put or evacuating. Lack of adequate preparation and provisions were a problem for those who stayed as well as for those who evacuated. The results of this study support reports from the lay press indicating that language, lack of information, lack of transportation, and poverty were significant barriers to evacuation among Latino residents. Our findings also highlight the role that health and health care access concerns played in deciding whether or not to stay or evacuate. A major challenge to local disaster preparedness and evacuation policies is to balance awareness of danger and the economic and social costs of preparedness to minority individuals, families, and communities, without running the risk of "crying wolf." Among Latinos, a lack of a preventive mentality and low expectations of formal assistance are formidable barriers to disaster preparedness.

In prior research with Puerto Rican disaster victims, Solomon and colleagues[24] hypothesized that victims with greater prior family responsibilities, specifically parents, would experience higher levels of emotional disability. They found single parents to be at particularly high risk for lack of emotional support in disaster situations. In our study, concern for the welfare of children was expressed by married and single parents and also by extended family and community members. An effective approach to reaching Latino communities with disaster preparedness interventions may be to capitalize on shared cultural valuing of children, family, and community rather than focusing on individual responsibility.

Practical, culturally appropriate information on feasible preparedness actions must be disseminated within minority communities. Public health preparedness plans and actions must take into consideration Latinos' perceived needs as well as their community resources, assets, and networks. The findings of this research point to resourcefulness and community solidarity among diverse Latino groups. It is necessary for local officials and health care providers to identify bilingual and bicultural liaisons who are able to reach and communicate with diverse Latino constituents and networks.

This research confirms common knowledge that disasters exacerbate existing restrictions and limitations to health care access among the poor and underserved. The fastest growing minority population,[27] Hispanics currently have the highest uninsured rates of any racial/ethnic group in the county.[28,29] In the aftermath of Katrina, even previously insured Latinos confronted economic and bureaucratic barriers to health insurance. Our findings suggest the few evacuees who were able to obtain public insurance in another state depended primarily on personal resourcefulness and advocacy and the good will of local providers. Federal and state policies for programs such as Medicaid and WIC should have automatic provisions for inter-state evacuees to facilitate access to all levels of care. Local service providers need training and education in order to ensure policies are implemented in culturally sensitive and appropriate ways.

In normal times, there is a tendency among the uninsured to forego primary care, often resulting in inappropriate utilization of emergency services. There is an urgent need for broader coverage for primary services, accompanied by culturally appropriate education of immigrants and limited-English-proficient Spanish speakers on how to access the U.S. health care system effectively and appropriately. Strengthening the knowledge and capacity of both users and the health care system is necessary for efficient, effective, and equitable service provision of health care during times of disaster.

Acknowledgment

This study was funded through a grant from the University of South Carolina Office of Research and Health Sciences.

Notes

1. Contreras J. Salvaban a blancos; a negros y latinos los dejaban morir. La Crónica de Hoy. 2005 Sept 7. Available at http://www.cronica.com.mx.

2. Gamboa S. Group: protect Katrina victim immigrants. AP. 2005 Sept 20. Available at http://www.sfgate.com/.

3. Kantor M. Katrina coverage brown-out. The Revealer. 2005 Sept 19. Available at www.therevealor.org/.

4. Ochoa S. Aiding Katrina's Latino victims: NCLR mobilizes its affiliates to assist victims of the hurricane disaster. La Prensa San Diego. 2005 Sept 9. Available at http://www.laprensa-sandiego.org/.

5. Radelat A. Katrina's hidden victims. Hattiesburg American. 2005 Sept 20.

6. Salinas ME. Latinos paid dearly after Katrina. Santa Maria Times. 2006 Mar 13. Available at http://www.santamariatimes.com/.

7. Cevallos D. Thousands of Latin American immigrants among Katrina's victims. Inter Press Service News Agency. 2005 Sep 5. Available at http://ipsnews.net/.

8. Donato K, Hakimzadeh S. The changing face of the Gulf Coast: immigration to Louisiana, Mississippi and Alabama. Migration Information Source. 2006 Jan 1. Available at http://www.migrationinformation.org/.

9. U.S. Census Bureau, 2005. American Community Survey. Table C03001, Hispanic or Latino Origin by Specific Origin. Available at http://factfinder.census.gov/.

10. U.S. Census Bureau, 2005. American Community Survey, Table C16006, Language Spoken at Home by Ability to Speak English for the Population 5 years and Over (Hispanic or Latino). Available at http://factfinder.census.gov/.

11. Muñiz B. In the eye of the storm: how the government and private response to Hurricane Katrina failed Latinos. Washington, DC: National Council of La Raza. 2006 Feb 28.

12. Shore E. Katrina victims denied aid and face deportation. New American Media. 2005 Sep 28. Available at http://news.ncmonline.com/.

13. Terhune C, Pérez E. Roundup of immigrants in shelter reveals rising tensions. Wall Street Journal. 2005 October 3:B1.

14. Hurricane Katrina Assessment Team Report. American Friends Service Committee, Southeastern Regional Office, Atlanta GA. Unpublished report, 2005 November 1.

15. Shore E. Katrina aftermath: Red Cross accused of evicting Latino victims. New American Media. 2005 October 19. Available at http://news.newamericamedia.org/.

16. Brodie M, Weltzien E, Altman D, et al. Experiences of Hurricane Katrina evacuees in Houston shelters: implications for future planning. Am J Public Health. 2006 Aug;96(8):1402–8.

17. Sandelowski M. Whatever happened to qualitative description? Res Nurs Health. 2000 Aug;23(4):334–40.

18. Strauss A, Corbin JM. Basics of qualitative research: grounded theory procedures and techniques. Newbury Park, CA: Sage, 1990.

19. Messias DKH, DeJoseph JF. Feminist narrative interpretations: challenges, tensions and opportunities for nurse researchers. Aquichan. 2004;4(4):40–9.

20. Norris FH, Perilla JL, Riad JK, et al. Stability and change in stress, resources, and psychological distress following natural disaster: findings from Hurricane Andrew. Anxiety, Stress and Coping. 1999;12(4):363–96.

21. Galea S, Vlahov D, Tracy M, et al. Hispanic ethnicity and post-traumatic stress disorder after a disaster: evidence from a general population survey after September 11, 2001. Ann Epidemiol. 2004 Sep;14(8):520–31.

22. La Greca A, Silverman WK, Vernberg EM, et al. Symptoms of posttraumatic stress in children after Hurricane Andrew: a prospective study. J Consult Clin Psychol. 1996 Aug;64(4):712–23.

23. Norris FH. Disaster research methods: past progress and future directions. J Trauma Stress. 2006 Apr;19(2):173–84.

24. Solomon SD, Bravo M, Rubio-Stipec M, et al. Effect of family role on response to disaster. J Trauma Stress. 1993 Apr;6(2):255–69.

25. Ibañez GE, Khatchikian N, Buck CA, et al. Qualitative analysis of social support and conflict among Mexican and Mexican-American disaster survivors. J Community Psychol. 2003 31(1):1–23.

26. Kaniasty K, Norris FH. Help-seeking comfort and receiving social support: the role of ethnicity and context of need. Am J Community Psychol. 2000 Aug;28(4):545–81.

27. U.S. Census Bureau. The Hispanic population: census 2000 brief. Washington, DC: U.S. Census Bureau, 2001. Available at http://www.census.gov/.

28. Doty MM, Holmgren AL. Health care disconnect: gaps in coverage and care for minority adults. Findings from the Commonwealth Fund Biennial Health Insurance Survey (2005). Issue Brief (Commonw Fund). 2006 Aug;21:1–12.

29. Flores G, Abreu M, Tomany-Korman SC. Why are Latinos the most uninsured racial/ethnic group of US children? A community-based study of risk factors for and consequences of being an uninsured Latino child. Pediatrics. 2006 Sep;118(3):e730–40.

Chapter 22
Emergency Preparedness: Knowledge and Perceptions of Latin American Immigrants

Olivia Carter-Pokras, PhD
Ruth E. Zambrana, PhD
Sonia E. Mora
Katherine A. Aaby, MPH, RN

There is an increasing recognition of the need to prepare the public for a wide range of hazards, from a terrorism incident to pandemic flu, natural disaster, or other emergency.[1] Although extensive infrastructure for emergency preparedness has been developed since 2001,[2] sparse information is available on the knowledge, attitudes, and views among low-income Latin American immigrants in the United States (U.S.) of what constitutes an emergency and how to respond to one. Racial and ethnic minorities are more vulnerable to disasters than non-Hispanic Whites for many reasons including, but not limited to, socioeconomic differences, language barriers, minority preference for particular information sources (e.g., family), and distrust of governmental authorities.[3-9] A survey of New Yorkers one year after the attacks of September 11th found African Americans and Hispanics, those with less education or income, and those more likely to flee, are also more fearful than their counterparts of future terrorist attacks.[10]

Low-income Latinos are often at particular risk following a disaster since they lack access to financial and material resources to recover their losses and cushion the impact of the disaster. Studies of earthquakes in California suggest that poor Latinos, undocumented immigrants, and monolingual ethnic groups are among the groups that encounter the most problems in acquiring resources and recovering.[11-12] Low-wage Latinos with fragile homes and livelihoods had limited access to post-disaster resources following Hurricane Andrew.[13] This chapter describes the level of public emergency knowledge and perceptions of risks among a group of Latin American immigrants, and their preferred and actual sources of emergency preparedness information (including warning signals).

Barriers to and facilitators of risk communication. Effective risk communication, or the "interactive process of exchange of information and opinion among individuals,

OLIVIA CARTER-POKRAS is an Associate Professor in the Department of Epidemiology and Bio-statistics at the University of Maryland College Park (UMCP). RUTH E. ZAMBRANA is a Professor in the Department of Women's Studies and Director of the Consortium on Race, Gender and Ethnicity at UMCP. SONIA MORA is Program Manager, Latino Health Initiative at the Department of Health and Human Services in Montgomery County, Maryland. KATHERINE AABY is Program Manager, Montgomery County Advanced Practice Center, Public Health Emergency Preparedness and Response Program at the Department of Health and Human Services in Montgomery County.

groups and institutions"[14] requires both knowledge of people from other cultures and respect for their diversity.[15] Cultural groups respond to risk and crisis communication on the basis of their perceptions and ways of thinking, and these differ from group to group.[16] Views are influenced by prior experiences, among other things. However, the lack of extensive research in the crisis and risk communication literature about differing cultural groups reveals a weakness in the potential use of the ten best practices of risk and crisis communication.[17] Latinos, who represent the largest minority group in the U.S., with high rates of recent immigration from Central and South America and residential concentration in large, urban, segregated areas are a population at risk in the event of an emergency. The lack of information on this group's risk perception, combined with barriers relating to language, literacy, and access, place them at a unique disadvantage.

Language barriers are known to be an important contributor to the ineffectiveness of disaster information dissemination and related problems, particularly in multicultural communities.[18-20] Disaster and hazard warnings in the U.S. are often broadcast only in English, leaving many ethnic minorities relatively susceptible to danger.[21-22] In addition to language and literacy issues, unfamiliarity with organizational structures and requirements pose serious access barriers to available public and private resources for many U.S.-born and immigrant Latinos. For vulnerable, low-income Latino immigrants, material and personal loss can be exacerbated by more recent aggressive stances by federal and state governments against the provision of social services.

Community-based organizations and grassroots Latino community members trained as volunteer community health workers or health promoters have successfully provided public health messages to low-income Latino communities. Health promoters serve as connectors between communities and the health care system, providing informal counseling and social support, and ensuring that people obtain the services that they need. Using participatory educational methods and interventions, they help community members put new knowledge into practice.[23] A growing body of literature establishes the unique role of health promoters. The use of health promoters in health intervention programs has been associated with improved health care access, prenatal care, pregnancy and birth outcomes, client health status, health- and screening-related behaviors, appropriate diabetes care, and reduced health care costs.[24-26] Although literature was not found on the role of Latino health promoters (*promotores*) in emergency preparedness, this exploratory study aimed to assess the knowledge level and perceptions of community members and *promotores* on emergency preparedness.

Methods

This qualitative study entailed focus groups to produce data and insights on perceptions on a defined area of interest through a planned discussion in a non-threatening environment; these data and insights might have never been attained without the interaction found in a group.[27-28] Focus groups have been increasingly used in social science and health disparities research to obtain preliminary findings where limited information is available.[29] Focus groups can be a useful tool in public health to assess needs, generate information, and develop plans and programs.[30] A strength of focus groups is that community members become part of and contribute to solutions to community problems as participants. In the area of risk communication, focus groups have been used to gain access to various cultural and social groups, raise unexpected issues for exploration, and identify perceived risks and reactions to those risks.[31-32]

Description of Montgomery County Latino community. In Maryland, Latinos are the fastest growing racial/ethnic minority group, now representing 5.8% of Maryland's and 13.7% of Montgomery County's population.[33] Maryland's Latino population differs from that of the entire United States in that the vast majority are recent immigrants, many of whom are from Central America. Among counties nation-wide, Montgomery County Maryland ranks 16th in the nation for the proportion of foreign-born.[34]

Development of discussion guide. In order to prepare for an expansion of an existing health promoter program to address emergency preparedness, Montgomery County Government (Advanced Practice Center for Public Health Emergency Preparedness and Response Program, and the Latino Health Initiative) and the University of Maryland collaborated to plan and conduct focus groups with low-income immigrant Latinos in Montgomery County, Maryland. All but one member of the research team were bilingual and bicultural.

The Latino Health Initiative's health promoter program is located in Montgomery County (a suburb of Washington D.C.). Established in 2000, Montgomery County Government's Latino Health Initiative (LHI) uses a multifaceted approach to develop new culturally and linguistically specific strategies and model programs, expand and improve health services and programs, improve data collection, and develop partnerships with organizations that focus on Latino health. The Montgomery County Public Health Emergency Preparedness and Response Program is one of eight Advance Practice Centers funded by the Centers for Disease Control and Prevention (CDC) and the National Association of County and City Health Officials (NACCHO) to develop cutting-edge tools and resources for local public health agencies nationwide to prepare for, respond to, and recover from major emergencies.

Guided by previous experience from the Latino Health Initiative's health promoter program and a review of the literature, the Montgomery County Government-University of Maryland research team collaboratively developed a sociodemographic questionnaire and guides for the moderator and note-taker. The purpose of the discussion guide was to elicit information on level of public emergency knowledge, perceptions of risks, and preferred and actual sources of information (including warning signals) among recently migrated Latinos residing in Montgomery County. Participants were asked questions to define an emergency, provide a list of emergencies, and identify signals they recognized as signs of emergencies and the sources of information that they were most likely to rely on in an emergency. To benefit from prior health education experiences of the health promoters, a few additional questions were asked of the participants in the health promoter focus group (one group) but not of the community members (five groups). These additional questions covered whether definitions of an emergency were thought to differ between the health promoters and the broader Latino community, key messages to motivate the community to take immediate action in the event of an emergency and who the messages should be directed to, the best format to educate the community about preparing for an emergency, and suggestions for supporting material for related talks in the community.

Five focus groups with Latino community members and one focus group with lay health promoters (*promotores*) were conducted between May and August 2006. Recruitment aims were 10 participants per group, for a total of 60 individuals. Latino adult participants at least 18 years of age were identified by LHI staff, health promoters, and the staff of three community-based agencies and clinics serving the target population (Camino de La Vida United Methodist Church, Community Ministries of Rockville, and CASA of Maryland).

Forty-five community members participated in five focus groups held at Camino de La Vida United Methodist Church in Gaithersburg, Twinbrook Baptist Church in Rockville, and CASA of Maryland in Wheaton. To solicit information from health promoters with similar background characteristics to those who would be trained in emergency preparedness for the program, one focus group was conducted with six health promoters at the Latino Health Initiative office in Silver Spring, Maryland. Since the purpose of the project was to plan an expansion of an existing health promoter program to include emergency preparedness, the number of focus groups was limited by the timeframe and amount of resources available for the assessment phase. Each participant received a $30 supermarket food certificate and a meal as an incentive for his or her participation. Childcare was provided to encourage participation. Prior approval was requested and obtained from the University of Maryland Institutional Review Board (IRB) and participants signed written consent forms in advance of their participation. The written consent forms in Spanish outlined the purpose of the focus groups: to help develop culturally appropriate materials and programs to meet the emergency preparedness needs of the community.

A Colombian bilingual (English/Spanish) facilitator, experienced in planning and conducting focus groups in Spanish, facilitated the focus groups and performed the initial content analysis of the data. All focus groups were facilitated in Spanish. Each session was tape-recorded to allow for analysis and the preparation of reports of the findings from the discussion. Audiotapes were destroyed following analysis per IRB-approved protocol. A note taker, fluent in Spanish, was trained to unobtrusively observe and take written notes using a note-taker's guide to recording participants' comments, as well as group dynamics and non-verbal communication (expressions, gestures, movements) that emphasized or supported points being made.

Notes and audiotapes were reviewed for each focus group and common themes mentioned across each focus group were identified using manual review in the original language. Audiotapes were transcribed and translated into English. Two bilingual/bicultural investigators reviewed the data and independently verified the themes. For purposes of accuracy, and to capture the cultural meaning of the response, we provide the original Spanish used by participants for key terms and concepts that are not easily translated into English. While data from each of the focus groups were analyzed separately, no significant differences emerged among the six groups with respect to thematic content or background. The findings are therefore presented as a summary of all groups.

Results

A total of 51 individuals participated in 6 focus groups: 30 women and 15 men in 5 focus groups of community members, and 6 women in a focus group of *promotoras*. Community participants came from 13 Latin American countries, including the Dominican Republic (1), Mexico (4), Central America [El Salvador (14), Guatemala (4), Honduras (1), Nicaragua (1), Panama (1)], and South America [Bolivia (5), Chile (1), Colombia (3), Ecuador (4), Peru (10), Venezuela (1)]. As shown in Table 1, 64.7% of participants had immigrated during the previous 5 years. Approximately half (52.9%) of the participants were employed, with an additional 17.6% working independently. Forty-three percent of participants had not completed high school in their country of origin or the U.S.

Perceptions of an emergency situation. One set of questions concerned perceptions of an *emergency situation*, definition of *an emergency*, and perceived emergencies in the United States. When the groups were asked, "When you think of an emergency situation, what situation(s) come to mind?" participants mentioned a wide variety of situations. These included natural disasters (earthquakes/tremors, hurricanes, snowstorms) as well as in-home fires, gangs (*maras*), terrorism, traffic accidents, and illnesses (e.g., heart attacks, flu). In four of the six groups, the majority of participants related emergency situations and stories that were common in their countries of origin or other parts of the U.S. where they had lived (e.g., earthquakes, hurricanes), although few had lived through one of these situations.

Participants had difficulty defining *emergency*, most often describing situations that put people at risk. One individual described an emergency as:

Anything that is happening that you don't have control over and that puts you in danger [*Cualquier cosa que este pasando que uno no tiene control y lo pone en peligro*]

Another participant suggested the following definition:

A silent monster that when it attacks you don't know it [*Un monstruo silencioso . . . cuando te ataca no lo sabes*]

Other terms used for *emergency* included: *alert, red alert, precaution, panic, chaos*, and *confusion*.

When participants were asked about emergency situations they believed we were at highest risk of encountering in the United States, and in the area, participants in four groups mentioned terrorism, making comments such as the following:

I know that bioterrorism is a problem, but I don't know very much about it [*Se que bioterrorism es un problema, pero no se mucho de eso*]

The terrorism that happened in New York and here in Washington [*El terrorismo que paso en Nueva York y aqui en Washington*]

Yes . . . I see a lot on TV . . . the terrorist danger [*Sí . . . veo mucho en la TV sobre el peligro de los terroristas*]

Table 1.

SOCIODEMOGRAPHIC CHARACTERISTICS OF PARTICIPANTS

Characteristic	%	(n)
Gender		
Male	29.4	(15)
Female	70.6	(36)
Country of origin		
Dominican Republic	2.0	(1)
Mexico	7.8	(4)
Central America	41.2	(21)
South America	47.1	(24)
N/A	2.0	(1)
Age range (years)		
18 to 25	15.7	(8)
26 to 35	19.6	(10)
36 to 45	33.3	(17)
46 to 55	19.6	(10)
56 to 65	11.8	(6)
Marital status		
Never married	27.5	(14)
Married or living with partner	54.9	(28)
Separated or divorced	17.6	(9)
Employment		
Employed	52.9	(27)
Working independently	17.6	(9)
Unemployed or unable to work	13.7	(7)
Housemate or student	15.7	(8)
Salary/week		
Less than $350	43.1	(22)
More than $350	33.3	(17)
Don't know or N/A	23.5	(12)
Formal schooling		
Less than high school	43.2	(22)
High school graduate	41.2	(21)
Technical school	7.8	(4)
Student	2.0	(1)
N/A	5.9	(3)
Years in U.S.		
Less than 1	19.6	(10)
1–3	13.7	(7)
3–5	31.4	(16)
6–10	19.6	(10)
More than 10	7.8	(4)
N/A	7.8	(4)

Other emergency situations that participants believed that we are at highest risk for in the U.S. included: bioterrorism (e.g., anthrax), avian virus (*virus de los pajaros, epidemia de pollo*), in-home fires and accidents (at work, in the car, personal), war, social risks such as gangs, natural disasters (e.g., no water), and the heat. Two focus groups were held in the late afternoon of a 100-degree day in rooms where the air conditioning systems were not working properly. Hence, many of the comments by the participants were framed around and referred to ambient heat as an emergency.

Participants, without exception, mentioned current immigration issues and the uncertain environment in this respect as representing an emergency situation and creating a sense of personal risk:

> I think that the problem of our legal status is a big emergency [*Creo que el problema de nuestro estatus legal es una emergencia muy grande*]

> We are frightened because we don't know what 's going to happen (with immigration) . . . this is an emergency [*Estamos asustados porque no sabemos lo que va a pasar (con imigracion)*]

> Some people don't even want to go out (of their house) [*Hay gente que no quiere salir (de su casa)*]

Crime, personal insecurity, gangs ("That gang thing has gotten uncontrollable and it's a real problem for all of us" [*Eso de las maras esta incontrollable y es un problema para todos*]); home/traffic accidents; home fires, environmental problems ("Pollution is a problem . . . in the air and water" [*La contaminacion es un problema en el agua y el aire*]) and snipers ("The sniper situation a few years ago created a real problem and emergency") were viewed as emergency risks for the area where they lived. The health promoters viewed emergency risks similarly:

> Yes, the people perceive emergency situations the same, but the difference is that the community is less informed . . . there's no help from the people above . . . the government [*Si la gente percibe las situaciones de emergencia igual, pero la diferencia es que no estan bien informados . . . no hay ayuda de la gente arriba del gobierno*]

> The problem is that they don't know how to express what they feel . . . they keep quiet. [*El problema es que no saben expresar lo que sienten . . . se quedan callados*]

What constitutes an emergency signal and response plan. Emergency signals that participants recognized and reported included alarms (smoke detectors, alarms at work); phone calls from family members or friends; police, ambulance or fire engine sirens; television and radio announcements; people running ("If people are running . . . each person is on their own" [*Si hay gente corriendo . . . salvase el que pueda*]); and church bells.

The vast majority of participants had not received information on emergency preparation.

We are not prepared, people don't think that it can happen from one moment to the other [*No estamos preparados, la gente no piensa en que puede pasar de un momento a otro*]

Information is lacking . . . we don't know anything. [*Hace falta información . . . no sabemos nada*]

Only four participants had an emergency plan, and those were incomplete ("I've told my kids that if something ever happened, we should meet in a central location . . . We haven't decided where"). Approximately half of parents with school-age children (about 80% of participants) had heard about an emergency plan in their children's schools from their children, but the vast majority was unable to describe it specifically:

I know that they are supposed to stay in the school if something happens, but I really don't know what else to do.

The information is not shared with the parents . . . the kids know, but they [the schools] don't tell us anything.

When asked why people don't have a plan, much of the discussion revolved around the lack of information or the fact that people were too busy working to make those types of plans. A general theme is that people wait until something happens to act ("The community reacts when it has already happened" [*La comunidad reacciona una vez les pasa*]). Some felt that there was no way to prepare for an emergency [*No hay forma de preparar*] and used this popular Hispanic saying: ". . . during an emergency there is no Saint Lucia that is worth anything" [*. . . durante una emergencia no hay Santa Lucia que valga*].

There was some confusion regarding the questions: "What steps would you take if you heard an emergency warning? What would be the first thing that you would do? Why?" and "How would you prepare to respond to an emergency situation? How would you prepare your family?" When specific examples of emergencies (snowstorm or terrorist attack) were provided by the facilitators, participants mentioned basic subsistence items, such as food, water, and blankets, as well as working channels of communication ("The first thing that I would do is make sure my cell phone and TV cable are working"), being calm and trusting God ("In a disaster everyone runs . . . they are not prepared because they haven't lived it before . . . you have to be calm and trust God"), and getting and disseminating information ("Investigate what type of an emergency it is and let the neighbors know").

Motivation to plan for an emergency and sources of information. Factors that would motivate the participants to prepare for an emergency and seek information included: *to stay alive, for my family, to be informed so we could help others,* and *feeling secure with knowledge.* The notion that it is difficult to get the community to think ahead of time about emergencies and planning was also expressed:

Latinos are lazy to read informational bulletins and go to meetings . . . sometimes the school holds the meetings to talk about things like this, but very few of us show up

. . . and they wait until it happens to react. [*Los latinos tienen pereza de leer boletines informativos . . . ir a reuniones . . . a veces las escuelas hacen reuniones pero pocos estamos ahí . . . esperan que les pase para reaccionar*]

Promotoras agreed that the focus of any educational effort on emergency preparedness in the community should be directed at all of the family, and stressed that it is important that the information provided be consistent.

As shown in Box 1, reported sources that are trusted to provide information on emergencies included firemen and police; the Red Cross; charismatic individuals who are well trained; doctors; community leaders; television and radio announcers; and Spanish-language newspapers. (It should perhaps be noted, however, that one participant remarked, "No one reads now a days . . . it's easiest to get information on TV or radio [when you're working].") The groups were unanimous in saying that whoever the person was, he or she should be well informed, should be Latino, and should speak Spanish. Participants noted that "Univisión and Telemundo don't transmit signs of alert" [. . . *no transmiten señales de alerta*], and that local cable television shows may not be accessible. The forms in which participants wanted to receive information included courses or seminars; television or radio programs; pamphlets, flyers, or manuals; and through simulations or practice ("We need to unite the theory with the practice").

There was general agreement that governmental entities are trusted sources of information ("If it's not the government . . . who else?" [*Si no es el gobierno . . . quien mas?*]), but a few participants expressed concern about how ready the government is to deal with an emergency ("We saw what happened in New Orleans . . . it's all the same"). Roles that participants said the government could play include: providing courses and training in churches, schools and work; making economic resources available; having doctors and hospitals ready; alerting the community; and orienting the community to what to do during different types of emergencies. *Promotoras* also saw a role that they could play by providing talks (*charlas*) in the community, but they emphasized that they must be well trained on how to educate the community for emergencies and how to prepare, and also that they need good support materials (such as manuals, videos, and handouts to distribute to the community).

Messages that participants said could be used to communicate with the Latino community included: be calm (*calma, calma, calma*), be alert (*estén atentos*), be united (*estén unidos*), and act (*actuar*), as well as messages reminding people to keep important telephone numbers handy and to prepare. *Promotoras* added the following messages: "Do you know how to distinguish emergencies?" [*Sabes distinguir una emergencia?*], "Let's reduce the risk . . . prepare yourself for an emergency" [*Reduzcamos el riesgo . . . prepárate para una emergencia*]. Materials that the *promotoras* suggested could be used when giving a talk in the community included pencils, bags with slogans on the side, flashlights, Band-aids, and other small gifts.

Discussion

This exploratory study reveals a consistent theme among the participants of a significant need to increase the Latino community's knowledge and preparedness with regard to

Box 1.

SOURCES OF INFORMATION AND PREFERENCES FOR RECEIPT OF EMERGENCY PREPAREDNESS INFORMATION

Reported most trusted sources of information (in rank order)
1. Firemen and police
2. Red Cross
3. Some one who is well trained with charisma
4. Doctors
5. Community leaders
6. TV and radio
7. Spanish-language newspapers

Reported preferences for receiving information (in rank order)
1. Courses or seminars
2. TV or radio programs
3. Pamphlets, flyers or manuals
4. Participating in simulations or practice

Perceptions of role government can play in preparing Latino community (in rank order)
1. Provide courses and training (e.g., churches, schools, work)
2. Make economic resources available
3. Have the doctors and hospitals ready
4. Alert the community
5. Orient the community on what to do

Reported messages to communicate to the Latino community
- Be calm (*calma*)
- Be alert (*esten atentos*)
- Be united (*esten unidos*)
- Act (*actuar*)
- Keep important telephone numbers handy and prepare

emergencies, including among community-based health promoters who serve as critical connectors to resources and information. Consistent with recent general population surveys,[35-36] few focus group participants had received information on emergency preparedness, and most did not have emergency plans. The mention of terrorism, anthrax, and avian virus as emergency situations that might arise in the U.S., suggests that participants are aware of current issues for which the federal government has invested resources to raise awareness. (For example, the federal government website, www.ready.gov, now has Spanish language materials and public service announcements.) In addition, the Washington D.C. area has directly experienced both anthrax and terrorism emergency situations.[37-38]

However, the matter of relative risk in comparison with other priority issues faced by the community should be considered. Additionally, although the focus of our research was on recent Latino immigrants residing in Montgomery County Maryland, the Latino community in the Washington D.C. metropolitan area is diverse in terms of birthplace/generation, national origin, English language ability, social class, race, and previous experience with natural disasters. These differences may matter a great deal for communication during emergencies. Prior experiences with emergencies influence one's response to a new one. In studies of responses to the Los Angeles earthquake, Bolin found that Mexican immigrants who experienced the Mexico city earthquake responded very differently from those without experience, and undocumented residents responded very differently from how U.S. citizens responded.[11-12]

A key new finding from our focus groups is that the topic of current immigration issues was clearly and significantly identified as an emergency by the participants and was perceived as a risk for the Latino community. Increased anti-immigrant sentiment and efforts to restrict immigrant access to driver's licenses, educational opportunities, health care, and other services have had ripple effects throughout the Latino community.[39-41]

Participants noted the need to identify a credible spokesperson to deliver a consistent and unified message around emergencies and preparedness. They consistently identified first responders (e.g., police, firefighters, ambulance, Red Cross) as trusted sources of information. There is increasing recognition of the need to have this cadre of workers fully trained (among other things, by including an adequate number of culturally competent, fluent Spanish-speakers in their ranks) to respond to the needs of the Latino community.[42]

Establishing interconnected networks of public health workers and other first response organizations is an important goal of emergency preparedness. Emergency personnel also must be informed of the fears of immigrants who do not have legal residence in the U.S., since the perception of immigration concerns as an emergency has important implications not only for emergency preparedness, but also for response, relief, and recovery. One study reported that, following Hurricane Katrina, undocumented immigrants avoided recovery assistance for fear of deportation, and some eligible Latinos who were legal residents did not receive correct information from Federal Emergency Management Agency (FEMA) regarding housing assistance due to confusion regarding eligibility.[9] In their testimony to Congress following Hurricane Katrina, Oxfam America and the Mississippi Immigrants Rights Alliance noted the importance of building trust prior to a disaster, maintaining that trust in the delivery of emergency services, knowing the communities, and developing plans from that knowledge.[43] The National Council of La Raza recommends that both public and private sectors do what is necessary to ensure that trained professional relief workers, volunteers from diverse communities, and managers are pre-positioned for the next disaster deployment.[9] In addition to receiving Latino-focused training, first responders should have an active and continuing role in the development and delivery of educational and informational messages to the community. These messages can be included in Spanish-language announcements on television and radio programs that low-income Latinos hear.

Limitations of these findings include their restriction to one geographic area, self-selection of the group of respondents (that may lead us to over-estimate or under-estimate the true level of emergency preparedness in the broader Latino community), and an inability to assess how participants would respond in an actual emergency. However, these data confirm the lack of emergency preparedness in a segment of the Latino population and suggest that additional inquiry by documenting the level of emergency preparedness among other Latino groups is warranted.

Implications and conclusions. The study results are being used to guide the design and development of specific emergency preparedness education concepts and messages (including terminology), and strategies to be incorporated into a culturally and linguistically appropriate training curriculum for health promoters. The information is also being used to guide the development of material(s) to support the health promoters' outreach and education efforts. Prior experience with *promotores* has demonstrated that simple, low-literacy materials focusing on a limited number of key messages are an effective means of delivering information to the target population by *promotores*.

Although not specifically mentioned as a credible source of information on public emergencies by community member participants, *promotores* have served as effective vehicles for health education in Montgomery County on other topics. Furthermore, a Florida study found that Latino homeowners are more likely than non-Latino homeowners to prefer to use friends and family as sources of disaster preparation information.[44] Latinos are also more likely than non-Latino Whites to use social networks and neighborhood meetings as communication channels for disaster and hazard information.[6,8,45] Grass-roots mobilization interventions by *promotores* and others can therefore complement television and radio to deliver messages. Once fully trained, *promotores* can conduct educational sessions at community-based organizations, churches, place of employment, and other sites. *Promotores* can organize community response teams to conduct simulations of emergencies, to review appropriate/inappropriate responses, and to emphasize practical steps for preparedness.

There is currently a pool of over 100 trained volunteer Latino health promoters providing effective education and outreach to the Latino population of Montgomery County in a wide range of areas (e.g., access to care, cancer screening services, pedestrian safety, HIV prevention and testing, tobacco-use prevention). These health promoters represent an important resource that can be developed to contribute to the overall, long-term goal of Montgomery County's public health emergency preparedness program. These data demonstrate the need to increase knowledge among Latinos of public health emergency threats and appropriate responses to them, knowledge of planning and preparing for public health emergencies (e.g., emergency preparedness kits, shelter-in-place [small interior room, with few or no windows to take refuge]). Thus, community-based participatory approaches can be effectively executed to develop culturally and linguistically appropriate emergency preparedness educational interventions, and to strengthen the existing infrastructure.

Developers of clear, prioritized messages regarding emergencies and emergency preparedness for the Latino community should recognize that prior experiences with emergencies in countries of origin may affect emergency preparation and responses of

Latino immigrants. Infrastructure development for emergencies is in its preliminary stages in many communities throughout the U.S. Thus, augmenting the capacity of health response workers is imperative and in the Latino community it would be wise to capitalize on the cadre of Spanish-speaking Latino professional relief workers, health promoters, and managers who are committed and ready to develop the knowledge and skills in emergency preparedness.

Acknowledgments

This research was supported by Cooperative Agreement Number U50/CCU302718 from the Centers for Disease Control and Prevention (CDC) to the National Association of County and City Health Officials (NACCHO). Its contents are solely the responsibility of the authors and do not necessarily represent the views of the CDC or the NACCHO.

Appendix A—Questions Used to Guide Focus Group Discussion

1. Perceptions

a. When you think about an emergency situation, what situation(s) comes to mind?
b. How would you define the word emergency? What other name or term would you use for an emergency?
c. In your country of origin, are emergency situations known by another name/term? Which?
d. What are the emergency situations that you believe we are at highest risk for in this country [the US]? How about in the area where you live? Why?
e. Of these situations which one(s) do you consider yourself personally at risk for?

For Promoters:

a. Do you believe that the Latino community sees (perceives) emergency situations the same way you do? Why? Why not?

2. Knowledge

a. How would you know that you are in an emergency situation?
b. Are you aware of any alert system that warns us that we are in danger of an emergency? Which one? What does it say?
c. Are you aware of any specific plans for emergencies in your children's school? What does it consist of?
d. Have any of you ever received information on how to prepare for an emergency? *[If someone has, ask the following:]* From where/whom? What did it say? What action did you take as a consequence of having received the information?

3. Preparation

a. Which steps would you take if you heard an emergency warning? What would be the first thing that you would do? Why?
b. How would prepare to respond to an emergency situation? How would you prepare your family?

c. Do you have a specific plan in case of an emergency? What does it consist of? *[If they don't, ask:]* Why not?

d. What would motivate you to prepare for an emergency and seek information on what to do during an emergency?

e. What do you think Latinos can do to become better informed about preparing for an emergency?

For Promoters:

a. Which message or messages would you use to motivate the community to take immediate action in case of an emergency? To whom should the message be directed? (parents, children, family) Why?

4. Trusted Sources and Information

a. Whom would you trust to talk to you about emergencies?

b. What source of information do you think are the most credible? Why?

c. How or in what form would you prefer to learn more about preparing for and handling an emergency? Why?

d. What do you think should be the role of governmental organizations in helping prepare for and handling an emergency? Would you trust governmental organizations?

e. If we wanted to share with the Latino community information on preparing for an emergency, what would the information consist of? What would be the best way to communicate the information?

f. What messages would you communicate to the community about preparing for an emergency?

For Promoters:

a. Based on your experience, which is the best form to teach to the community about preparing for an emergency? What would be the most effective message(s) to teach the community what to do in case of an emergency?

b. If you were to give a talk (charla) in the community, and were to use materials to support you, what materials do you believe would be most effective in the community? What characteristics would the materials have that you would consider most effective?

Is there anything else you would like to share?

Notes

1. United States Government Accountability Office. Hurricane Katrina: GAO's preliminary observations regarding preparedness, response, and recovery. Statement of David M. Walker, Comptroller General of the United States. Testimony before the Senate Homeland Security and Governmental Affairs Committee. (GAO-06-442T.) Washington, DC: Government Accountability Office, 2006. Available at http://www.gao.gov/.

2. Geberding JL. Protecting health—the new research imperative. JAMA. 2005 Sep 21; 294(11):1403–6.

3. Kasperson RE, Golding D, Tuler S. Social distrust as a factor in sitting hazardous facilities and communication risks. J Soc Issues. 1992;48:161–87.

4. Perry HS, Lindell MK. The effects of ethnicity on decision-making. Int J Mass Emerg Disasters. 1991;9(1):47–68.

5. Phillips BD. Cultural diversity in disasters: sheltering, housing, and long term recovery. Int J Mass Emerg Disasters. 1993;11(1):99–100.

6. Perry RW, Mushkatel AH. Minority citizens in disaster. Athens, GA: University of Georgia Press, 1986.

7. Vaughn E. The significance of socioeconomics and ethnic diversity for the risk communication process. Risk Anal. 1995;15(2):169–80.

8. Phillips BD, Ephraim M. Living in the aftermath: blaming process in the Loma Prieta earthquake. (Working Paper no. 80.) Boulder, CO: University of Colorado, IBS, Natural Hazards Research and Applications Information Center, 1992.

9. Muniz B. In the eye of the storm: how the government and private response to Hurricane Katrina failed Latinos. Washington, DC: National Council of La Raza, 2006. Available at http://www.nclr.org/.

10. Boscarino JA, Figley CR, Adams RE. Fear of terrorism in New York after the September 11 terrorist attacks: implications for emergency mental health and preparedness. Int J Emerg Mental Health. 2003 Fall;5(4):199–209.

11. Bolin R, Stanford L. The Northridge earthquake: community-based approaches to unmet recovery needs. Disasters. 1998 Mar;22(1):21–38.

12. Bolin R. The Northridge earthquake: vulnerability and disaster. New York: Routledge, 1998.

13. Morrow BH, Peacock WG. Disasters and social change: Hurricane Andrew and the reshaping of Miami? In: Peacock WG, Morrow BH, Gladwin H, eds. Hurricane Andrew: ethnicity, gender and the sociology of disasters. New York: Routledge, 1997; 226–42.

14. Committee on Risk Perception and Communication, National Research Council. Improving risk communication. Washington, DC: National Academies Press, 1989.

15. Samovar LA, Porter RE, McDaniel ER. Communication between cultures. Wadsworth Publishing, 2006.

16. Lindell MK, Perry RW. Communicating environmental risk in multiethnic communities. Thousand Oaks, CA: Sage, 2004.

17. Seeger MW. Best practices in risk and crisis communication: an expert panel process. J Appl Commun Res. 2006 Aug;34(3):232–44.

18. Fothergill A, Maestas EG, Darlington JD. Race, ethnicity and disasters in the United States: a review of the literature. Disasters. 1999 Jun;23(2):156–73.

19. Peacock WG, Girard C. Ethnic and racial inequalities in hurricane damage and insurance settlements. In: Peacock WG, Morrow BH, Gladwin H, eds. Hurricane Andrew: ethnicity, gender and the sociology of disasters. New York: Routledge, 2000.

20. Perry RW, Nelson L. Ethnicity and hazard information dissemination. Environ Manage. 1991 Jul;15(4):581–7.

21. Aguirre BE. The lack of warnings before Saragosa tornado. Int J Mass Emerg Disasters. 1988 Mar;6(1):65–74.

22. Lindell MK, Perry RW, Greene MR. Race and disaster warning response. Seattle, WA: Battelle Human Affairs Research Centers, 1980.

23. Wiggins N, Barbon A. Core roles and competencies of community health advisors. In: Rosenthal EL, Wiggins N, Brownstein JN, et al. Final report of the National Community Health Advisory Study: weaving the future. Tucson, AZ: University of Arizona Press, 1998.

24. Community Health Worker and Promotora de Salud Workgroup, CDC Division of Diabetes Translation. Community health workers/promotores de salud: critical connection in communities. Atlanta, GA: Centers for Disease Control and Prevention, 2003.

25. Earp JA, Eng E, O'Malley MS, et al. Increasing use of mammography among older, rural African American women: results from a community trial. Am J Public Health. 2002 Apr;92(4):646–54.

26. Rosenbach M, Ellwood M, Czajka J, et al. Implementation of the State Children's Health Insurance Program: synthesis of state evaluations. Background for the report to Congress. Cambridge, MA: Mathematica Policy Research Inc., 2003;123–7.

27. Morgan DL. Focus groups in qualitative research. Newbury Park, CA: Sage, 1988; 12.

28. Krueger RA. Focus groups: a practical guide for applied research. Newbury Park, CA: Sage, 1988;18.

29. Ruff CC, Alexander IM, McKie C. The use of focus group methodology in health disparities research. Nurs Outlook. 2005 May–Jun;53(3):134–40.

30. Marshall C, Rossman GB, Designing qualitative research, 3d ed. Thousand Oaks, CA: Sage Publications, 1999;115.

31. Blanchard JC, Haywood Y, Stein BD, et al. In their own words: lessons learned from those exposed to anthrax. Am J Public Health. 2005 Mar;95(3):489–95.

32. McGough M, Frank LL, Tipton S, et al. Communicating the risks of bioterrorism and other emergencies in a diverse society: a case study of special populations in North Dakota. Biosecur Bioterror. 2005;3(3):235–45.

33. U.S. Census Bureau. 2005 American Community Survey. Selected social characteristics. Washington, DC: U.S. Census Bureau, 2006.

34. U.S. Census Bureau. Table 2: County ranking—percent of population that is foreign born. Washington, DC: U.S. Census Bureau, 2003 Sep. Available at http://www.census.gov/.

35. National Center for Disaster Preparedness. Where the American public stands on terrorism, security and disaster preparedness: five-years after September 11, one-year after Hurricane Katrina. New York: Columbia University, 2006 Sep. Available at http://www.ncdp.mailman.columbia.edu/.

36. JKV Research, LLC. Washington County Community Health & Emergency Preparedness Survey. Fond du Lac, WI: Quad Counties Public Health Consortium, 2006. Available at http://www.co.washington.wi.us/.

37. Centers for Disease Control and Prevention (CDC). Update: Investigation of bioterrorism-related anthrax and interim guidelines for exposure management and antimicrobial therapy, October 2001. MMWR. 2001 Oct 26;50(42):909–19.

38. National Commission on Terrorist Attacks Upon the United States. The 9/11 Commission report: final report of the National Commission on Terrorist Attacks Upon the United States. Washington, DC: Government Printing Office, 2004.

39. Donato KM, Massey DS, Wagner B. The chilling effect: public service usage by Mexican migrants to the United States. Presented at: Annual Meeting of the Population

Association of America, Los Angeles (CA), Jan 2006. Available at http://paa2006 .princeton.edu/.

40. Pupovac J. Local immigration measures raise a host of new concerns. The New Standard. 2006 Oct 24. Available at http://newstandardnews.net/.

41. Anti-defamation League (ADL). The Ku Klux Klan today. Washington, DC: ADL, 2007. Available at http://www.adl.org/.

42. Dell'Orto G. First responders learning Spanish. Associated Press. 2006 Nov 27. Available at https://www.mmrs.fema.gov/.

43. Chandler B, Gamboa G. Hurricane Katrina response and immigrants. Written testimony for the record to the Select Bipartisan Committee to Investigate the Preparation for and Response to Hurricane Katrina. Boston, MA: Oxfam America, 2006 Dec 6. Available at http://www.oxfamamerica.org/.

44. Peguero AA. Latino disaster vulnerability: the dissemination of hurricane mitigation information among Florida's homeowners. Hisp J Behav Sci. 2006;28(1):5–22.

45. Blanchard-Boehm D. Risk communication in southern California: ethnic and gender response to 1995 revised, upgraded earthquake probabilities. Research report. Boulder, CO: University of Colorado, Natural Hazards Research Center, 1997.

Chapter 23
The Resuscitation of a New Orleans Substance Abuse Treatment Agency after Hurricane Katrina

Paul J. Toriello, RhD
Patricia Morse, PhD
Edward V. Morse, PhD
Patricia Kissinger, PhD
Else Pedersen-Wasson, BA

On August 28th, 2005, Hurricane Katrina (Katrina) closed the entire New Orleans substance abuse treatment system, leaving people in need of treatment, including those in the treatment already, without services. Since then, the New Orleans substance abuse treatment system has re-opened in a flurry, with staff members attempting to establish order with what resources exist.[1] The period of reconstruction after Katrina presents an opportunity to examine how substance abuse treatment agencies have begun to operate in new ways. This report describes Katrina's impact on the clinical operations of the largest residential substance abuse treatment facility in New Orleans. Specifically, our intent is to briefly delineate how this facility operated clinically before Katrina, and how the concepts of therapeutic community were introduced into this facility to mitigate the stressors associated with a post-Katrina environment.

Previous disaster research. Post-disaster research suggests that Katrina may have had major effects on people in New Orleans with substance abuse problems.[2-5] As a result, treatment agencies may have to modify operations and resource allocation to accommodate a post-Katrina clientele with significant potential for increased impairment that may necessitate more intensive and longer treatment. For example, research has shown that providing health care in a post-disaster environment may lead to (a) a reduction in staffs' ability to address clients' post-disaster treatment needs, as well as (b) an increase in staffs' own post-traumatic stress symptoms.[6-7] Thus, substance abuse agencies may see an increase in staff taking sick leave,[2] physical and/or emotional exhaustion and low morale,[8] as well as regression to less effective intervention techniques.[9] During recovery from Katrina, New Orleans' substance abuse agencies face the unprecedented task of rebuilding a treatment system and treating a potentially more severely impaired and chronic clientele with potentially unstable staff.

PAUL TORIELLO *is an Assistant Professor of Rehabilitations Studies at East Carolina University.* PATRICIA MORSE *and* EDWARD MORSE *are Associate Professors of Clinical Psychiatry at Louisiana State University Health Sciences Center.* PATRICIA KISSINGER *is a Professor of Epidemiology at Tulane University.* ELSE PEDERSEN-WASSON *is the Associate Executive Director of the Bridge House Corporation.*

Bridge House: Pre-Katrina. Bridge House, Inc. is Louisiana's largest residential substance abuse treatment program. Bridge House has treated New Orleans's indigent residents with substance abuse problems since 1957. Bridge House is a not-for-profit (501.c.3) organization that, prior to Katrina, employed 80 staff members and had the capacity to treat 130 adult men. Approximately 75% of Bridge House funding was generated through in-house businesses (e.g., used car sales, thrift stores). Six years ago, Bridge House operated from a traditional treatment philosophy where counselors routinely used a confrontational approach by pressuring clients to accept themselves as *alcoholics/addicts*. If clients did not commit to one year of treatment and remain abstinent from substance use, they would receive ultimatums from counselors that led to the withdrawal of services for non-compliance. This clinical approach was not idiosyncratic to Bridge House, but representative of traditional substance abuse treatment.[10-11]

Bridge House also operated from a loose organizational structure; it lacked the infrastructure and characteristics that organizational research has shown to be key to effective and sustained organizational change.[8] Improvement efforts were unstructured and haphazard. Moreover, counselors and clients were minimally involved in the improvement process, and they typically viewed improvement efforts as a separate function within the organization. Thus, organizational improvement efforts were fragmented and their effects were unclear and difficult to sustain.

However, by August 2005, Bridge House was an example of an improving organization. The transition began in 2000 when Bridge House was awarded a grant to support the implementation of an evidence-based relapse prevention treatment curriculum. The model became the core treatment curriculum at Bridge House. Subsequently, Bridge House participated in a Center for Substance Abuse Treatment project. This project facilitated the adoption of motivational interviewing, an evidence-based counseling style.[10] Motivational interviewing (MI) replaced the traditional confrontational approach as the core clinical style at Bridge House. Bridge House also implemented a client database including the Drug Evaluation Network System software.[12] Finally, for the past three years, Bridge House has participated in the national Network for the Improvement of Addiction Treatment, an alliance of 40 drug abuse treatment programs using a Rapid Cycle Change model to increase early treatment retention and admissions/utilization, as well as to reduce treatment wait-time and no-shows.[13]

These changes at Bridge House were not singular events but components of a gradual shift toward organizational operations based on continuous quality improvement technology. However, on August 28th, 2005, Katrina put a halt to this development. The Bridge House facilities sustained wind and water damage; moreover, the Bridge House businesses (used car lots, multiple thrift stores) were flooded, looted, and vandalized.

Bridge House: Post-Katrina. During the six weeks following Katrina, Bridge House existed without electricity, gas, water, or sewage service. A majority of the buildings constituting the Bridge House campus had sustained significant hurricane-related damage. There were no clients and the staff had dropped from 80 to 3 people. In early October 2005, Bridge House administrators met with external consultants to discuss whether Bridge House could be resuscitated. The consultants proposed that the current Bridge House situation might be an appropriate time to reassess the strengths and weaknesses of the Bridge House program and might present an opportunity to introduce a major change into the organization's structure. After a discussion of this proposal, the program director was asked to consider allowing the future post-Katrina clients to take primary responsibility for their own self-governance by having them develop their own formally constituted therapeutic community.

Eventually, Bridge House administrators decided to reopen, believing that the benefits to be derived from making the client component of the organization into a semi-autonomous subsystem, while relatively simple, would significantly enhance overall Bridge House treatment. For example, clients would be led to assume significant responsibility for supervision of their own actions and the behaviors of the group as a whole. Second, clients would have the opportunity through social interaction to develop their self-esteem and self-efficacy. As a result, the behaviors of clients, both open and clandestine, would be monitored much more closely. The expectation was that such dynamics would facilitate a cohesive community where clients operate with respect for self and others, as well a sense of responsibility for the recovery of self and others. Bridge House administrators believed a strong sense of community was critical to helping clients cope with the additional stressors of receiving treatment in a post-Katrina environment.

To work, the seed ideas spelling out the desired characteristics of a client community were initially provided to a small number of clients, who formed the nucleus of the community group. These clients were then asked to formulate a set of community policies and procedures to cover all major categories of community and individual client interactions. The materials developed were then assembled into a logical sequence of topics, codified, and made into a handbook. The clients were then instructed to meet together each day and work out the details of their community. This enabled the nascent community's social capital to accumulate slowly enough that it was molded and reshaped under the watchful eyes of both the clinical staff and the consultants. The clinical staff and consultants modeled their interactions with the clients after the tenets of the aforementioned motivational interviewing (MI).

The acceptance of the therapeutic community model by Bridge House was eased by the fact that the administration had been working over the previous three years to introduce changes using the Rapid Cycle Change (RCC) model techniques to improve various organizational and clinical processes and outcomes. The RCC model is based on five actions that research has shown to distinguish organizations that successfully change and improve versus those that do not: (a) select key problems, (b) involve the client, (c) involve outside experts, (d) use rapid cycle testing, and (e) pick a powerful change leader.[13]

The first step for an agency using the RCC model to guide their improvement involves answering the following question: *What are we trying to accomplish?* In this case, the answer was *implementation of a therapeutic community*. From this point, agency clients and staff were integrally involved in planning, implementing, and evaluating the progress of the therapeutic community. This involvement included the community meetings mentioned above, as well as focus groups facilitated by clinicians. Regular solicitation of feedback from key stakeholders provided the community leaders with valuable information that was used to adjust community policy and procedures. Additionally, external consultants helped the community's progress by identifying ways to customize the community policy and procedures optimally. When appropriate, the external consultants also provided technical assistance and training to support the identified changes. The importance of involving outside experts was to learn from their successes and failures. Outside experts were often able to take a comprehensive view of the situation, a perspective that fostered fresh ideas for community improvement within a post-Katrina environment. Changes to community policy and procedures identified through the above process were implemented in a rapid cycle (2 to 4 four weeks). Thus, the community used rapid cycle testing as long as the changes were resulting in desired outcomes (e.g., fewer rule infractions, increased group attendance). Finally, at the heart of the RCC model is the *change leader*. A change leader is a person who will serve as a champion or "cheerleader" for a programmatic change or set of changes. A change leader, in this case the clients leading the community, facilitated the RCC process from a position of pro-social influence and respect within the client community.

This process began on November 16th, 2005 when Bridge House reopened its doors to clients. During the first two weeks, the average daily census counted five clients. All clients followed the same daily routine, rising at 6:00 am, eating, engaging in silent meditation, and then being transported to a Bridge House retail outlet where they worked for eight hours a day sorting inventory, stocking shelves, and/or working sales. Upon returning each evening, clients ate dinner and then held a one-hour community meeting, first with the consultants and clinicians present. The consultants shared with the clients the basic attributes of what a client-based therapeutic community would look like structurally, and how it would function on a day-to-day basis. The clients were provided model handbooks and asked to develop a handbook of policy and procedures that they would use to govern their community. Since then, clients have continued with the community development process; Bridge House has been steadily admitting clients since November 2005.

Bridge House: Today. Currently, Bridge House has the capacity to treat 75 adult men at one time. Post-Katrina Bridge clients who also attended Bridge House programming prior to Katrina have consistently stated that the new Bridge House is a significantly better program, a program that is more client-centered. Clients have stated they feel more empowered and more responsible for their recovery due to the structure of the therapeutic community. Many clients have expressed the sense that the Bridge House client community provides a *safe place*, away from all the post-Katrina stressors in the city. The therapeutic community has proven helpful for traumatized clients, including one who was having difficulty dealing with the "image of dead bodies floating in Katrina's floodwater." Finally, Bridge House recently subsumed another New Orleans based residential treatment agency that was unable to restart operations after Katrina. As a new subsidiary of Bridge House, this facility is now fully operational. Thus, in addition to serving 75 men, Bridge House now serves 25 women.

Bridge House is one of the few New Orleans' substance abuse treatment providers that have successfully resuscitated themselves since Katrina. Natural disasters are not a question of *if* but a question of *when*. Substance abuse treatment agencies can learn from Bridge House about the barriers and facilitators to surviving in a post-disaster environment, and about the opportunities for improvement they may present.

Acknowledgments

Preparation of this chapter was supported in part by an award to the Council on Drug and Alcohol Abuse for Greater New Orleans from the Center for Substance Abuse Treatment (5QBITI15651-02), as well as awards from the Robert Wood Johnson Foundation (046876), and the National Institute on Drug Abuse (R01 DA018282).

Notes

1. Mallak LA. Putting organizational resilience to work. Industrial Management. 1998; 40(6):8–13.

2. Norris FH, Friedman MJ, Watson PJ, et al. 60,000 disaster victims speak: Part I. An empirical review of the empirical literature, 1981–2001. Psychiatry. 2002 Fall; 65(3):207–39.

3. North CS, Kawasaki A, Spitznagel EL, et al. The course of PTSD, major depression, substance abuse, and somatization after a natural disaster. J Nerv Ment Dis. 2004 Dec;192(12):823–9.

4. Freedy JR, Kilpatrick DG. Everything you wanted to know about natural disasters and mental health (well, almost). National Center for PTSD Clinical Quartertly. 1994;4(2).

5. Norris FH. Risk factors for adverse outcomes in natural and human-caused disasters: a review of the empirical literature. (Fact Sheet.) Washington, DC: National Center for PTSD, 2005.

6. Benight CC, Ironson G, Durham RL. Psychometric properties of a hurricane coping self-efficacy measure. J Trauma Stress. 1999 Apr;12(2):379–86.

7. Benight CC, Ironson G, Klebe K, et al. Conservation of resources and coping self efficacy predicting distress following a natural disaster: a causal model analysis where the environment meets the mind. Anxiety Stress and Coping. 1999;12(2):107–26.

8. Clark HW. Traumatic events and substance use: demands on the substance abuse treatment delivery system. Rockville, MD: Substance Abuse and Mental Health Services Administration, 2004.

9. Diamond MA. Innovation and diffusion of technology: a human process. Consulting Psychology Journal: Practice and Research. 1996 Fall;48(4):221–9.

10. Miller WR, Rollnick S. Motivational interviewing: preparing people for change. Second Ed. New York: Guilford Press, 2002.

11. Schneider RJ, Casey J, Kohn R. Motivational versus confrontational interviewing: a comparison of substance abuse assessment practices at employee assistance programs. J Behav Health Serv Res. 2000 Feb;27(1):60–74.

12. Carise D, Gurel O. Benefits of integrating assessment technology with treatment—the DENS Project. In: Sorensen JL, Rawson RA, Guydish J, et al., eds. Drug abuse treatment through collaboration: practice and research partnerships that work. Washington, DC: American Psychological Association, 2003 Feb;181–95.

13. Gustafson DH. Designing systems to improve addiction treatment: the foundation. Alcohol & Drug Abuse Weekly. 2002;14(42):1–2.

Chapter 24
Hurricane Readiness and Environmental Risks on the Bayous—an NIEHS Community-Based Pilot Project in South Terrebonne–Lafourche Parishes, Louisiana

John Sullivan

After Hurricane Rita devastated the western Louisiana and east Texas Gulf coasts, the National Institute of Environmental Health Sciences (NIEHS) Community Outreach and Education Core (COEC) at the University of Texas Medical Branch (UTMB) responded by delivering medical supplies to Larose, Louisiana, and deploying an outreach survey team that videotaped a series of interviews with public health advocates, environmental activists and citizens involved in rescue and recovery efforts. Between October 4th and December 17th, 2005, this team asked respondents to identify and prioritize perceived environmental health risks due to storm damage, and to suggest outreach strategies that would assist recovery and increase community readiness for future storms.

Questions posed to survey respondents included:

- What significant damage did your region sustain during or because of hurricanes Katrina and Rita?
- What is the most significant threat to human health in your area, post-Katrina (or Rita)?
- How has the hurricane evacuation, reentry, and recovery process disrupted the social fabric of your area, and Louisiana generally?
- What environmental health projects—involving collaborations among environmental scientists, health care and social service providers, and communities—do you think are most important to safeguard the health of people and the environment in your region and the state?
- Describe your organization's response to this disaster. How have you modified your mission to make an effective response? How have these modifications affected your organization's capacity to realize your original mission? [only asked in interviews with staff or members of environmental organizations]

The results of this video survey were compiled and edited (with an emphasis on suggestions for collaborative projects among, researchers, clinicians, and communities)

JOHN SULLIVAN is the Co-Director of Public Forum and Toxics Assistance at the Sealy Center for Environmental Health & Medicine/NIEHS Center in Environmental Toxicology at the University of Texas Medical Branch at Galveston.

for presentation in November 2005. The footage was further edited, with the title that it now has, ". . . *after the wind, child, after the water's gone* . . . ;" the full film is available from the author upon request. The URL for excerpts is listed in the appendix to this volume.

In April 2006, the UTMB-NIEHS COEC's Public Forum and Toxics Assistance Division received funding for an NIEHS pilot project to create and implement a site-specific community environmental risk curriculum that incorporates major areas of concern identified in the survey with a primary focus on the health consequences of large storms. Analysis of video transcripts identified the following responses as significant (by frequency and emphasis):

- exposure to mold: concentrations, direct exposure effects, possible immuno-suppression and recommended precautions;
- extent of threat from pathogens in water; ongoing monitoring of pathogen levels in bayou surface water and major bodies such as Lake Salvador; rashes and lesions as consequences of immersion in flood water;
- flooding/overflow risk to surface water from Resource Conservation and Recovery Act exempt waste pits and compromised sewage treatment facilities;
- dispersion patterns and health effects of toxic releases from submerged automobiles, agricultural chemicals, non-petrochemical industrial sites;
- levels of metals, diesel, and hydrocarbon residues in desiccated sludge, and change in levels over time;
- respiratory and other health effects of wind-borne sludge dust (*Katrina cough*);
- transport patterns of petrochemical toxicants and metal residues moved from previously contaminated areas by storm surges;
- need for specific re-entry safety gear not clearly indicated, lack of information on re-entry procedures, safety equipment unavailable, price-gouging;
- effects of damage to coastal marsh on subsistence food supply and health of the estuarine eco-system;
- massive loss of marsh and wetlands, loss of marshland's hurricane dampening effect;
- depression, disorientation, post-traumatic stress effects of disaster;
- effects of disaster stressors on the most vulnerable segments of the population: children, the elderly, people with low incomes, disabled individuals.

The project's organization, education, and outreach derive from a merger of two survey suggestions for collaborative disaster preparedness projects that were mentioned with some frequency, and also fit the parameters of our available infrastructure and limited funding:

- Conduct a comprehensive survey of industrial and hazardous waste sites in affected area to assess extent of structural damage to facilities, especially as damage might affect fugitive emissions, seepage, or emergency flaring procedures; and
- Develop a comprehensive, but site-specific, disaster management plan and procedures that incorporate environmental health, state and local environmental risk

communication, and hazardous situation preparedness training for community-based environmental organizations.

The project also addresses the wide personal variations in risk perceptions and degree of acceptable risk observed by the survey team. Because risk anxiety affected municipal and regional response plans and personal re-entry decisions alike, the meaning of risk, and the ways in which environmental sampling decisions, economic pragmatism, and scientific benchmarks converge to create official risk estimates, formed part of the curriculum.

The targeted area for this intervention was south Terrebonne and Lafourche Parishes. This part of Louisiana is home to the United Houma Nation, others of Louisiana Cajun culture, and numerous small-scale commercial shrimp fishermen. The area hosts several active oil and gas operations, and some of these facilities are vital conduits for national energy supplies. Port Fourchon, for example, lies at the southern tip of Lafourche Parish. Booster pumps at Fourchon convey huge quantities of crude oil from the Louisiana Offshore Oil Port for storage in underground salt domes near Galliano, Louisiana, and storm damage at this site could carry particularly catastrophic consequences for coastal communities. Terrebonne and Lafourche Parishes received a number of Houma and other evacuees from towns and villages in Plaquemines Parish, severely damaged by the full brunt of Katrina. Several families from Jefferson, St. Bernard, and Orleans Parishes also sought refuge there, and the local recovery infrastructure was challenged by the rapid influx. This is also one of the few regions (outside of Alaska) where subsistence fishing, trapping, and hunting are still significant factors in the local economy, and anxieties over the health of estuaries and surrounding marshlands were high. The COEC outreach team chose this region for the pilot project because storm surge from Hurricane Rita caused significant environmental damage in the area, the concentration of potential industrial hazards is high, most respondents in the original survey lived there, and a number of local organizations expressed enthusiasm and offered logistical support for the project.

Les Reflections du Bayou, a grassroots gulf restoration group, emerged as the local organizational anchor. Since this project employs a community-based research and intervention model, several planning sessions with a network of local organizations were convened; this interactive process yielded fresh ideas and urgency stemming from years of local experience with storms, recovery and coastal loss. The final themes and topics reflect community priorities as well as the environmental health focus of the NIEHS. The network co-created a handbook for workshop participants, and devised a 15 hour intensive training program titled, *Hurricane Readiness: a Way of Life on the Bayous,** which covered the following topics:

- **the rate of wetlands loss and coastal subsidence**: an overview of how local geology, hydrology, the Corps of Engineers management plan for the Mississippi River, past land use and channel construction by the energy industry, and possible

---

* The project is officially designated on the pilot project application as Community Environmental Health & Risk Outreach (CEHRO).

outcomes of global warming may affect the safety and longevity of humans and nature in Louisiana's southern parishes;

- **evacuation safety**: stressing the importance of timing, routes, and flooding patterns from past storms and future projections, with some mention of effective risk communication;
- **toxic exposures and medical outcomes of storm disasters**: a site-specific overview of a) exposure pathways for pathogens, industrial toxics, heavy metals, and Persistent Organic Pollutants (POP) residues; b) pathogen-borne diseases, neurotoxic exposure effects of industrial/agricultural products, and other adverse health outcomes; c) respiratory effects possibly related to concentrated mold spore exposure or desiccated storm sludge; c) redeposit of toxic sludge displaced by storm surges; d) pre-storm containment of household toxics; and e) typical types of injuries sustained at different points in the disaster response.
- **storm-related mental health issues**: particularly, though not exclusively, abandonment and personal safety issues in cases of displaced children (based on behavioral observations after the fact of the original survey by child care workers and school personnel in Terrebonne-Lafourche);
- **risk communication**: an adaptation of the NIEHS-UTMB Augusto Boal Forum theatre-based *Tox & Risk* curriculum was employed to offer a non-technical introduction to understanding community risk perceptions and rehearsing effective models of risk communication;
- **community hazard assessment**: a survey of point and secondary toxic hazard locations throughout south Terrebonne-Lafourche parishes guided by a checklist (which has since expanded in response to suggestions from workshop participants), materials later improved as locations were identified more precisely during the public forum as Wilma Subra presented specific maps of local hazardous waste facilities, classified by category of waste, type of construction and current level of activity.

Les Reflection du Bayou coordinated the training from September 8th through September 12th, 2006. The process consisted of an intensive weekend training workshop, hosted by the South Planning District in Gray, Louisiana, geared toward representatives of local groups. In addition, the training group presented two public forums: one in Terrebonne Parish (at Houma), the other in Lafourche Parish (at Galliano). Guest presenters included a mix of local and academic research expertise, including co-facilitation of training process and public forum (Rochelle Ste. Marie/Inner Works, Inc.), coastal/wetlands deterioration (Windell Curole/South Lafourche Levee District), local clinical medicine (Michael Robichaux, MD / Mathews, Louisiana), disaster epidemiology (Sharon Petronella, PhD/UTMB), and community hazard assessment (Wilma Subra, MS/analytic chemist). The workshop participants met for a second phase of training in March 2007, covering characteristics of vulnerable populations, advanced community storm hazard identification and risk assessment, effective advocacy for coastal restoration, and achieving sustainable outcomes (maintaining the Terrebonne-Lafourche network and funding future programs).

Louisiana communities actively represented in this project include: Larose, Lockport, Galliano, Golden Meadow, Cut Off, Pointe-aux-Chenes, Montegut, Dulac, Chauvin, Houma, Mathews, New Iberia, Isle de Jean Charles and Grand Bois. Partner organizations contributing to this project encompassed a wide range of social service, public health, emergency services, and educational organizations (such as South Lafourche Levee District, South Lafourche Unified School District, United Houma Nation Vocational Rehabilitation, Bayou Grace, Louisiana Spirit, Catholic Social Services, Knights of Columbus, Les Reflections du Bayou, Barateria-Terrebonne National Estuary Programs, Bayou Interfaith Shared Community Organizing, Inner Works, Inc., and the Gulf Restoration Network).

Acknowledgments

Key local personnel for this project were Rochelle Ste. Marie (Inner Works, Inc.), Gregory Harding (Louisiana Spirit), Warren Sapp (Bayou Grace), Windell Curole (South Lafourche Levee District), Lanor Curole (United Housma Nation Vocational Rehabilitation Services), Courtney Pellegrin (Bayou Grace), Michael Robichaux, MD (group practice clinician), Wilma Subra (Subra Company, Inc.), and Bryan Parras (T.e.j.a.s.).

Key university research/outreach personnel were Jennifer Gorenstein (MD Anderson Cancer Center/University of Texas (UT) Smithville), Robin Fuchs-Young (MD Anderson/UT-Smithville), Ray Kay Santa (University of Texas Medical Branch at Galveston (UTMB-G)), Albert J. Chavarria (UTMB-G), John Sullivan (UTMB-G), Sharon Petronella (UTMB-G), and Pamela Diamond (UTMB-G).

Chapter 25
Re-establishing a Home after Katrina: A Long and Winding Road

Muriel J. Harris, PhD, MPH
Monica H. Powell, RN
Elvin Stampely, MBA

S triking the Gulf Coast as a Category 3 storm, 2005's Hurricane Katrina was the worst storm that the people of New Orleans had experienced in many years. The aftermath of the hurricane was widespread flooding of the city that resulted from the breaching of the levees. Eighty percent of the city and surrounding parishes were damaged and 4.9 million people were affected.[1] It was one of the strongest Atlantic hurricanes ever recorded and it left 1,464 people dead in Louisiana alone.[2] Many of those who survived were forced to flee their homes, often going to other states. Approximately 1,400 found their way to Kentucky, most of whom staying in Louisville.

This narrative presents the experiences of two people who lived to tell their stories after Hurricane Katrina struck on August 29, 2005. The report has three central purposes: 1) to describe the effects of Hurricane Katrina on two individuals; 2) to demonstrate the attitudes, beliefs, and skills that helped two people in their survival and recovery; 3) to illustrate the social, emotional, and economic supports they harnessed for their recovery. Fifty-four year old Angela* lived in Bogalusa, 60 miles north of New Orleans. Married and non-Hispanic White, Angela is a registered nurse who was disabled nine years ago. Before Katrina she was very involved in a literacy program and provided home health to other disabled residents in her community. Angela stayed in her residence, which flooded, through the hurricane. After holding on for as long as she could to keep herself above water, Angela agreed to go to a shelter, but when it closed following Hurricane Rita and the residents were told to go north, she, her husband, and her dog went to Louisville, although they knew no one in Kentucky. Angela now works as a volunteer for local organizations and is being trained to be a member of an emergency response team.

Sam lived with his wife and his five-year old son in the 9th Ward of New Orleans. Thirty-five year old Sam is African American; he had just returned from active duty in the U.S. Army when the storm began threatening. His family had already left its home

---

* Both names used in this report are pseudonyms.

MURIEL HARRIS *is an Assistant Professor at the University of Louisville in the School of Public Health and Information Sciences.* **MONICA POWELL** *and* **ELVIN STAMPELY** *both also reside in Louisville, where they have been involved in the Katrina recovery efforts.*

to go to New Iberia, Louisiana, where his wife's family lived. After some thought, he picked up his bags and fled, first to New Iberia, where he spent a few days, then to Louisville, at the urging of an old college friend who offered him the opportunity to start over. He was soon able to reunite his family and they stayed with his friend for the first two months. He currently works as a career advisor for Katrina evacuees in Louisville.

The authors had heard parts of Angela's and Sam's accounts of the hurricane and its aftermath, and in spring 2006 both agreed to tell their stories more formally. Sam agreed to be interviewed, while Angela preferred to write down her experiences in the quiet and privacy of her home. Each described the experience of the hurricane and being displaced as overpowering. Angela called it "overwhelming, massive, too big to comprehend." Referring to the alienation he felt, Sam said, "I was no longer a short drive from my extended family, i.e., mother, father, sister, aunts, uncles, cousins, in-laws." What follows are their stories.

In the aftermath of the storm, Sam said, "Levees were breached, flood waters were everywhere, [I was in] a state of emotional loss. I have a sincere love for my home-town—the food, the culture, the music, the visitors, the beautiful architecture—all changed with the hurricane." Angela had also lost her home, but her reflections were different. Her first realization was of "being homeless, vulnerable and totally lost in the figurative and literal sense." They both expressed feelings of alienation and, while Sam was familiar with living in a city, Angela had only lived in rural Louisiana and the city frightened her. "I had lived in a rural setting and now I was in an apartment in a city. I was afraid of everything and everyone. There was little reason to live. My friends were gone, and everything that made me real was gone." They were both now in a Midwestern culture with "different ways of interacting, socializing, working, eating foods, entertaining," [Sam] a long way from what was recognizable and from the New Orleans accents they both yearned to hear.

Angela and Sam were not prepared for Katrina even though they had experienced previous hurricanes. Angela said, "All that experience did not prepare me in any way to cope with this. I have never been in this position and have no frame of reference." In addition to her frustration with her new situation, Angela agonized about family and friends who had stayed behind, and the upsetting situation in which they found themselves. She said, "Everyone I know was traumatized." The hurricane took away the ability of individuals to make independent choices and to feel joy. It took away jobs and livelihoods. Angela said, "Since August 29, 2005 not one thing has been our choice. All choices are made on the basis of survival. I am making an effort to restart my life. It is necessary, but a lot died that day and it is gone forever." She said that the love of her husband and the kindness and patience of the therapist she found in Louisville gave her the will to live.

Angela and Sam had come a long way from their cultures and traditions, and they mourned their losses. Sam said, "I will always be that person with Louisiana customs. Eating seafood—that is important. Seafood is not only eaten on Fridays during the Easter season, rather it's eaten every Friday if not more often than that." Angela felt a strong need to keep her dialect, saying, "I pray I do not lose my accent." For Angela and Sam the road to recovery is long, but it is one they have both begun. They are committed to moving forward even though doing so is difficult. In a thoughtful moment, Angela said, "[We] decided at the outset that we would move forward and we just kept moving. [We] set a goal for that day, like take a shower, or eat, or try to read. It was months before we could listen to music or laugh or meet people." Being in a new city, it was important to be able to find one's way around; Sam accomplished that by using a mnemonic. For the route he took from the emergency services to the local library (to use a computer to look for a job) Sam's mnemonic went like this, "At the MAIN Street MARKET there was a fight between JEFFERSON and MUHAMMAD ALI. They are fighting for LIBERTY. The fighter discussed the size of the purse . . . CHESTNUTS! Forget the fight, let's go down BROADWAY."

Sam's wife played an important role in reestablishing a life for his family. He said, "My wife and I made a big celebration about picking out lamps we could appreciate, and that was a big accomplishment." His new coworkers also supported his transition. He said, "Coworkers from my first employment donated a computer desk, chairs, a sofa, toys, a bike, and local magazines and the churches provided economic assistance." Less concrete supports for Angela included, "the countless people who smiled, hugged, and wiped our tears." Sam also thought that his relocation was made easier by his being able to get a job and identify with familiar things. He said, "Getting a job and having access to the services. It was also the familiar names like Veaux Carré that sounded so French and so much like it was misplaced from New Orleans and the celebration of Mardi Gras. The bridge downtown also reminds me of New Orleans." Relocation was made easier for Angela by moving into a house and having a personal space, being offered full-time employment, meeting evacuees and establishing support systems. It included being able to plant flowers in the back yard, which symbolized ownership and stability, and having options and choices again.

Adapting to a new city and a new way of life requires determination, fortitude, and an ability to cope with very different situations. Both Angela and Sam exhibited these qualities and adopted various ways of coping. Angela reached acceptance after initially being very depressed and contemplating suicide. She said, "I guess my way of adapting is accepting that everything I knew and loved is gone. I can never go home and this will never be home but I can make a life and one day I will feel safe." Sam, on the other hand, found his motivation in his confidence in creating a new home for his son. He said, "I will achieve. Now I have to share new experiences in raising my son. I have to open the door of opportunity. I take on the challenge every day and make it my business so he can see opportunity." Adapting also means, "learning a new way of life, a new culture, and a new environment—the weather, the highways, the terrain, as well as all the new names!" [Sam]. It means, "celebrating the small victories as well, like finding lamps for a new apartment" [Sam].

Even though Sam had left behind his culture, it was that culture that made him strong. This is what Sam said: "What I used mostly was inside of me, my upbringing that I was taught not to give up, the pride was the burden, that what does not kill you makes you better and being angry is destructive. I had the strength to figure out what I needed to survive."

Like others in situations like theirs, Angela and Sam required community supports in the form of such necessities as safety and protection; shelter; employment opportunities;

community resources; and a wide range of services. Becoming stable meant having a job, since in Angela's words, "to have a job awards membership into the community and employment quickly associates with self esteem." She also identified the important need for a sense of belonging and acceptance from the larger adopted community.

Given their experiences of being evacuees, Angela and Sam suggested that communities respond to people who relocate to their cities following a major disaster by keeping their residents continually informed of their needs, and fostering opportunities for employment and the development of a compassionate community. Angela pointed out the importance of training caregivers, and ensuring a comprehensive database for reuniting families, friends, and the displaced community. She emphasized the importance of ensuring that agencies' efforts are well coordinated and that there is simple concise information available to evacuees. This could include lists of services that are available in the community such as bus routes, doctor's offices, dentists, stores, pharmacies, churches, police stations, fire departments, schools, the Department of Motor Vehicles, and taxicabs. Ongoing personal or e-mail contact were also suggested as ways of keeping evacuees connected.

Home is a reality that differs for Angela and Sam, yet for both the place they call home is where they strive to make a living and exist peacefully. People who are displaced may be forced to accept a rambling existence and the ever-changing identity it implies. In order to soften the impact of such blows, however, public health professionals and others in the health professions must develop expandable structures, services, and trained staff to support individuals and their families in the aftermath of disasters. A critical element of recovery is moving forward from the initial shock, disbelief and hurt, to acceptance and a sense of purpose. This requires material support that only communities and institutions can provide.

Notes

1. U.S. Census Bureau. Census bureau estimates nearly 10 million residents along Gulf Coast hit by Hurricane Katrina. Washington, DC: U.S. Census Bureau, 2005 Sep 2. Available at http://www.census.gov/Press-Release/www/releases/archives/hurricanes_tropical_storms/005673.html.

2. Louisiana Department of Health and Hospitals (DHH). Reports of missing and deceased. Baton Rouge: DHH, 2006 Aug 6. Available at http://www.dhh.louisiana.gov/offices/page.asp?ID=192&Detail=5248.

Chapter 26
Cultural Competency in Disaster Recovery: The Lessons of Hurricane Katrina for Serving Marginalized Communities

Jennifer Seidenberg, JD

Following the great earthquake and fire of 1906, Chinese residents of San Francisco found themselves shunted to a far corner of the city, denied relief assistance afforded the White population, and arrested for attempting to re-enter their homes in Chinatown.[1] San Francisco's ruling elite took advantage of an opportunity to reclaim Chinatown for White business interests and formulated a plan to move the refugee Chinese population south of the city to Hunter's Point.[1] In the wake of Hurricane Andrew, the Red Cross placed ethnic minority populations within ghettoized districts of tent cities where Latino survivors encountered taunting and hostility from other ethnic groups.[2] We may lament these events as falling within a familiar pattern of America's failed poverty policy, as many lament our health, welfare, and housing systems. The disaster context presents, however, unique, discrete situations wherein government at all levels may actually find an opportunity to respond directly to the position of vulnerable populations, potentially transforming their experience of our social safety net.

In this chapter, I argue that the Federal Emergency Management Agency (FEMA), in coordination with state governments, should rely more than they presently do on partnerships with locally based government and community social services organizations in long-term recovery efforts. To create real cultural empathy within the bureaucracy, providers of relief must have substantial connections with the affected community. This chapter focuses on the long-term recovery efforts that follow the first few weeks of a disaster and continue at least for the following year. This phase of recovery is aimed at returning survivors to relative financial security, stable housing, and access to services for health and general welfare. For purposes of definition, *marginalized populations* refers to a broad spectrum of citizens who depend on social services, often live below the poverty line, often have mental or physical disabilities, sometimes lack English language proficiency, and may endure low social standing due to lack of education or job opportunity.[3] *Cultural competency* refers to a high level of sophistication within organizations' interactions with diverse populations; it is "a set of values, behaviors, attitudes, and practices . . . that allows people to work effectively across cultures" (p. 12).[4]

Jennifer Seidenberg *is a litigation associate at Rossmann and Moore, LLP, in the practice of public interest environmental law. Ms. Seidenberg organized the Boalt Hall Katrina Relief Project and traveled to New Orleans in the winter of 2005 to provide legal services to residents affected by Hurricane Katrina.*

First I review social science findings regarding marginalized populations in disaster recovery, demographic characteristics of New Orleans relating to Katrina survivors' experiences after the hurricane, and the traditional recovery system after Katrina as it has served middle-class recovery yet failed to move poor and marginalized communities toward long-term stability. I go on to propose reforms to create cultural competency within government recovery efforts and conclude by examining congressional efforts at reform, policy considerations, and the potential legal obstacles to needed reform.

The Problem: Marginalized Groups Fall Further Behind during Disaster Recovery

Well before Hurricane Katrina made landfall on August 29, 2005, the geography and demography of New Orleans placed its poor and minority populations in a state of "social vulnerability," leaving them at severe risk of harm from natural disaster.[5]* In Louisiana, 21.4% of the population in hurricane-damaged or flooded areas lived below the poverty line, in comparison with 19.6% of the Louisiana population overall and 12.4% of the U.S. population.[6] Poverty was even more widespread in New Orleans, where 28% of people pre-Katrina lived in poverty, most of them (84%) African American.[7] A significant portion of those affected by the hurricane were African American citizens living below the poverty line, predictably given the long-standing traits of the region.

New Orleans's history of racial division produced a city where, in 2005, African American and White communities were largely segregated from one another. The lowest-lying areas of New Orleans most likely to be inundated by water were neighborhoods such as the Lower Ninth Ward, where 98% of the population was African American.[7] Homeownership, not long-term residency or community ties, has proven to be a key factor aiding recovery from the disaster.[8]† Sadly, the proportion of residents of areas most severely affected by Katrina who were homeowners was smaller than average (55% compared with the national average of 66%).[6] Renters of single family homes in the Lower Ninth Ward did have long-term ties to the area, many having rented the same property for more than a decade.[6] These citizens, who were certainly part of and contributed to the community, still held no tangible property rights in the neighborhood.

---

*Cutter explains that, in addition to housing and financial concerns, *social vulnerability* involves intangible elements, many of which SAMHSA and social scientists studying disasters have discussed.[4,5] Cutter includes within this intangible list "the basic provisions of health care, the livability of places, overall indicators of quality of life, . . . capital, and political representation."[5]

---

†See discussion below, on middle-class solutions including FEMA's *Blue Roof* program and trailer allocation, which has allowed some homeowners to establish stability sooner than others. Notably, working class homeowners are less likely to reap these advantages; while they have "acquired some of the trappings associated with economic success, they may lack the 'defense in depth'—the economic security, political and social influence, and personal power of the professional classes, which can be especially crucial in times of disaster" (p. 152).[8]

Cultural differences and social networks in the context of disaster. Marginalized populations are not only more likely to be vulnerable to disasters due to self-evident problems of geography and resources, but are also considerably disadvantaged by less obvious social and cultural phenomena. Social scientists studying minority populations within modern disaster recovery efforts have produced a substantial literature detailing the outcomes of federal programs seeking to aid these groups.[9]

At-risk citizens are likely to have had experience previous to a disaster with the social welfare system, yet this experience may not help them in navigating the massive federal bureaucracy in charge of provisioning aid following a disaster; in fact, negative associations may impede their willingness to approach government authorities.[9]* Perhaps due to this skepticism toward government bureaucracy, non-White survivors of disasters are "more likely than Whites to cite churches and the Red Cross as helpful sources of information during recovery" (p. 163).[9] Despite this phenomenon, during the Katrina recovery FEMA continued to operate its Disaster Relief Centers (DRCs, information and aid processing sites) with khaki-clad private security guards who wore Blackwater security T-shirts and were outfitted with weapons.[10]† In a *New York Times* study of recovery seven months after the hurricane, about half of all African American evacuees surveyed "called race a major factor in the government's slow response."[11]‡

The Hurricane Andrew experience in 1992 taught federal agencies and charities alike that maneuvering within the aid process requires education, time, and skills that low-income people often lack.[8] Numerous families in South Florida never entered the relief system and were living with the effects of the disaster long after the deadline to register for FEMA assistance had passed.[8] In contrast, upper-middle-class survivors may be better equipped to navigate the governmental system and better able to perform bureaucratic tasks such as filling out forms and providing relevant information to disaster personnel,[9] all of which makes them more likely than marginalized populations to receive federal disaster aid.

Social networks also play a key role in disaster recovery, as survivors are able to rely upon neighborhood, workplace, and kinship ties for temporary housing, emotional support, and access to other practical resources such as transportation and communication.[12] New Orleans's tradition of voluntary organizations (such as the Mardi Gras crews) and multi-generational families within the same neighborhoods might have made Katrina survivors' social networks a strength in disaster recovery. Instead, the

---

* As Perry and Mushkatel write, "Another aspect of cultural differences is that some minority members perceive authority figures—particularly uniformed government representatives—differently from majority group members. Amongst members of some urban/ethnic racial minority groups in the United States, public safety personnel . . . are not necessarily viewed in positive terms or as sources from whom to expect help and protection" (p. 154).[9]

† Many of Blackwater USA's personnel who worked in DRCs following Katrina had recently returned to the United States from security work in Iraq.

‡ For the study reported in the *New York Times*, 337 respondents were selected randomly from a Red Cross Katrina survivor database. Contrasting with African American perspectives on the government response, "almost three-quarters of the White evacuees said race was not a factor at all."[11]

population's wide dispersal across the United States after Hurricane Katrina through government evacuation efforts—including the dispersal of members of a single-family household to different locations and different states—meant that indigent survivors probably had a much more difficult time staying connected with these potentially critical social networks, difficulties compounded by these survivors' widespread lack of telephones and e-mail.[12] Future efforts at disaster recovery should be sensitive to maintaining low-income families' social networks (and their ability to return), to the extent practicable, by allowing survivors to stay closer to home and facilitating contact among those who must be displaced. (See discussion below of Catholic Charities' Operation Starfish.)

Discrimination by design? The bipartisan congressional committee that investigated the failed response to Hurricane Katrina aptly titled its report "A Failure of Initiative," lamenting that, although the nation had anticipated the disaster and even planned for it, those who were supposed to implement the plan proved unable to do so. Though committee members examined the minutiae of the failed leadership response, they seemed unable to put their finger on exactly what had accounted for this lack of leadership. Grasping for a general explanation, they concluded simply that "we again encountered the risk-averse culture that pervades big government" (p. 2).[13]

Offering an alternative explanation to a merely risk-averse government bureaucracy, sociologist Harvey Molotch suggests that, among bureaucratic actors in the context of disasters, "a little bit of racism can go a long way."[14] Molotch argues that African Americans in New Orleans were sufficiently outside White middle-management's social milieu to disable any impulse to take extraordinary action outside bureaucratic norms to aid survivors.[14] Molotch's observation sounds a familiar theme in critical race scholarship, where scholars often assess the role of race in the arena of social welfare and affirmative action programs. Discussing the cycle of grinding poverty that produces crime and drug abuse in the African American community, Professor Derrick Bell argues, "Few Whites are able to identify with Blacks as a group—the essential prerequisite for feeling empathy with, rather than aversion from, Blacks' self-inflicted suffering" (p. 4).[15]

The connection between empathy and action may be most dramatic when we think of the failure of the federal government to respond in the days following Hurricane Katrina's landfall. It is hard to understand why the national military were not mobilized while images were broadcast on television of African American families stranded on rooftops and waiting inside the Superdome. The persistent failure of initiative that hobbled the government's long-term disaster recovery program in New Orleans exemplifies a troubling symmetry between race and access to social welfare resources. The problems evident during and after Hurricane Katrina—ineligibility for government resources, misinformation from official sources, and poorly tailored programs—sprang from practices dating back to the roots of the U.S. social welfare system in the New Deal.

Discrimination by design,[16]* or the construction of government programs primarily to favor middle-class White Americans over their minority counterparts, is deeply

---

* The term *discrimination by design* has been used by various authors for different types of social critiques. The term as I use it points to government programs and other systems that, though neutral on their face, yield results with disparities along racial and/or class lines. The term has also been used in analysis of gender and public space.[16]

embedded in the history of social welfare legislation and accompanying regulations. In the 1930s, programs were tailored to fit the outlines of White, but not African American, poverty. For example, federal agricultural assistance benefited White farmers by enabling them to keep their farms with financial aid; African American farmers, who were short on capital and had poorer access to banks, did not see their farm holdings increase with the new provisions of government aid.[17] The obstacles faced by minority survivors of Hurricane Katrina as they worked to rebuild their lives and recover property losses echo this early history.

Another example of discrimination by design comes from the Social Security Program of 1940, which excluded scores of African American workers because they had previously worked as farm workers or domestic servants, categories that did not qualify under the act.[17] This difference persists to the present day for many off-the-books workers with respect not only to Social Security but also to Medicare. In the Katrina context, the *single-household* rule, discussed below and challenged in the courts,[18] limited the number of applicants living under the same roof who could apply to FEMA for disaster grants. Just as the categories established by the Social Security Act directly disadvantaged African Americans based upon the nature of work available to them, FEMA's definition of a household was squarely in conflict with the interests of citizens living in multi-family and multi-generational households who could not squeeze into a program designed for nuclear families.

Ira Katznelson, investigating welfare policies in the New Deal South, notes that African American citizens consistently received fewer benefits in relation to their needs than did Whites and argues that such a system was deliberately designed to ensure the supply of cheap African American labor.[17] These discriminatory underpinnings of public welfare were made possible by the discretionary power available to state and local officials;[17] for most of the twentieth century, *localism* in America meant racism, and states' rights initiatives were thinly disguised vehicles for pursuing discriminatory policies.

Below, however, I argue for a partially local approach to disaster recovery in order to serve minority and other marginalized citizens more effectively. Although localism may have once had exclusively negative racial connotations, in present-day urban America, where minority populations are concentrated, often with a good deal of political power, devolution of power to the local level for disaster recovery may prove fruitful. Marginalized survivors of disasters will probably fare better during recovery if they are reliably assisted at the local level by minority leaders, advocates, and nonprofit organizations with charitable missions, rather than if they approach a massive agency such as FEMA alone.

The politics of social welfare have continued to be imbued with racial biases since the second half of the twentieth century. Racial stereotypes regarding social welfare programs have long been used as political weapons, as they were during the debates over welfare reform in the mid-1990s, when politicians emphasized the need to push against abuse of benefits, which they constructed as an African American pathology.[19]

This need for "responsibility" in the African American community served as justification for cutting benefits.[19]*

In the immediate aftermath of Hurricane Katrina, numerous commentators noted the racial dynamics of the disaster.[14,20] More subtle, however, has been the unwillingness of FEMA to design adequate ways of serving the marginalized and primarily African American population displaced from New Orleans. This failure of initiative has now persisted for years.

Middle-Class Solutions Fail Marginalized Communities

On a visit to New Orleans in March 2006, while touring the Lower Ninth Ward, the president implored African American residents to return home,[21] apparently unaware that many former residents of the neighborhood were hundreds of miles away as a result of the haphazard post-Katrina evacuation of people without private transportation and without the resources to return home. Failure to understand low-income evacuees' plight after the storm was also evident in the federal government's lopsided approach to rebuilding New Orleans, an approach that has had lasting consequences.

A comparison of recovery in the Lower Ninth Ward with that in upper-middle-class Lakeview and working-class St. Bernard Parish provides a lens for evaluating the effectiveness of the ongoing government response to the plight of low-income survivors of Hurricane Katrina. Since the initial deluge, the three communities have moved in starkly different directions, two steadily toward recovery while the third's future existence remains a question mark as a result of the interplay between socioculturally specific responses and government's inadequate efforts to serve marginalized populations. Practical solutions, such as blue roofs and trailer programs, though well intentioned, may work for middle-class communities with private resources, stable social networks, and property rights, but not for those with less.

African American survivors surveyed in a March 2006 *New York Times* study "were having the most difficulty returning" to New Orleans and were also "more likely to have had their homes destroyed or to have lost a close friend or relative."[11] In contrast, Whites were far more likely to have returned to the area and to have kept their old jobs or found new ones.[11] In the Lower Ninth Ward, where comparatively low numbers of residents owned homes but most rental properties were owned by African Americans, Louisiana ACORN (a non-profit agency) and other local organizations had to fight in court to stop bulldozing that was scheduled without notice or consultation with residents and homeowners.[22] Despite FEMA's stated desire "to keep you as close to your home and as comfortable as possible,"[23] the agency found it impossible to locate travel trailers for African American families within wealthier neighborhoods of New Orleans.[24] Neither did the federal government make any concerted effort to clean up, restore basic services, and move trailers into the Lower Ninth Ward and other African

---

*Republican efforts at welfare reform in the mid-1990s, such as its Contract with America, included explicit references to African American behavior as demonstrating the need to cut aid. See proposed Personal Responsibility Act, which was passed by the house but vetoed by President Clinton in 1995, available at www.house.gov/house/Contract/persrespb.txt (last visited Sept. 8, 2008).

American neighborhoods to facilitate the return of African American citizens in the immediate aftermath of the disaster.*

St. Bernard Parish, a close-knit working class community, was the hardest hit area outside of Orleans Parish. An estimated 65,000 residents (97% of the parish's total population) were affected by flooding, and a portion of the parish was exposed to toxic floodwaters from the Murphy Oil Refinery spill.[6] Despite this extensive damage, within a few months of the disaster the parish was humming with construction activity. Numerous St. Bernard homeowners were living in trailers from FEMA or in ones they had paid for themselves in front of their damaged homes, working to rip out rotted material and begin structural repairs.[27] A backdrop of stronger individual financial resources, coupled with the response of citizen groups such as the St. Bernard Citizens Recovery Committee, allowed the community to move forward quite rapidly.[28] In contrast with developments in the Lower Ninth Ward, the local government has allowed the community to influence how it will rebuild, without the threat of bulldozers (though a majority of the land mass in St. Bernard Parish is reclaimed and below sea level).[28]

The Lakeview neighborhood of Orleans Parish is also on a fast track to recovery, even though the area was subject to massive flooding from a breach of the 17th Street Canal levee.[29] Overwhelmingly White and middle-class, "an estimated 400 to 500 families have moved back . . . most are living in government-issued trailers while gutting their homes."[29] FEMA's Blue Roof program, which installed heavy-duty plastic coverings, also allowed many Katrina survivors to stay in their moderately damaged homes during the recovery period.[30†]

Readily available FEMA resources such as blue roofs[30] and trailers have thus allowed the middle class to stay within the community and rebuild; most of the indigent community, in contrast, remains far from home, unable even to begin the process of reconstructing their lives. Louisiana legislators recognized the importance of rebuilding the community from the inside out, urging FEMA to re-work its trailer system so that "parish residents are given priority for housing in FEMA trailers located within their parish."[31‡] Senator Sharon Broome introduced Senate Concurrent Resolution No. 7 urging FEMA, as well as the U.S. Department of Housing and Urban Development, to consider providing funds for modular housing, recognizing the need to "move people out of shelters and into longer term housing . . . that would allow families the privacy

---

* Progress in rebuilding the Lower Ninth Ward, once home to 30,000 residents, has been slow to non-existent. Most of the area is still unpopulated and desolate, with no new home building or available community services. Non-profit groups such as ACORN and Common Ground Relief have had the most visible impact in the community, rebuilding a few homes, restoring a community church, and working to re-plant wetlands near the neighborhood.[25,26]

† Following Hurricanes Katrina and Rita, 82,000 blue roofs were installed in Louisiana. The blue roof program was administered by FEMA, but the U.S. Army Corps of Engineers operated the program on the ground, hiring contractors and coordinating volunteers.

‡ The Louisiana legislature recognized the importance of on-site housing to maintaining the viability of New Orleans's local African American communities by passing at least three resolutions in the First Extraordinary Session of 2006; House Concurrent Resolution No. 39 specifically cites the importance of "allow[ing] parish residents to reestablish themselves in or near their own communities, to return to their jobs, and to settle their children back into their schools."[31]

needed to re-establish some sense of normalcy (p. 1)."[31] As late as mid-February 2006, approximately 27,000 families remained displaced in hotel rooms across the nation, facing imminent eviction.[31] While middle-class and working-class families were able to stay in their own neighborhoods, closer to jobs, their childrens' schools, and what remained of their social networks, low-income survivors of Katrina remained isolated and unable to re-establish their lives long after the storm. A lack of personal financial resources as well as dramatic increases in rental rates in New Orleans prevented these evacuees from returning home, and FEMA never proposed any viable alternative.

Instead, low-income families were shuffled from one temporary living situation to another, facing the loss of whatever normalcy they had created for their children in attending school regularly or obtaining new work. In March 2007, 58 families were given only 2 days of notice before they were suddenly moved from their trailer park in Hammond, Louisiana (about an hour from New Orleans), to a crime-ridden trailer park an hour away in Belle Chasse.[32]

In a different political context (perhaps with the spirit of President Johnson's War on Poverty),[17] we might have seen the government issuing grants to families to rebuild, spending millions of dollars on contractor work to construct new single-family homes rather than to assemble, shuffle, and relocate trailer parks.[33] Minority residents of disaster-struck regions who lost their jobs might have been employed to help rebuild their own cities at respectable wages.[34]* Instead, FEMA and the rest of the federal government took an arms-length approach that exacerbated rather than mitigated the effect of race and class on Katrina survivors' recovery from the disaster.

Minorities and the Market Recovery Approach

Low-income and minority survivors of disasters are in great need of federal financial assistance, as they often are uninsured and lack significant financial reserves. Peculiarly, however, government aid programs are more likely to be successfully accessed by middle-class and upper-class survivors. W. G. Peacock notes that the United States has adopted a largely "market-based approach" to disaster recovery, wherein individuals are expected to rely upon private insurance payments and financial reserves, with government and charity funds potentially "filling in some of the gaps" (p. 26).[35] Government responses rooted in such assumptions of the possibility of market-based recovery for a majority of citizens "tend to magnify the consequences of these conditions [poverty, discrimination and other cultural factors], placing minority households at greater risk of failing to recover" (p. 27).[35] A great many of Katrina's poorest survivors, both homeowners and renters, lacked flood insurance.[36] Already disadvantaged by the market recovery system, these families turned to the federal government for the most basic assistance.

One of the foundational government disaster programs meant to provide for very low-income people are federal disaster loans through the Small Business Administration of the Department of Agriculture (SBA loans).[37] SBA loans offered in the Katrina

---

*The workers who were in fact employed were recruited from Central America by contractors paid by the federal government; these workers' suffering of human rights abuses goes beyond this account. See International Human Rights Law Clinic (Univ. of California at Berkeley, Boalt Hall) Report.[34]

recovery provided up to $200,000 to homeowners to repair or replace damaged real estate; renters were eligible for up to $40,000 to replace personal property.[37,38] These seemingly generous loans are combined with excellent interest and repayment terms, but members of minority groups are often ineligible for SBA loans and unsuccessful obtaining other federal grant funding from FEMA.[39] In South Florida in 1992 after Hurricane Andrew, middle-class Homestead faired significantly better than did Florida City, many of whose residents live in poverty.[39] In Homestead, 20% of homeowners were approved for SBA loans, compared with only 5.5% in Florida City.[39] The difference also extended to Individual Assistance (IA) and Individual Family Grants (IFGs) granted directly by FEMA; in Homestead, 88.1% of these were approved, as opposed to only about 30% in Florida City.[39]

In the aftermath of Hurricane Katrina, without the advantage of equity in homeownership and other forms of credit and collateral, minority renters received little to no "direct rebuilding assistance from the federal government" (p. 1).[32] Indeed, the SBA's application is market-based, relying upon survivors' work history, credit scores, and collateral (required for any loan over $10,000).[40] Thus, the same factors that are likely to influence marginalized citizens' ability to obtain insurance, home loans, and other forms of equity leave them out of the running for recovery assistance. Among the key variables explaining differences in economic recovery between African American and White survivors of disasters, Robert Bolin noted nearly 20 years before Katrina struck, is the circumstance that SBA loans "figured prominently among the White subsample but not among Blacks. This reflects the fact that many Blacks could not qualify for SBA disaster loans."[41]

While federal disaster recovery programs may not be able immediately to address the underlying factors aggravating minority communities' unduly heavy burdens in disasters, federal authorities are well aware of the issues (as they re-appear in disaster after disaster). Recovery programs must not re-create the same barriers to progress that stood in the way of marginalized citizens prior to the disaster. Rather, recovery projects present an opportunity to create new functional processes in communities starting anew. Although a system of grants, or loans with more generous eligibility standards, would be preferable to the current terms offered, government also has the responsibility to respond to marginalized survivors in a manner that helps rather than hinders their access to financial and housing relief intended to fill the gaps in our market recovery system.

Disastrous Bureaucracy: Two Case Studies

Ronald Perry and Alvin Mushkatel's extensive work on minority citizens' reactions to disasters suggests that official information is relied upon across ethnic boundaries (p. 83).[42] Considering this reliance, coupled with marginalized populations' educational disadvantages, the capacity of the federal government to communicate information to survivors becomes crucial. Two federal court cases brought in the aftermath of Hurricane Katrina, *McWaters v. FEMA*[18] and *ACORN v. FEMA*,[43] illustrate the severely dysfunctional interaction between the government and marginalized survivors of the disaster.

McWaters v. FEMA. In late 2005, residents of New Orleans who had been displaced by the hurricane and the Lawyers Committee for Civil Rights brought suit against FEMA to force the agency to clarify its procedures toward survivors regarding housing benefits, the relation of FEMA awards to SBA loans, and the "single-household rule" for applying for benefits.[18] The plaintiffs argued in federal district court that FEMA had failed its mandate and also violated hurricane survivors' due process rights by denying benefits and misleading survivors about how to obtain funds.[18] Though the court did not find any due process violations and held that sovereign immunity precluded many of the plaintiffs' claims, it did find that FEMA violated mandatory requirements regarding information and that its decision to cut off housing aid was arbitrary and dangerous.[18] The case reveals a pattern of mis-information, changing information, and abrogation of responsibility that continues to exacerbate the position of Hurricane Katrina survivors.

McWaters v. FEMA was a class action suit comprising thirteen named plaintiffs who, as late as November 10, 2005, had received no disaster assistance whatsoever from FEMA, despite having lost their homes in the hurricane.[18] The suit told the story of Katrina survivors who had received a preliminary payment of $2,358 but were not adequately informed that the money was restricted to use for housing and had spent the funds on other necessities, thereby becoming ineligible for further FEMA benefits.[18*] Additionally, FEMA officials at DRCs confused potential beneficiaries and probably left many without benefits by requiring survivors to register for SBA loans before receiving FEMA benefits, contrary to the explicit language of the relevant federal legislation. Here, the court found the agency had "violated a mandatory duty through the mis-communication or inartful communication of the protocol for receiving Temporary Housing Assistance" (p. 232).[18]

Under the single-household rule, Katrina survivors were required to file for FEMA benefits as members of a household rather than as individuals. Numerous disaster survivors were denied FEMA assistance because they "shared the same address or phone number as another applicant" (p. 226).[18] The rule ignored the social reality of many Katrina survivors who lived in multiple family or multi-generational units, as well as considerations of gender inequality wherein single mothers supporting children had to battle their estranged husbands for benefits.[†] Adding to the frustration of survivors, FEMA attempted to change the rule to accommodate families separated during the evacuation process. Even the federal court in *McWaters* could not ascertain the actual rule in place until after "systematically questioning the parties in several conferences"

---

* FEMA issued a Memorandum allowing beneficiaries who had spent the funds on non-housing needs to fill out forms requesting to be "recertified" for benefits. FEMA's waiver of the restriction was not widely understood, nor was the process for recertification clearly defined.

† Studying the Hurricane Andrew disaster recovery process for minority survivors, Yelvington noted that, "given the complex ethnic, cultural, and class makeup of South Dade, official policies often did not match the realities of victims' lives" (p. 109–10).[2] Advocacy groups responding to the disaster similarly bemoaned the single-household rule: "Maria Escobar, with the South Dade Immigration Association, said, 'The reality is that the households are not Mom and Dad and three kids. These people rent rooms and part of rooms'" (p. 109–10).[2]

(p. 230).[18] The court found that FEMA's actions regarding the single-household rule were not severe enough to overcome sovereign immunity, but this was after the parties to the lawsuit had achieved an agreement about future dissemination of information.[18*] Critics charge that the system still fails to protect those most vulnerable: people whose claims remain pending because the federal bureaucracy has not yet been able to reach them.[44] A combination of FEMA's narrowly envisioned financial aid programs and its capacity for under-informing and misinforming disaster survivors has thrown up major roadblocks to recovery for underserved populations.

ACORN v. FEMA. On August 29, 2005, exactly one year after Hurricane Katrina made landfall, a coalition of Katrina survivors, housing rights advocates, and public interest lawyers filed suit against FEMA, as the agency moved to discontinue housing assistance for tens of thousands of evacuees.[43] At the time, FEMA seemed to be utilizing the transition from "essential assistance" to longer-term housing in order to declare thousands of Katrina survivors ineligible for continued housing aid.[43] Although longer-term housing aid does impose stricter eligibility requirements,[43] the agency's preference for cutting off benefits to survivors was evident in its inscrutable communications as well as its decision to cut off payments to thousands of evacuees despite a court warning that it could be ordered to reimburse them for back payments.[43]

The D.C. District Court found that FEMA's notice provisions in their letters to evacuees were "unconstitutionally vague and uninformative" (p. 16).[43] The court found that the risk to plaintiffs of damage through official action was high, balanced against the administrative burdens of more effective communication.[43] The key finding was an analysis of the "risk of erroneous deprivation" based upon inadequate notice (p. 13).[43] Here, the court detailed the FEMA process, which included letters to evacuees using code terms and referral to a separate Applicant Guide, which was said to explain such codes (p. 14).[43] Plaintiffs also detailed for the court attempts to contact FEMA in order to clarify their eligibility and their receiving of a different answer from each representative they were able to contact.

The obfuscation caused by the letters bordered on intentional misrepresentation; it begs the question of whether the agency designed such communications to dissuade evacuees from pursuing long-term housing. For example, Mr. Joseph Douglas, a New Orleans evacuee, received a letter from FEMA in August 2006 stating: "Determination ENC- Eligible- No change on appeal, original eligible status stands . . . Total Grant Amount: $0.00" (p. 8).[43] The court found that the evacuees faced "considerable risk of erroneous determinations caused by vague and cryptic explanations" (p. 16).[43] FEMA had argued, in its defense, that despite the encoded, computer-generated form letters sent to evacuees, the appeals process for long-term housing aid served to mitigate such a risk.[43] The court disagreed, citing precedent for the common-sense finding that, without proper notice and explanation of a denial, an appeal hearing could serve no purpose.[43]

The question that lingers after the decision in *ACORN v. FEMA* is why the agency seems determined to withhold aid from the very people it was created to serve. Civil

---

*Lawyers for survivors agreed to tracking codes, so that FEMA would be able to create a system to evaluate survivors' housing needs more accurately. This system was finally rolled out in early January 2006.

rights lawyers would like to press this question, yet case law as it stands today is not prepared to address issues of discrimination in the design of federal aid programs.

Opportunities for Reform

A problem the courts cannot solve. Legal remedies such as those discussed briefly above are unlikely to solve the problems inherent in the structure of the federal government's provision of aid to marginalized communities, in part due to a legal provision for sovereign immunity, which was held to protect FEMA from much liability in the *McWaters* case.[18,45] While plaintiffs may succeed in obtaining *ad hoc* injunctions correcting agency action (as was the case in *ACORN v. FEMA*), they are unlikely to achieve the deeper structural reforms necessary to improve the provision of recovery services.

The case for structural reform. Local charities, particularly those with long-standing relationships within the community, were better able than FEMA to serve marginalized communities during and after Hurricane Katrina. The methods of de-centralized organizations, including Catholic Charities and other community-based organizations, effectively answered social science calls for greater sensitivity to the particular needs of minority and low-income populations. The success of these groups suggests a larger role for them in disaster response, their integration into disaster response plans, or the adoption of their methods by government entities. Each of these opportunities is tempered by the reality of government bureaucracy, as well as legal concerns.

The failure of federally managed charitable operations. Although FEMA provides the staff for DRCs and administers many programs (such as emergency grants, blue roofs, and trailers), the government also leans heavily on quasi-private national charities to do much of the work. Unfortunately, many of these coordinated operations have picked up some of the same bad habits as FEMA in their dealings with the marginalized survivors of disasters. The National Response Plan (NRP) attempts to integrate the efforts of local charities with those of the federal government and FEMA. In its heavy-handed efforts, however, federal management has spoiled some of the very elements it sought to encourage.

Under the NRP, the American Red Cross is responsible for coordinating federal services during a disaster, including mass care, housing, and human services, in coordination with FEMA.[46] Though the Red Cross is a non-governmental organization (NGO), it is also government-chartered, and the federal government relies heavily upon it to deliver disaster services. The Red Cross was widely critiqued by Louisiana politicians and local service providers, as well as rather forcefully in Congress's final Katrina report.[13] Louisiana Representative Jim McCrery described numerous situations in which local churches and *ad hoc* relief groups took on responsibilities when the Red Cross was unable to provide staff, supplies, or management.[13] He also noted that, "[w]hile the Red Cross could barely manage its own network of shelters, the organization offered little assistance to struggling independent shelters" (p. 350).[13] The Red Cross explained that, although it is the only NGO included directly in the government's emergency planning, its absence in New Orleans was due to its own procedure, which demanded that the Red Cross not staff refuges "of last resort," including the Superdome (p. 350).[13] The organization also agreed with federal officials not to enter New Orleans until it was safe (p. 351).[13] Working largely with the federal government, the Red Cross faced severe criticism that it failed to coordinate its efforts with local charities and religious groups; it now plans to share funds and training with these groups.[47]

Although it is also a nationally based organization, the Salvation Army was comparatively well regarded by hurricane survivors for its appropriate and timely response. Observers on the scene noted that the Salvation Army was able to respond to individual problems rather than being overly burdened by programmatic planning.[48] The organization was also willing to coordinate with other service providers and the government.[48] The failure of the Red Cross after Hurricane Katrina suggests that federal partnership with only one large bureaucratic, nationally based charity cannot adequately serve the needs of marginalized survivors of disasters. A more nimble approach, utilizing the skills of local charities and social service providers, may provide much-needed relief.

During Hurricane Katrina, National Voluntary Organizations Active in Disaster (VOAD, an umbrella group for charities formed under the NRP in 1992) commenced conference calls that purported to coordinate the efforts of the Red Cross and FEMA with smaller organizations.[46] Charity representatives complained that the conference calls were ineffective; with more than 40 groups on the calls, the conversations "often ran long or dealt with issues that may not have been of interest to the whole group" (pp. 8–9).[46] Although top-down coordination from the government served to smother the creative energy of small, flexible organizations, only the federal government has the ability to coordinate information on a mass scale, a service critical to meeting the needs of marginalized populations.

After the attacks of September 11, 2001, the General Accounting Office (GAO) advised FEMA to encourage information-sharing among charitable groups.[46] In the aftermath of Katrina, charities did use the Coordinated Assistance Network (CAN) to share information about clients, reducing the need for survivors to give the same information again and again to different groups.[46] Whether this system worked depends on whom one asks: charities reported that putting data into the computer database took time and often did not happen because of failures of electricity or stable Internet connections, while officials in charge of the CAN program emphasized its usefulness for longer-term recovery efforts.[46] While the CAN project may need time to develop and evolve, the program does directly address the position of marginalized citizens lacking information resources and savvy.

Far more successful was the dissemination of information through coordinated nongovernmental efforts. While survivors often complained about busy FEMA information lines and inaccurate FEMA-supplied information, a little-known program made some headway. The 2-1-1 program, coordinated by the United Way, began in 1997 in Atlanta and is now operating in 38 states.[49] Analogous to the 4-1-1 directory and 5-1-1 traffic information systems, 2-1-1 provides callers with social services information.[49] Although the system was not fully operational in Louisiana when Hurricane Katrina made landfall, the system fielded many calls: the United Way reports that calls to the Texas system rose from 2,000 to about 18,000 per day in the weeks following Katrina.[50] Working with centralized repositories of information, volunteers at the 2-1-1 centers were able to assist Katrina survivors facing multi-layered dilemmas. One circumstance is illustrative:

Caller needed medication, didn't have prescriptions, but did have empty medicine bottles. I called the local Walmart Pharmacy, verified that they would supply meds for evacuees in this situation . . . the caller, who was very grateful . . . said "I've been calling for three days and you're the first live person I've spoken with" (p. 102).[51]

In other situations callers turned to the call center for FEMA information. Volunteers acting as advocates were able to respond nimbly to their requests.[51]*

Locally-based organizations' success aiding Katrina survivors. In contrast to the performance of the Red Cross, Catholic Charities, another national organization, was far more effective delivering services to populations affected by Katrina. Its mission statement includes this summary: "Our long-term goal is to raise the family above prior conditions and not rebuild poverty."[52] Catholic Charities has the critical advantage of a local angle on the problems facing Orleans Parish. Since the group's primary organizational structure is at the local level, it has experience with and an entrée into the community. In the months following the storm, Catholic Charities set up shop within DRCs, allowing the group to reach clients where they were seeking help most immediately from FEMA and other agencies. The organization provided services ranging from mental health care and crisis counseling to financial and material assistance, as well as assistance with housing and navigating through the FEMA bureaucracy.[52]

More significant than its position in the community is Catholic Charities' willingness to respect marginalized communities' unique cultural needs. Recognizing the importance of empowering individuals with the ability to navigate difficult bureaucratic systems, the group offered trainings to church parishes on how to assist survivors with post-traumatic stress and FEMA assistance.[52] Catholic Charities' Operation Starfish responded directly to cultural differences recognized by social scientists; for example, Operation Starfish was designed with the recognition that African American and Latino populations tend to rely on family members for shelter and support, while White families may rely on friends and co-workers to a greater degree.[42,52] Understanding the importance of re-establishing social networks in disaster recovery, Operation Starfish coordinated and paid for more than 1,500 evacuees to be flown or driven to stay with relatives around the country.[53]† Key to Catholic Charities' success after Katrina was its ability to stay responsive and flexible, as its local groups were able to reorient their focus to recovery efforts: "The relief and response activities of Catholic Community Services have varied week-to-week, day-to-day, based on a changing landscape."[54]

Recommendations for Creating Cultural Competency in Disaster Recovery

Structural reforms. The effectiveness of Catholic Charities and the United Way suggest that a de-centralized, flexible organization located within the community may be the

---

*For example: "A woman called looking for a list of services—she asked for information about unemployment, storage, FEMA and basic needs. I listened to her requests and took her through the available resources as well as suggesting the best course of action in each circumstance" (p. 102).[51]

†Catholic Charities also made an effort to limit shelters to fewer than 100 people.

best vehicle for serving marginalized populations during disaster recovery. Congress's report on the failures of FEMA highlighted the agency's inability to respond to actual, local situations in an *ad hoc* manner due to structural inefficiencies. For example, faced with the urgent need to disperse funds, FEMA workers lacked such authority because "the FCO [federal coordinating officer], by doctrine, is the individual that is supposed to be in charge of all federal response operations, and only the FCO has the authority to obligate federal funds" (p. 189).[13] Structural reforms proposed by the bipartisan Senate report urge that FEMA be scrapped entirely and replaced with a "National Preparedness and Response Authority," which would include "a stronger national preparedness system with regional coordinators" (p. A03).[55] Congress should re-work the structure of FEMA or put another disaster response agency in its place to devolve decision-making authority to regional and local workers; in doing so, they could encourage flexibility and creativity in the rapid response time necessary during a disaster. The extent to which government bureaucracies may be so reformed is limited, however, and solutions using existing local resources may be equally effective and more easily achieved.

Contracting with local non-profit organizations. Numerous non-profit organizations, in addition to the Red Cross, contract with FEMA to provide hurricane relief services, yet these services are not always most effectively targeted to affect communities at the local level. FEMA can easily establish such contracts at the local level before a disaster. FEMA, as well as state and local authorities, can establish relationships with NGOs and draft contracts that specifically guarantee the provision of services during a disaster and reimbursement following an event.[3] California's Office of Emergency Services (OES) suggests utilizing current contracts between local governments and providers to supplement programs such as social services and including within those agreements clauses ensuring participation during disaster recovery.[3]

Drawing from government's internal strengths. Another significant opportunity for reform may exist within government social services. The effectiveness of Catholic Charities' various service providers was born out of their experience with the needs of the community; some similar experience exists within government social service agencies. FEMA could, in effect, deputize local federal (and potentially state) Social Security, Veterans' Affairs, housing, welfare, health care, and other social service workers. These workers are likely to have the right training to interact with people in need effectively and in a culturally sensitive manner. Transferring professional social workers temporarily from their branch offices to work at DRCs would greatly strengthen FEMA's ability to address the needs of already-vulnerable populations in the aftermath of a disaster.

The practice of FEMA in staffing their DRCs in the aftermath of Katrina was either to commandeer federal workers from other federal departments,[13] with little social service background, or simply to take out want ads for clerical workers (author's interview with workers at Chalmette Disaster Relief Center, December 31, 2005). Louisiana Attorney Jamie Campbell, who worked at FEMA DRCs, suggests that important skills include the ability to ask the right questions of low-income survivors, to be sensitive to unfamiliar family structures, and to carefully attend to inter-personal relations during times of crisis, when empathy is at a premium.[48] These are part of a social worker's presumed skill set but not that of federal workers untrained in these areas. While FEMA and state agencies should emphasize cultural competency training programs for all contract employees, in the midst of an emergency they must be able to call on workers who already have these skills.

Planning with community leaders. Charity representatives reported to the GAO that despite FEMA's attempts to coordinate charity endeavors, their attempts "were not as important to coordination efforts as pre-existing relationships" (p. 9).[46] California's OES suggests that, in addition to contracting with NGOs, government at all levels must involve NGOs in disaster preparedness planning, willingly take advice from local groups, and include NGOs and local groups in disaster exercises.[46]

In addition to formal contract relationships, FEMA and coordinating governments should establish relationships with community leaders and neighborhood organizations in order to facilitate cooperation in an emergency but, more importantly, to build cultural competency within its own ranks.[4]* Following the 1989 Loma Prieta earthquake, the Watsonville Red Cross recruited members of the local community to undergo Red Cross training and also had its own employees join local Latino organizations.[56] Such "inter-organizational cooperation fostered awareness, reduced friction, and created a pool of trained personnel for the next disaster."[56] Such interactions demonstrate the strengths of local minority communities and show disaster recovery officials tapping into networks with which they might otherwise have no contact. Even the Red Cross is following suit. Under fire for failing to work effectively with minorities, the organization "hired a vice president of diversity who should see to it that more minorities—including Spanish speakers—work the front lines."[47]

Provide survivor advocates. The General Accounting Office noted that providing survivors with case managers in New York and Washington, D.C., after the attacks of September 11, 2001, as numerous charitable organizations did, was one of the most effective ways to "help survivors find out what assistance is available and ease their access to that aid through a central, easy-to-access clearinghouse of private and public assistance."[46] This suggests that FEMA should employ workers in disaster recovery not as disinterested processors of applications but as advocates for obtaining maximum aid for eligible survivors. Advocates are key to filling the information gap into which so many low-income survivors fall due to linguistic, cultural, and social patterns.

FEMA's interest in conserving federal resources and preventing fraud gives its bureaucrats incentives to obfuscate the aid process, provide misinformation, and issue standardized denials to possibly worthy claimants.[43] Advocates can serve as a critical counter-balance to this phenomenon. Furthermore, there may be surprising efficiency benefits to such an approach for the agency itself. Advocates are likely to save the government time and money by ensuring that applications submitted by disaster survivors are clear and correct.

Behavioral solutions to cultural incompetence. To address fundamental cultural differences, FEMA and state organizations should make a concerted effort to hire

---

* SAMHSA's guide notes, "Cultural competence training programs work particularly well when they are provided in collaboration with community based groups that offer expertise or technical assistance in cultural competence or in the needs of a particular culture. Involving such groups not only enables program staff to gain firsthand knowledge of various cultures, but also opens up the door for long-term partnerships" (p. 27).[4]

members of minority communities as managers at the regional level.[4] At the local level, government has the opportunity within the course of a year-long disaster recovery process to employ members of the local community to provide services to their peers. In 1998, Ventura County, California, implemented such a program in the wake of severe storms that had produced flooding in migrant worker communities.[4] The county hired farm laborers to go into migrant worker camps and communicate with leaders: "[T] hese were the first 'government' workers in recent memory to be allowed in the farm workers' camp" (p. 26).[4]

Removing Roadblocks to Reform

Congress's response. In the months after Hurricane Katrina, significant public and media attention highlighted the failure of FEMA to serve the recovery needs of Gulf Coast communities. Congress reacted with a number of legislative reforms, some of which directly address the particular issues of marginalized communities raised in this chapter and others that address instances of federal mismanagement through which survivors of the disaster were unfairly punished.

Reorganization of FEMA took center stage. For our purposes, several measures were significant, including the development of regional offices, as well as a high-level disability coordinator.[57] The Post-Katrina Emergency Management Reform Act of 2006 also calls for the development of a Surge Capacity Force, which would allow Department of Homeland Security employees who are not directly supervised by FEMA, as well as other federal employees, to be deployed to manage disaster recovery efforts.[57] These personnel would serve mainly in higher-level leadership capacities; as suggested in the previous discussion of the role of advocacy in recovery, FEMA should also consider deputizing ground-level social services personnel who know the community and will be the first to make contact with its members.

In addition to organization and personnel, FEMA reform did directly address some of the unique problems of marginalized communities that came to the forefront of national attention as ineffective recovery assistance dragged on for over a year and a half preceding congressional action. The Post-Katrina Act attempts to address the significant problem of family separation by establishing a National Emergency Family Registry and Locator system and the Child Locator Center.[57] It is unclear whether these information systems will also enable the practical reunification of low-income families with transportation and housing obstacles (as Catholic Charities' Operation Starfish does), though the act does authorize the president to provide transportation services to return survivors of disaster to their original residences. The Post-Katrina Act's national disaster housing strategy calls for establishing a plan to address low-income and special needs populations but does not provide any articulation of the goals of such a plan or the resources that will be dedicated to implement it.[57]

Perhaps most responsive to the needs of marginalized citizens, part of the Stafford Act was amended to include funding for case management services:

> The President may provide case management services, including financial assistance, to State or local government agencies or qualified private organizations to provide such services, to victims of major disasters to identify and address unmet needs.[45]

Although recognizing the need for case management services is a major step forward, the language of the amended act is not mandatory, and thus is no guarantee that survivors will receive such case management or advocacy services. FEMA should elevate the significance of this provision by identifying case management service providers for every region in advance of the next major disaster recovery effort.

The policy of NGOs as providers of entitlements. Delegation to the private sector of what were once thought to be exclusively governmental functions (such as the regulation of environmental compliance,[58] the administration of prisons, and the carrying out of foreign warfare) has become commonplace at the beginning of the twenty-first century. Similarly, the provision of social services has also been turned over in some states from the federal government to administration by state, as well as private non-profit and for-profit entities. For example, private contractors manage significant portions of Wisconsin's welfare system, including determining applicants' eligibility as well as "sanctioning beneficiaries for noncompliance with program requirements" (p. 1367).[59] These developments arouse significant concerns regarding the potential loss of public law values of transparency, public participation, and accountability when a private actor supplants a traditional government function. However, within the temporary context of disaster recovery, these concerns may be mitigated by a number of factors suggesting that some privatization would better serve marginalized communities.

The ideological commitments and guiding missions of local non-profit and charity organizations provide the key justification for looking toward them as alternatives to federal bureaucracies such as FEMA. In the welfare context, Metzger notes, "Government-run welfare programs are often characterized by abusive procedures designed simply to keep individuals off the rolls, whereas privatization may mean services are provided by nonprofits with ideological commitments more allied with beneficiaries' interests" (p. 1387).[59] In her extensive research on corporate versus government and non-profit management of hospitals, Jill Horwitz found that data confirmed "objective theories" that non-profit firms "are more likely than for profits to adopt public goals" (p. 4).[60]

While some commentators on the FEMA debacle in managing Hurricane Katrina recovery argue for broad delegation to private for-profit business at the higher levels of management and decision-making, I have argued that privatization at the *local* level is most efficient for marginalized communities.[61] A moderate level of privatization at the local level is likely to yield significant results. Matthew Diller argues that the long process from congressional mandate to local application that attends significant policy decisions on social welfare means that "administration, particularly at the ground level, assumes a role of great importance" (p. 1130).[62] This is especially true in the wake of welfare reform, wherein programs emphasize lower-level worker discretion and replace the uniformity and predictability of the old central system (p. 1219).[62] It is just this discretion on the part of lower-level FEMA employees that went awry in the aftermath of Hurricane Katrina, giving rise to working-family tragedies by way of misinformation, badly tailored relief programs, and cultural misunderstanding. Local charities and non-profits—by virtue of their experience in the community, access to local leaders, and cultural competency—are better situated to exercise discretion for the benefit of marginalized survivors of disasters.

Although there are serious concerns about the privatization of government functions,[63] they do not wholly justify dismissing privatization as a means of aiding marginalized communities. This is especially true where contracts are made with non-profit organizations, are carried out at the local level, and ensure that the government includes safeguards to guarantee proper procedure.

First Amendment concerns over the establishment of religion also come into play when religious groups such as Catholic Charities, the Salvation Army, and local churches are engaged to provide disaster recovery services. The sort of contracting I am advocating in disaster recovery is unlikely to prove problematic in this respect, since the provision of tangible services such as housing and financial assistance is a straightforward matter (in comparison with more tangled domains such as education).[64-67]* To avoid legal objections to privatization such as those just mentioned, FEMA must establish guidelines regarding the separation of relief funds from funds for religious activities. Where contracting with NGOs may require real-time decisions by government officials, disaster plans should include lists of pre-approved organizations that have been vetted for their willingness to adhere to strict separation of religious from social service functions. The balance desired is a delicate one between ensuring procedural safeguards without replicating the problems of bureaucracy that strategies for cultural competence seek to address.

Conclusion

Privatization does not usually rise to the top of the list of progressive solutions to problems of low-income, minority communities in their dealings with the federal government. It suits the unique context of disaster recovery, however, when local non-profit and charitable organizations offer the advocacy, cultural sensitivity, and local knowledge that disaster survivors so desperately need. The temporary nature of the disaster recovery process minimizes the associated risks. Core governmental functions should be retained by the federal government, and only not-for-profit organizations should take on duties at the local level, dissuading private interests from seeking benefit at the expense of the most vulnerable disaster survivors.[61] Public law values such as transparency, due process, and public participation may be explicitly written into government contracts to guarantee accountability by those undertaking disaster relief responsibilities.

Notes

1. National Park Service. Presidio of San Francisco: Chinese displacement. San Francisco: National Park Service, U.S. Dept. of the Interior. Available at www.nps.gov/prsf/history/1906eq/chinese.htm (last visited Sept. 14, 2008).

---

* Notably, President Bush's office of Faith-Based and Community Initiatives promised it would only reimburse funds to those churches and religious organizations that had been asked by FEMA to help following the disaster.[64] Additionally, First Amendment claims where government contracts with the Salvation Army for the provision of social services were judged to be religion-neutral were dismissed in court.[67]

2.   Yelvington KA. Coping in a temporary way: the tent cities. In: Peacock WG, Morrow BH, Gladwyn H, eds. Hurricane Andrew: ethnicity, gender, and the sociology of disasters. New York: Routledge, 1997;103–5.

3.   California Governor's Office of Emergency Services (OES). Meeting the needs of vulnerable people in times of disaster: a guide for emergency managers. Sacramento, CA: California Governor's Office of Emergency Services, 2000. Available at www.oes.ca.gov/Operational/OESHome.nsf/PDF/Vulnerable%20Populations/$file/Vulnerable%20Populations.PDF (last visited Sept. 14, 2008).

4.   U.S. Department of Health and Human Services, Substance Abuse and Mental Health Services Administration (SAMHSA). Cultural competence in disaster mental health programs: guiding principles and recommendations. Washington, DC: DHHS, 2003. Available at mentalhealth.samhsa.gov/publications/allpubs/sma03-3828/default.asp (last visited Sept. 14, 2008).

5.   Cutter S. The geography of social vulnerability: race, class and catastrophe. In: Kaufman SB, Dill N, Rauscher E, eds. The Hurricane Katrina social science research database and hub. New York: Social Science Research Council, 2005–present. Available at understandingkatrina.ssrc.org/(last visited Sept. 14, 2008).

6.   Congressional Research Service. Hurricane Katrina: social-demographic characteristics of impacted areas, RL33141; November 4, 2005.

7.   Center for Progressive Reform. An unnatural disaster: the aftermath of Hurricane Katrina, CPR Publication #512. Edgewater, MD: CPR, September 2005.

8.   Morrow BH. Stretching the bonds: the families of Andrew. In: Peacock WG, Morrow BH, Gladwyn H, eds. Hurricane Andrew: ethnicity, gender, and the sociology of disasters. New York: Routledge, 1997.

9.   Fothergill A, Maestas EG, Darlington JD. Race, ethnicity and disaster in the United States: a review of the literature. Disasters. 1999;23(2):156–73.

10. Witte G. Private security contractors head to Gulf. Washington Post, September 8, 2005.

11. Dewan S, Connelly M, Lehren A. Evacuees' lives still upended seven months after hurricane. New York Times, March 22, 2006.

12. Hurlbert JS, Beggs JJ, Haines VA. Bridges over troubled waters: what are the optimal networks for Katrina's victims? In: Kaufman SB, Dill N, Rauscher E, eds. The Hurricane Katrina social science research database and hub. New York: Social Science Research Council, June 11, 2006. Available at katrinaresearchhub.ssrc.org/ (last visited September 14, 2008).

13. Congressional Reports: H. Rpt. 109–377, A failure of initiative: final report of the Select Bipartisan Committee to Investigate the Preparation for and Response to Hurricane Katrina. Available at www.gpoaccess.gov/serialset/creports/katrina.html (last visited Sept. 10, 2008).

14. Molotch H. Death on the roof: race and bureaucratic failure. In: Kaufman SB, Dill N, Rauscher E, eds. The Hurricane Katrina social science research database and hub. New York: Social Science Research Council, 2005–present. Available at understandingkatrina.ssrc.org/Molotch/ (last visited Sept. 8, 2008).

15. Bell D. Faces at the bottom of the well: the permanence of racism. New York: Basic-Books, 1992.

16. Weisman LK. Discrimination by design: a feminist critique of the man-made environment. Champaign, IL: University of Illinois Press, 1994.

17. Katznelson I. When affirmative action was White: an untold history of racial inequality in twentieth-century America. New York: W.W. Norton, 2005.

18. *McWaters v. Federal Emergency Management Agency*, 408 F. Supp. 2d 221 (E.D. Louisiana, 2005).

19. Roberts D. Killing the Black body: race, reproduction and the meaning of liberty. New York: Vintage, 1997.

20. Fletcher MA. Katrina pushes issues of race and poverty at Bush. Washington Post, September 12, 2005.

21. Pear R. Bush visits Gulf region as it struggles to rebuild. New York Times, March 8, 2006.

22. Association of Community Organizations for Reform Now, Inc. (ACORN). 9th Ward ACORN members win bulldozing settlement. New Orleans: ACORN, January 23, 2006. Available at www.acorn.org (last visited Sept. 14, 2008).

23. FEMA. Katrina Recovery Times. Vol. 1. Mississippi: U.S. Department of Homeland Security/FEMA and the Mississippi Emergency Management Agency, October 7, 2005. Available at www.fema.gov/txt/rt/rt_1604_100705.txt (last visited Sept. 14, 2008).

24. Martin A. Hitches show in FEMA trailer plan; $2 billion program for hurricane homeless moving slowly, critics say. Chicago Tribune, November 6, 2006.

25. Nossiter A. In New Orleans, progress at last in the Lower Ninth Ward. New York Times, February 23, 2007.

26. Terdiman D. The ignored nonrecovery of New Orleans, CNET News, 2008 July 2. Available at: news.cnet.com/8301-13772_3-9982575-52.html (last visited Sept. 8, 2008).

27. Louisiana Recovery Authority. Louisiana speaks. Baton Rouge: LRA, 2006–present. Available at louisianaspeaks.org.

28. Bazile KT. St. Bernard gets recovery going: council gives nod to planner's big ideas. Times-Picayune, March 22, 2006.

29. Zucchino D. In Katrina's ruins, a land of opportunity; residents, new buyers and real estate agents await a neighborhood's rebirth. Los Angeles Times, March 2, 2006.

30. FEMA. Blue roof program reaches lofty goals (press release). Washington, DC: FEMA, March 9, 2006. Available at www.fema.gov/news/newsrelease.fema?id=24103 (last visited Sept. 14, 2008).

31. House Concurrent Resolutions Nos. 3 and 39, Senate Concurrent Resolution No.7 (First Extraordinary Session of 2006). Baton Rouge: Louisiana State Legislature, 2006. Available at www.legis.state.la.us (last visited Sept. 14, 2008).

32. Whoriskey P. We called it Hurricane FEMA: trailer park was quickly emptied, Washington Post, March 12, 2007.

33. NewsHour report. Controversy continues over post-Katrina spending on trailers. Washington, DC: Public Broadcasting Service, aired April 9, 2007. Available at www.pbs.org/newshour/bb/weather/jan-june07/katrina_04-09.html (last visited Sept. 14, 2008).

34. International Human Rights Law Clinic and the Human Rights Center at the University of California, Berkeley and the Payson Center for International Development at Tulane University. Rebuilding after Katrina: a population-based study of labor and human rights in New Orleans. Berkeley and New Orleans: UC Berkeley and Tulane University, July 7, 2006. Available at hrc.berkeley.edu/us.html (last visited Sept. 14, 2008.)

35. Peacock WG with Ragsdale AK. Social systems, ecological networks and disasters: toward a socio-political ecology of disasters. In: Peacock WG, Morrow BH, Gladwyn H, eds. Hurricane Andrew: ethnicity, gender, and the sociology of disasters. New York: Routledge, 1997.

36. Birch EL, Wachter SM. Rebuilding urban places after disaster: lessons from Hurricane Katrina. Philadelphia: Univ. of Pennsylvania Press, 2006.

37. USDA Rural Development. Disaster recovery guide for people and communities. Obtained in New Orleans, December 2005. On file with author. Also see www.rurdev.usda.gov/la.

38. U.S. Small Business Administration. Disaster assistance: federal disaster loans for homeowners, renters and businesses of all sizes (flyer). Obtained in New Orleans December 2005. On file with author.

39. Peacock WG, Morrow BH, Gladwyn H, eds. Hurricane Andrew: ethnicity, gender, and the sociology of disasters. New York: Routledge, 1997.

40. U.S. Small Business Administration. Disaster loans—fact sheet declarations 101176/10177, 10203/10204 & 10205/10206 (flyer). Obtained in New Orleans December 2005. On file with author.

41. Bolin, R. Disaster impact and recovery: a comparison of Black and White victims. Int J Mass Emergencies Disasters. 1986;4(1):35–50.

42. Perry RW, Mushkatel AH. Minority citizens in disasters. Athens, GA: Univ. of Georgia Press, 1986.

43. *Association of Community Organizations for Reform Now, Inc. (ACORN) v. Federal Emergency Management Agency (FEMA)*, 463 F. Supp. 2d 26 (D.D.C. 2006) Complaint for declaratory and injunctive relief. Available at www.citizen.org/ (last visited Sept. 14, 2008).

44. Rapp KT. Equal justice society. Presented at Après le deluge: rebuilding a sustainable city after Katrina, a legal charette, University of California at Berkeley School of Law, Jan. 19, 2006.

45. The Stafford Act, 42 U.S.C. § 5189d (2008).

46. Government Accountability Office. Statement of Cynthia Fagnoni, managing director, education, workforce and income security issues. Hurricanes Katrina and Rita: provisions of charitable assistance. Testimony before the Subcommittee on Oversight, Committee on Ways and Means, House of Representatives, Dec. 13, 2005 GAO-06-297T. Washington, DC: Government Accounting Office, 2005.

47. Editorial. Rescuing the Red Cross. Christian Science Monitor, April 5, 2006. Available at: www.csmonitor.com/2006/0405/p08s02-comv.html (last visited Sept. 10, 2008).

48. Telephone interview by the author with Jamie Campbell, managing attorney at Southeast Louisiana Legal Services, Covington, LA (April 18, 2006).

49. The Alliance of Information and Referral Systems (AIRS) and the United Way. 2-1-1 Information and referral search. Fairfax, VA: AIRS, 2008. Available at www.211.org/ (last visited Sept. 14, 2008).

50. Gallagher BA. Brian Gallagher's Web Log [president and CEO of United Way of America]. Virginia: United Way of America, 2006. Available at national.unitedway.org/katrina/BAGweblog_2.cfm (last visited April 11, 2006).

51. Marin M and Walker M. 2-1-1 California Partnership, Business Plan. Alameda CA: 2-1-1 Los Angeles United Way Silicon Valley, 2005 October. Available at www.211california.org (last visited Sept. 14, 2008).

52. Catholic Charities USA. Local agency recovery efforts in response to Hurricanes Katrina and Rita. Alexandria, VA: Catholic Charities USA, 2006.

53. Catholic Charities. Houma LA: Catholic Services of Houma-Thibodaux LA, 2006.

54. Catholic Community Services. Baton Rouge: Catholic Charities of the Diocese of Baton Rouge, 2006.

55. Hsu SS. Senate report urges dismantling of FEMA: a new agency, with more funding and authority, would be built in Homeland Security Department. Washington Post, April 27, 2006. Available at www.washingtonpost.com (last visited Sept. 10, 2008).

56. Phillips B. Cultural diversity in disasters: sheltering, housing and long term recovery. Int J Mass Emergencies Disasters. 1993 Mar;11(1):99–110.

57. CRS Report. Federal emergency management policy changes after Hurricane Katrina: a summary of statutory provisions, Nov. 15, 2006. RL 33729.

58. Seifter S. Rent-a-regulator: design and innovation in privatized governmental decisionmaking, 33 Ecology L.Q. 4 (2006).

59. Metzger GE. Privatization as delegation, 103 Colum. L. Rev. 1367, 1367 (2003).

60. Horwitz JR. Does corporate ownership matter? Service provision in the hospital industry, National Bureau of Economic Research (NBER) Working Paper Series #11376. Universitad Complutense Madrid: NBER, May 2005.

61. Sobel RS, Leeson PT. Flirting with disaster: the inherent problems with FEMA. Policy Analysis. 2006 July 19;No. 573, CATO Institute.

62. Diller M. The revolution in welfare administration: rules, discretion, and entrepreneurial government, 75 N.Y.U. L. Rev. (2000).

63. Bamberger KA. Regulation as delegation: private firms, decisionmaking, and accountability in the administrative state. 56 Duke L.J. 377, 399 (2006).

64. *Morning Edition: Faith-based groups to receive Katrina funds,* National Public Radio broadcast, September 29, 2005.

65. *Mitchell v. Thomas,* 530 U.S. 793 (2000).

66. *Bowen v. Kendrick,* 487 U.S. 589 (1988).

67. *Lown v. Salvation Army, Inc.,* 393 F. Supp. 2d 223 (S.D.N.Y. 2005).

Appendix: Films and Notable Books on the Hurricanes of 2005

Associated Film Documentaries

After the Wind, Child, After the Water's Gone
John Sullivan
url: *www.communityarts.net*

Voices of the Storm: Six Months after Katrina
Jackie Judd, The Kaiser Family Foundation
url: *www.kff.org/uninsured/voices.cfm*

Voices of the Storm: One Year after Katrina
Jackie Judd, The Kaiser Family Foundation
url: *www.kff.org/uninsured/voices.cfm*

Notable Books on the Hurricanes of 2005

Brinkley DG. The Great Deluge: Hurricane Katrina, New Orleans, and the Mississippi Gulf Coast. New York: William Morrow & Co., 2006.

Bryan B. The Storm: What Went Wrong and Why during Hurricane Katrina: The Inside Story from One Louisiana Scientist. New York: Viking Books, 2006.

Cooper C, Block R. Disaster: Hurricane Katrina and the Failure of Homeland Security. New York: Times Books, 2006.

Dallas Morning News. Eyes of the Storm: Hurricanes Katrina and Rita: The Photographic Story. New York: Taylor Trade Publishing, 2006.

Dyson ME. Come Hell or High Water: Hurricane Katrina and the Color of Disaster. New York: Basic Books, 2006.

Horne J. Breach of Faith: Hurricane Katrina and the Near Death of a Great American City. New York: Random House, 2006.

Reed B, ed. Unnatural Disaster: The Nation on Hurricane Katrina. New York: Nation Books, 2006.

Rich F. The Greatest Story Ever Sold: The Decline and Fall of Truth from 9/11 to Katrina. New York: Penguin, 2006.

Tidwell M. The Ravaging Tide: The Strange Weather, Future Katrinas, and the Coming Death of America's Coastal Cities. Washington, DC: Free Press, 2006.

Trout DD, ed. After the Storm: Black Intellectuals Explore the Meaning of Hurricane Katrina. New York: New Press, 2006.

Index